Cases on Diversity, Equity, and Inclusion for the Health Professions Educator

Chasity Beth O'Malley
Wright State University Boonshoft School of Medicine, USA

Arkene Levy
Nova Southeastern University Dr. Kiran C. Patel College of Allopathic Medicine, USA

Amanda Chase
Nova Southeastern University Dr. Kiran C. Patel College of Allopathic Medicine, USA

Samiksha Prasad
Nova Southeastern University Dr. Kiran C. Patel College of Allopathic Medicine, USA

A volume in the Advances in Medical Education, Research, and Ethics (AMERE) Book Series

IGI Global
PUBLISHER of TIMELY KNOWLEDGE

Published in the United States of America by
IGI Global
Medical Information Science Reference (an imprint of IGI Global)
701 E. Chocolate Avenue
Hershey PA, USA 17033
Tel: 717-533-8845
Fax: 717-533-8661
E-mail: cust@igi-global.com
Web site: http://www.igi-global.com

Library of Congress Cataloging-in-Publication Data

Names: O'Malley, Chasity (Chasity Beth), 1979- editor. | Johnston, Arkene Levy, 1979- editor. | Chase, Amanda (Amanda J.), 1976- editor. | Prasad, Samiksha, 1988- editor.
Title: Cases on diversity, equity, and inclusion for the health professions educator / edited by Chasity Beth O'Malley, Arkene Levy Johnston, Amanda J Chase, Samiksha Prasad.
Description: Hershey, PA : Information Science Reference, [2022] | Includes bibliographical references and index. | Summary: "The purpose of this book is to provide educators with cases in topics such as racism, mental health stigma, classism, etc., for use in case-based learning across the healthcare professions. The chapters will each include two to three cases with components of background information on the topic, a case frame for discussion, questions and answers, and an epilogue"-- Provided by publisher.
Identifiers: LCCN 2022046931 (print) | LCCN 2022046932 (ebook) | ISBN 9781668454930 (hardcover) | ISBN 9781668454978 (paperback) | ISBN 9781668454947 (ebook)
Subjects: LCSH: Discrimination in medical care--United States. | Sex discrimination in medicine--United States. | Transcultural medical care--United States. | Cultural competence--United States. | Medical education--United States.
Classification: LCC RA563.M56 C37 2022 (print) | LCC RA563.M56 (ebook) | DDC 362.1089--dc23/eng/20221122
LC record available at https://lccn.loc.gov/2022046931
LC ebook record available at https://lccn.loc.gov/2022046932

This book is published in the IGI Global book series Advances in Medical Education, Research, and Ethics (AMERE) (ISSN: 2475-6601; eISSN: 2475-661X)

British Cataloguing in Publication Data
A Cataloguing in Publication record for this book is available from the British Library.

For electronic access to this publication, please contact: eresources@igi-global.com.

Advances in Medical Education, Research, and Ethics (AMERE) Book Series

ISSN:2475-6601
EISSN:2475-661X

Mission

Humans are living longer now than ever as a result of advances in the medical field. Having the tools available to train knowledgeable and ethical future generations of doctors and medical researchers is essential to continuing to advance our understanding of the human body and develop new ways of treating and curing sickness and disease.

The **Advances in Medical Education, Research, and Ethics (AMERE)** book series highlights publications pertaining to advancements in pedagogical practice for developing future healthcare professionals, research methods, and advancements in the medical field, as well as moral behavior and practice of healthcare professionals, students, and researchers. Featuring research-based book publications that are highly relevant to the healthcare community, this series is ideally designed for library inclusion at medical universities and research institutions as well as personal use by medical professionals, researchers, and upper-level students entering the field.

Coverage

- Clinical Research
- Conflicts of Interest
- Ethics in Medicine
- Healthcare Pedagogy
- Medical Curricula
- Medical Simulation
- Patient Data
- Professional Development
- Research Methods
- Scientific Misconduct

IGI Global is currently accepting manuscripts for publication within this series. To submit a proposal for a volume in this series, please contact our Acquisition Editors at Acquisitions@igi-global.com or visit: http://www.igi-global.com/publish/.

The Advances in Medical Education, Research, and Ethics (AMERE) Book Series (ISSN 2475-6601) is published by IGI Global, 701 E. Chocolate Avenue, Hershey, PA 17033-1240, USA, www.igi-global.com. This series is composed of titles available for purchase individually; each title is edited to be contextually exclusive from any other title within the series. For pricing and ordering information please visit http://www.igi-global.com/book-series/advances-medical-education-research-ethics/132365. Postmaster: Send all address changes to above address.

Titles in this Series

For a list of additional titles in this series, please visit: www.igi-global.com/book-series

Contemporary Issues in Global Medicine and Moving Toward International Healthcare Equity
Nick Comninellis (University of Missouri-Kansas City, USA) and Steven D. Waldman (University of Missouri-Kansas City School of Medicine, USA)
Medical Information Science Reference • © 2022 • 463pp • H/C (ISBN: 9781799884903) • US $325.00

Simulation and Game-Based Learning for the Health Professions
Rachel Umoren (University of Washington, USA)
Medical Information Science Reference • © 2022 • 275pp • H/C (ISBN: 9781799843788) • US $270.00

Handbook of Research on Developing Competencies for Pre-Health Professional Students, Advisors, and Programs
Rohini Ganjoo (The George Washington University, USA) and Lisa S. Schwartz (The George Washington University, USA)
Medical Information Science Reference • © 2022 • 492pp • H/C (ISBN: 9781668459690) • US $470.00

Handbook of Research on Improving Allied Health Professions Education Advancing Clinical Training and Interdisciplinary Translational Research
Rui Pedro Pereira Almeida (University of Algarve, Portugal)
Medical Information Science Reference • © 2022 • 409pp • H/C (ISBN: 9781799895787) • US $435.00

Handbook of Research on Advising and Developing the Pre-Health Professional Student
Lisa S. Schwartz (The George Washington University, USA) and Rohini Ganjoo (The George Washington University, USA)
Information Science Reference • © 2022 • 390pp • H/C (ISBN: 9781799896173) • US $470.00

Instructional Design Exemplars in eHealth and mHealth Education Interventions
Suha R. Tamim (University of South Carolina, USA)
Medical Information Science Reference • © 2022 • 323pp • H/C (ISBN: 9781799894902) • US $325.00

Technological Adoption and Trends in Health Sciences Teaching, Learning, and Practice
Samuel Marcos-Pablos (University of Salamanca, Spain) and Juan Antonio Juanes-Méndez (University of Salamanca, Spain)
Medical Information Science Reference • © 2022 • 387pp • H/C (ISBN: 9781799888710) • US $380.00

IGI Global
PUBLISHER of TIMELY KNOWLEDGE

701 East Chocolate Avenue, Hershey, PA 17033, USA
Tel: 717-533-8845 x100 • Fax: 717-533-8661
E-Mail: cust@igi-global.com • www.igi-global.com

Table of Contents

Detailed Table of Contents

The American Psychological Association defines racism as a construct that is 'structural, institutional, interpersonal, and internalized.' The marginalization of persons of color due to blatant racism is a pervasive social issue that has historically held negative consequences for the health of these individuals, and evidence links racism to the higher levels of morbidity and mortality, seen especially among Blacks/African Americans (Paradies, 2015). The effort and movement to reduce marginalization of minorities through healthcare professional education is upon us. Providing health professional learners and practitioners with tools to understand manifestations and implications of racial acts and microaggressions in the healthcare setting is imperative, as is training medical professionals to recognize and mitigate their biases. This chapter highlights cases of varying levels of racism from the healthcare professionals' view and experience in the clinical setting.

Healthcare and cultural competency are intimately intertwined concepts. Understanding how to provide the latter when caring for patients translates to better care. Transitioning between cultures and overcoming linguistic barriers can be challenging for healthcare workers. Differences in cultural norms can often be the cause of irritation and discontent for both patients and healthcare professionals, impeding the ease with which we are able to communicate and connect with our patients. Insufficient education and training on culturally competent care for patients renders our healthcare team unprepared for the challenges faced when practicing in culturally diverse clinical environments. In this chapter, the authors will explore how medical interpretation is vital to the care of patients with limited English-speaking proficiency (LEP), how healthcare professional's beliefs can affect their practice, and how to navigate working with healthcare professionals of various cultural backgrounds.

cases highlight examples of unintentional institutional classism in healthcare that provide learners and practitioners with the tools to identify institutional classism or procedural blind spots in the healthcare setting and its implications. It is important for healthcare learners and institutions to be educated on actions, procedures, and strategies to mitigate classism in healthcare.

This chapter addresses gender bias, gender performativity, and sexual harassment in the clinical setting. The prevalence of gender disparities and bias is well documented in fields such as orthopedic surgery, urology, radiology, neurosurgery, and plastic surgery. Marginalized groups are more frequently impacted by these negative behaviors. Notably, in the field of urology, female residents comprise less than 30% of the demographic and often face bias. Gender performativity may play a role in the stereotyping seen for males in the nursing profession. Traditional views of masculinity and femininity may limit a supervisor's ability to see the potential in clinical staff members and cause conscious or unconscious limitations for professional growth. The interactions represented in these cases offer an opportunity for discussion of the prevalence and impact of gender bias and associated microaggressions in medicine. Various strategies to effectively mitigate gender bias in the clinical and academic environment are also discussed.

Three scenarios involving LGBTQI+ populations are presented. Case 1 highlights an in-class interaction between a faculty member and two students. A female-to-male transgender student is misgendered by a faculty member in front of the class, resulting in the student leaving the session. A second student acts as an ally when approached by the faculty member about the situation. Case 2 involves a professional development session focused on creating inclusive environments for LGBTQI+ students. One faculty member presents her approach of avoiding knowledge of students' personal lives as an effective tool for protecting students and faculty. Case 3 involves an inclusivity training session that doesn't connect as intended with the audience, resulting in students who are disengaged. Prompt questions promote reflection on what transpired, its impact, and institutional resources to help faculty in building inclusive environments. Readers will consider how to address what transpired both immediately and in the future.

Microaggressions are commonly encountered in the clinical learning environment. Although microaggressions may be subtle and/or unintentional, it has been well established that microaggressions can have significant negative impacts on healthcare workers, patients, and patient care, contributing to health inequities. Microaggressions are difficult to address in the clinical learning environment for many reasons. This chapter will provide health professions educators with a framework to effectively teach learners how to recognize and address microaggressions in the clinical learning environment in a non-accusatory way that will build relationships. It will also discuss common barriers to addressing microaggressions in medicine and provide potential solutions.

A light review of historical practices can provide what some may consider a superficial evolution of higher education and its practices. Specifically, in the field of health professions, a shift that is easily identifiable is the move from black and white photos of white male physicians in coats and nurses in starched white dresses to a more diversified student body adorned with white coats. However, are the current systems in place supportive of the individual needs and beliefs of these students or are students inadvertently being required to alter who they are to fit into systems not supportive of their individuality, especially as it relates to their religious beliefs? How do we undo the practices of a one-size-fits-all approach to educating students and move towards a goal of inclusivity for all faiths by providing students educational environments and curriculums purposefully designed to support students of different religions?

It is well-established that medical students and practicing physicians alike continue to suffer from extreme burnout, despite growing efforts to attend more closely to wellness. This often takes the form of mindfulness practices, community activities, transparency around work expectations, mentor and support groups, and the like. However, less attention is paid to how efforts towards inclusive learning experiences can themselves support wellness. This chapter will explore how to build a truly inclusive and justice-oriented environment in the service of student wellness by looking at three key moments of the medical education journey, exploring where things often go awry, and offering possible solutions to enhance them. Specifically, the cases will leverage the didactic experience as a student, clinical encounters as a resident, and physician educator encounters with colleagues to illustrate how enhancing inclusive dialogue, environments, and practices in these spaces can also support practitioner wellness.

Preface

Diversity, Equity, and Inclusion (DEI) are concepts that have become the focal point of strategic planning for higher education institutions in the United States over the past few years. In health professions education where the goal is to provide culturally responsive education and training, DEI is a critical strategic priority in improving the quality of education of learners in order to equip them to care for an increasingly diverse population. By definition, diversity is a term that captures every unique aspect of human differences and is defined by the National Institute of Health (NIH) as "the range of human differences, including but not limited to race, ethnicity, gender, sexual orientation, age, social class, physical ability or attributes, religious or ethical value system, national origin, and political beliefs" (NIH, 2017). Therefore, we attain diversity through the recognition and dismantling of practices that are discriminatory toward any individual or group. Traditionally, when discussing diversity in the health professions, race and ethnicity are the focal points of these conversations. This is because, by 2043, the demographic of the USA is expected to become a majority-minority population with Black Indigenous and people of color (BIPOC) individuals constituting the majority (Bernstein, 2012). This shift heightens the need for closing the health disparities gap which has historically held deleterious consequences for BIPOC individuals largely because of inequities in structural racism and educational and socioeconomic status (CDC, 2013). Inclusion is defined by the NIH as "involvement and empowerment, where the inherent worth and dignity of all people is recognized" (NIH 2017). Within the learning environment, Doughtery and colleagues define inclusion as "making sure that all students and employees feel welcome and their unique learning and working styles are attended to and valued (Doughtery & Kienzl, 2006). Equity in the context of healthcare can be defined as "the absence of systematic disparities in health, or in the major social determinants of health, between groups with different levels of underlying social advantage or disadvantage" (Braveman, 2003).

Connecting DEI to learning in health professions education is critical in bridging the health equity gap that currently exists for marginalized populations. This requires more robust and innovative curricular approaches to enhance existing diversity-related education in a manner that will translate into equitable actions by future health professionals (Institute of Medicine, 2004). For example, medical schools are currently being guided in their curricular innovations by the recent DEI competency framework released by the AAMC (AAMC, 2022) and this holds the potential to inform new curricular approaches that will foster the development of more targeted curricular materials to enhance learner knowledge and competencies around DEI, which will ultimately translate into better care for all patients. Similar curricular innovations are warranted for other health professions programs especially those that leverage active learning and interprofessional education in a manner that truly represents the lived experiences of patients, families, and community members (Parsons, 2021; McElfish, 2018).

Health professions programs are therefore challenged to orient learners to the existing disparities in healthcare in the USA, which are numerous and systemic and hold serious consequences for varying groups of individuals. For example, BIPOC individuals face several disadvantages in their access to healthcare and the quality of care they receive because of race and ethnicity, income and education, and disability status (CDC, 2013). People of color have a higher prevalence of infant mortality, pregnancy-related deaths, and chronic conditions when compared to their White counterparts, and Black people have a life expectancy that is four years lower than White people (Ndugga, 2021). Most recently these disparities were amplified by the COVID-19 pandemic which resulted in an increase in rates of illness and death for American Indians, Alaskan Natives, and Black and Hispanic populations. Additionally, the mental health of LGBTQIA+ individuals has been disproportionately impacted by the pandemic (Ndugga, 2021).

In developing new curricular materials, it is critical to examine the health professions education literature to identify curricular gaps that can be addressed to allow us to maximize the opportunities to integrate DEI by expanding the modalities through which students are able to learn about DEI and health disparities. Although a significant component of every individual's overall health is influenced by socio-economic and environmental factors, the topic of health equity which addresses some of these concerns is underrepresented in core health professions curricula (Hood, 2016). In medical education especially, both faculty and students have reported a general lack of satisfaction with the current healthcare disparity curricula, especially in undergraduate medical education (Doobay-Persaud, 2019). In other health professions programs such as nursing, governing bodies such as the National League for Nursing (NLN) have also acknowledged that the social determinants of health are not well integrated into undergraduate and graduate nursing education (NLN, 2021). For example, education and training to address the health needs of Lesbian, gay, bisexual, queer, intersex, and asexual, (LGBTQIA+) individuals were found to be lacking in nursing curricula, and one survey of nursing faculty in undergraduate programs found that 23–63% of the faculty had not taught LGBT health-related topics in the past 2 years (Lim, 2015). In Pharmacy programs in the USA, educational standards mandate that curricula include the teaching of health disparities and cultural competency as well as their longitudinal assessment, but several studies have identified that more needs to be done to holistically integrate training on these topics in a manner that will improve the knowledge and skills of pharmacy graduates around DEI (Drame, 2022; Okoro, 2012).

The topic of racism and incorporating antiracism training into health professions education curricula is often a difficult topic to navigate but it is critically important to orient learners and faculty and all members of the learning community to the impact that racism has on the healthcare system both historically and currently. Since the pandemic and following the George Floyd incident most health professions programs have made efforts to highlight racial discrimination and the consequences of race as a social determinant of health. In medical education for example, the DEI competency framework released by the Association of American Medical Colleges (AAMC) has directly outlined educational objectives and assessment outcomes for incorporating antiracism education into curricula for learners at different points in their training (AAMC, 2022). This type of framework is adaptable across other health professions programs to guide curricular innovations.

Many approaches have been used to address curricular gaps related to DEI and health equity such as diversifying curricular materials and leveraging diverse individual experiences as teaching tools to demonstrate inequities in both patient care and the learning environment (Boelen, 2012; Roberts, 2020). Broad guidance for developing educational materials for improving health disparities education has been provided by stakeholder groups such as the Society of General Internal Medicine (SGIM) Health Equity Commission (Ross, 2010). Recommendations from the SGIM include ensuring that educational approaches allow for an understanding of attitudes such as implicit bias and stereotyping and their impact on the clinical encounter, providing knowledge of the prevalence of health disparities, and facilitating the acquisition of cross-cultural skills by learners that will help them to effectively communicate with diverse individuals (Ross, 2010). For example, antiracism training can be facilitated through various pedagogical approaches including open discussion across various social groups and self-reflection (Diffey, 2017). Recognizing and employing strategies to mitigate implicit bias is key to promoting fairness and equity. In this book, the cases were designed to amplify the voices of marginalized groups and individuals through the incorporation of scenarios that counter stereotyping, magnify the discriminatory practices prevalent in healthcare and allow for reflection by the audience.

The overall goal of this publication is to provide an educational resource focused on representing the diverse medical needs, health inequities, and health system challenges facing marginalized populations. The character actions represented in the cases derive from diverse patient experiences that highlight structural barriers, disrespectful attitudes, and discriminatory treatment that limit or prevent marginalized individuals from receiving optimal patient care. The cases and their prompt questions were developed with the goal of not only fostering the development of cultural and structural competencies in health professions learners, but also to shift assessment practices towards the evaluation of biases and behaviors that can perpetuate health inequities. With this book, a case-based approach has been used to generate robust discussions centered around topics in diversity, equity, and inclusion.

Health professional educators with diverse backgrounds from across the United States have come together to develop cases that reflect the breadth and depth of DEI topics that are relevant to healthcare and healthcare education. The case authors bring a wealth of experiences in health professions education. The editors were intentional in engaging a diverse group of individuals with diverse perspectives and experiences to ensure that the cases are inclusive and will resonate with a broad readership. Our hope is that the cases will serve as a tool to enhance structural and cultural competencies of learners in the health professions. There is a critical need to integrate diversity and inclusion into health professions curricula and to diversify educators' approaches to teaching. To address these inequities, it is important to promote diversity and inclusion in thought, practice, and curricular content. Social and cultural experiences uniquely influence the learning experience, so a plurality of perspectives should be represented in educational material seen in the classroom. This case book will engage both learners and educators in the health professions in robust discussions that will serve to enhance their awareness and knowledge around these issues with the expectation that knowledge will translate into practice that eventually reduces health inequities. The publication can be utilized in a variety of classroom-based and community settings. Overall, the case book was designed to achieve the following educational outcomes:

1. Integrate diversity and inclusion into health professions curricula by providing a variety of cases that represent diverse patient experiences.
2. Provide opportunities for health professions learners and educators to acquire the knowledge, skills, and tools to contribute to equitable health outcomes for vulnerable individuals.
3. Promote discussion on critical topics around health disparities and health equity.
4. Enhance the cultural and structural competencies of health professions learners.

We hope a diverse audience will take advantage of this publication including health professions educators and learners, health professionals, and community stakeholders. The cases are relevant to higher education institutions, hospitals, and community-based centers and can be utilized in a variety of settings including educational and professional development sessions. The unique case scenarios facilitate understanding and self-reflection to build cultural competence in health professions learners and add more diversity to existing thought-provoking resources that address DEI.

For educators, we envision this book to be a resource that can be leveraged in all health professions programs. In addition to being used in individual programs, the cases and their discussion points can be utilized during interprofessional educational activities to promote team building and allow learners to critically reflect on assumptions of themselves and other members of healthcare teams and how this can impact patient care, especially those from underrepresented groups. The cases present a unique opportunity to utilize an active learning format to engage learners and educators in discussion on more non-traditional topics and facilitate the depth and breadth of self-reflection and understanding that effectively cultivates cultural competence for both learners, educators, and practicing health professionals.

For leadership in health professional organizations, higher education, and community groups, the importance of DEI to institutional missions and strategic planning cannot be overemphasized. This publication is a resource that holds immense potential to not only enhance educational experiences and educational outcomes but also to contribute in a tangible way to achieving institutional missions and strategic goals around DEI. Many unique and underexplored topics are addressed in the various chapters, and this presents opportunities that leaders can build on, when designing strategic goals around belonging and DEI.

There are eighteen chapters in this book that span various topics relevant to health disparities, bias, cultural competency, and cultural humility. Each chapter addresses unique perspectives, and some may interrelate with topics in other chapters, which we consider a strength of the book.

Chapter 1, "Mental Health Stigma," focuses on how the stigma associated with mental health can impact access to appropriate care not only for patients but also for healthcare providers. Through these cases, different ways are highlighted in which implicit biases can impact the delivery of quality care to patients with mental illness.

Chapter 2, "Ableism in Medicine: Disability-Related Barriers to Healthcare Access," puts a lens on ableism which, due to its entrenchment in medicine, significantly impacts persons with disabilities via ableist attitudes and actions. Twenty-five percent of individuals in the US self-identify as having a disability and it is therefore important to ensure that persons with disabilities receive culturally competent healthcare and that healthcare educators teach about disability. This chapter illuminates many of the medically related structural barriers that persons with disabilities face and sets the stage for learners to have intentional discourse around the importance and immediate need to improve the delivery of quality care to these individuals.

Chapter 3, "Size Inclusivity in Medicine: Barriers to Healthcare Access for Patients With Obesity," portrays examples of weight stigma and bias in the healthcare system and the consequences that it has on the person. The 2 cases aim to equip health professions learners and practitioners with the tools to identify and reduce weight bias.

Chapter 4, "Ageism: Care at the Extremes of Life," focuses on the stereotypes, prejudice, and discrimination arising from ageism that affects both young and old age groups. The 3 cases aim to enhance empathy, dispel misconceptions about different age groups, and reduce prejudice by catalyzing discussion of the causes and consequences of ageism. Furthermore, this chapter provides health professions learners and practitioners with the tools to recognize ageism and strategies to reduce or eliminate its effects in the healthcare system.

Chapter 5, "Race and Racism and the Healthcare Professional Perspective," delves into racism and proactive anti-racism in healthcare. Three cases highlight unique situations in which a person's race affects their treatment. Discussion questions highlight the importance of recognizing and dismantling racism.

Chapter 6, "Cultural Competency by and for the Healthcare Professional," presents a look into cultural competency and its relationship to health professions. The three cases presented cover language barriers, religious or moral beliefs, and interprofessional relationships involving foreign medical graduates. Discussion questions and suggested responses accompany each case to encourage readers to reflect on the case scenarios. Through the cases and discussions, the complexity of cultural competency is revealed and prompted for discussion.

Chapter 7, "Language Barriers in Healthcare," emphasizes on the existing literature and language barriers that can lead to miscommunications between healthcare professionals and patients, contributing to reduced satisfaction among both groups, decreased quality of care, and reduced patient safety. Through the cases, an understanding of the health impacts of suboptimal language and the ethical obligation of linguistic equity is highlighted with respect to providing competent healthcare.

Chapter 8, "Healthcare in Patients With Limited English Proficiency and Linguistic Diversity in Medicine," includes cases that highlight the appropriate use of and loopholes in medical interpreter services, patient-provider language concordance to bypass language barriers, and relevance of medical translation to improve understanding of health, disease, and medication adherence.

Chapter 9, "Classism: Navigating the Hierarchy," presents the ethical elements of classism. Both ends of the spectrum are touched on, with cases related to low income and high-income individuals, as well as a look into the foster system, through 3 case presentations and discussion questions.

Chapter 10, "Gender Bias and Performativity," focuses on gender bias, gender performativity, microaggressions, and sexual harassment in clinical settings. The interactions represented in the 2 cases aim to equip health professions learners and practitioners with the skills to recognize and navigate gender bias and associated microaggressions within clinical and academic environments.

Chapter 11, "Lesbian, Gay, Bisexual, Transgender, Queer, Intersex, and Others (LGBTQI+): Providing Comprehensive Care Across the Spectrum," addresses challenges faced by lesbian, gay, bisexual, transgender, queer, and intersex persons. The 3 cases aim to prompt discussion and self-reflection about microaggressions and microinvalidations experienced by the LGBTQI+ community in academic and clinical settings. Additionally, this chapter presents strategies to enhance LGBTQI+ cultural competencies and create a safe and affirming learning environment.

Chapter 12, "Addressing Microaggressions in the Clinical Environment," utilizes a unique approach to present the negative impacts that microaggressions can have on patients and healthcare workers. The three cases provide learners with opportunities to apply a framework to recognize and respond to microaggressions in the clinical environment.

Chapter 13, "Making Room for Religion in Health Education: Institutional Discrimination and Dismantling the Framework," focuses on the intersection of religion with health professions education and clinical practice. Recognizing that there are both formal and informal barriers that prevent health professions learners from integrating their religious beliefs into their professional identities, readers are oriented to the importance of moving away from a one size fits all approach towards implementing supportive systems that accommodate the individual needs of learners especially as it relates to their religious beliefs. Faith inclusivity in both the learning environment and patient care is a focal point for the cases in this chapter.

Chapter 14, "Inclusion for Wellness: Fostering Wellness Through Inclusive Dialogue, Environments, and Practices," provides an overview of how healthcare professionals are at high risk to suffer from extreme burnout, despite growing efforts towards wellness. The cases in this chapter highlight the need for more attention for efforts towards inclusive learning experiences to support wellness. This chapter will explore how to build a truly inclusive and justice-oriented environment in the service of student wellness, by looking through different points during a student's healthcare professional training to explore how enhancing inclusive dialogue, environments, and practices in these spaces can also support practitioner wellness.

Chapter 15, "Work-Life Integration in Medicine: Unlearning Medical Culture and Establishing Boundaries," highlights barriers to work-life balance in medicine, particularly the impact of burnout on the delivery of quality health care. Fifty percent of healthcare workers in the United States report burnout at some point in their careers and this has likely been amplified by the COVID-19 pandemic due to increased physical and emotional workload demands. The chapter also discusses strategies to achieve work-life balance based on the personal goals of different individuals and the importance of this in preventing moral injury.

Chapter 16, "Cultivating Wellness and Cultural Humility Through Self-Awareness and Self-Reflection: The Practice of Physician Cultural Responsibility," presents the concept of Physician Cultural Responsibility. Through two diverse cases, the importance of Physician Cultural Responsibility is highlighted through a discussion on providing unbiased care to patients from other cultures and gender bias/stereotyping of patients. Reflection through the Physician Cultural Responsibility framework is supplemented by discussion questions for each case.

Chapter 17, "Curiosity, Humility, and Accountability: Key Elements to Advance a Culture of Diversity, Equity, and Inclusion in Health Professions Education," presents key factors for advancing a culture of belonging, equity, diversity, and inclusion in health professions education. Cases are structured to engage educators in reflecting on their teaching materials. The scenarios provide insights into strategies that have been effectively employed to mitigate unintended discrimination within health professions curricula such as decreasing bias in case presentations and explaining racial health disparities in the context of longstanding structural racism. The prompt questions leverage resources to advance health equity in health professions education.

Chapter 18, "Increasing Diversity in Medical Education: A Case Study," presents a unique twist to the view of diversity, equity, and inclusion in the health professions by examining how a health network sought to increase its diversity to attract a more diverse population of learners. The authors discuss the changes implemented and the outcomes from two different perspectives.

This book underscores the importance and benefits of diversity, equity, and inclusion in health professions education. The editors employed an evidenced-based approach in conceptualizing and enacting the content considerations for the cases. In reviewing the literature, we identified key topics related to cultural competency and DEI that are integral in guiding training outcomes in health professions education. The unique attributes of this scholarly work lay within underexplored topics that are addressed head-on in the various chapters. For example, mental health stigma is tackled at the beginning of the book, as stereotypes related to mental illness in the healthcare system and among healthcare providers is a critical barrier to healthcare for vulnerable patients and even for health professionals themselves. Chapter 1 highlights the need for mental illness stigma reduction initiatives to improve patient experiences. Similarly, in chapter 13, the role that religion and spirituality play in medical decision-making for patients in the clinical setting and learners in health professions programs are discussed.

Understanding that there are many instructional approaches for teaching learners about the social and structural determinants of health and assisting with skills acquisition for enhancing cultural competency, our case book specifically leverages case-based learning as a tool to facilitate critical reflection. Doobay-Persaud and colleagues describe critical reflection as a process where "the learner becomes aware of their own assumptions and preconceived notions through assessing, questioning, criticizing their actions and the experience with the goal of reframing perspective and using this analysis to inform future behavior" (Doobay-Persaud, 2019). The cases within this publication provide learners with thought-provoking scenarios that stimulate self-consciousness and reflection toward assumptions and conceptions. The cases also relate content about health inequities and structural barriers in healthcare to attitudes, thoughts, and actions in professional practice. Our hope is that this book will serve as a driver for transformative change in a way that will positively impact learning in health professions education and contribute to more culturally sensitive care for all patients. We thank every contributing author, many of whom tapped into their own personal and professional experiences to construct the cases presented in this publication.

Chasity Beth O'Malley
Wright State University Boonshoft School of Medicine, USA

Arkene Levy
Nova Southeastern University Dr. Kiran C. Patel College of Allopathic Medicine, USA

Amanda Chase
Nova Southeastern University Dr. Kiran C. Patel College of Allopathic Medicine, USA

Samiksha Prasad
Nova Southeastern University Dr. Kiran C. Patel College of Allopathic Medicine, USA

REFERENCES

AAMC. (2022). *Diversity, Equity, and Inclusion Competencies Across the Learning Continuum*. https://www.aamc.org/data-reports/report/diversity-equity-and-inclusion-competencies-across-learning-continuum

Bernstein, R. (2012). U.S. Census Bureau Projections Show a Slower Growing, Older, More Diverse Nation a Half Century From Now. United States Census Bureau, Public Information Office. CB12-243.

Boelen, C., Dharamsi, S., & Gibbs, T. (2012). The social accountability of medical schools and its indicators. *Education for Health*, *25*(3), 180.

Braveman, P., & Gruskin, S. (2003, April). Defining equity in health. *Journal of Epidemiology and Community Health*, *57*(4), 254–258. doi:10.1136/jech.57.4.254 PMID:12646539

CDC. (2013). *Health Disparities & Inequalities Report (CHDIR) Minority Health*. Centers for Disease Control and Prevention. https://www.cdc.gov/minorityhealth/chdireport.html

Diffey, L., & Mignone, J. (2017). Implementing anti-racist pedagogy in health professional education: A realist review. *Health Edu Care, 2*.

Doobay-Persaud, A., Adler, M. D., Bartell, T. R., Sheneman, N. E., Martinez, M. D., Mangold, K. A., Smith, P., & Sheehan, K. M. (2019). Teaching the Social Determinants of Health in Undergraduate Medical Education: A Scoping Review. *Journal of General Internal Medicine, 34*(5), 720–730.

Dougherty, K. J., & Kienzl, G. S. (2006). It's Not Enough to Get through the Open Door: Inequalities by Social Background in Transfer from Community Colleges to Four-Year Colleges. *Teachers College Record, 108*(3), 452–487. doi:10.1111/j.1467-9620.2006.00658.x

Drame, I., Gibson, C. M., Nonyel, N. P., Addo-Atuah, J., Butler, L., Riley, A., Kebodeaux, C., Henson, B., & Borja-Hart, N. (2022). Article. *American Journal of Pharmaceutical Education, 86*(3).

Hood, C. M., Gennuso, K. P., Swain, G. R., & Catlin, B. B. (2016). County health rankings: Relationships between determinant factors and health outcomes. *American Journal of Preventive Medicine, 50*(2), 129–135.

Lim, F., Johnson, M., & Eliason, M. (2015). A national survey of faculty knowledge, experience, and readiness for teaching lesbian, gay, bisexual, and transgender health in baccalaureate nursing programs. *Nursing Education Perspectives, 36*, 144–152.

McElfish, P. A., Moore, R., Buron, B., Hudson, J., Long, C. R., Purvis, R. S., Schulz, T. K., Rowland, B., & Warmack, T. S. (2018). Integrating Interprofessional Education and Cultural Competency Training to Address Health Disparities. *Teaching and Learning in Medicine, 30*(2), 213–222.

Ndugga, N., & Artiga, S. (2021). *Disparities in Health and Health Care: Five Key Questions and Answers*. Kaiser Family Foundation. https://www.kff.org/racial-equity-and-health-policy/issue-brief/disparities-in-health-and-health-care-5-key-question-and-answers/

NIH. (2017). *NIH Glossary*. National Institutes of Health. https://diversity.nih.gov/find-read-learn/glossary

NLN. (2021). *NLN Launches New Program to Raise Awareness with Nursing Educators of Societal Inequities Affecting Health & Welfare of Communities of Color*. NLN. http://www.nln.org/newsroom/news-releases/news-release/2021/05/12/nln-launches-new-program-to-raise-awareness-with-nurse-educators-of-societal-inequities-affecting-health-welfare-of-communities-of-color

Okoro, O. N., Odedina, F. T., Reams, R. R., & Smith, W. T. (2012). Clinical cultural competency and knowledge of health disparities among pharmacy students. *American Journal of Pharmaceutical Education, 76*(3), 40.

Parsons, A., Unaka, N. I., Stewart, C., Foster, J., Perez, V., Jones, N. Y., Kahn, R., Beck, A. F., & Riley, C. (2021). Seven practices for pursuing equity through learning health systems: Notes from the field. *Learn Health Syst., 5*(3), e10279.

Roberts, L. W. (2020). Belonging, respectful inclusion, and diversity in medical education. *Academic Medicine, 95*(5), 661–664.

Ross, P. T., Wiley Cene, C., Bussey-Jones, J., Brown, A. F., Blackman, D., Fernandez, A., Fernandez, L., Glick, S. B., Horowitz, C. R., & Jacobs, E. A. (2010). A strategy for improving health disparities education in medicine. *Journal of General Internal Medicine*, *25*(Suppl 2), S160–S163.

Thistlethwaite, J. E., Davies, D., Ekeocha, S., Kidd, J. M., MacDougall, C., Matthews, P., Purkis, J., & Clay, D. (2012). The effectiveness of case-based learning in health professional education. A BEME systematic review: BEME Guide No. 23. *Medical Teacher*, *34*(6), e421–e444.

Treacy-Abarca, S., Aguilar, M., & Vassar, S. D. (2021). Enhancing existing medical school curricula with an innovative healthcare disparities curriculum. *BMC Medical Education*, *21*, 613.

Acknowledgment

The editors would like to acknowledge the help of all the people involved in this project and, more specifically, to the authors and reviewers that took part in the review process. Without their support, this book would not have become a reality.

First, the editors would like to thank each one of the authors for their contributions. Our sincere gratitude goes to the chapter's authors who contributed their time and expertise to this book.

Second, the editors wish to acknowledge the valuable contributions of the reviewers regarding the improvement of quality, coherence, and content presentation of chapters. Most of the authors also served as referees; we highly appreciate their double task. The editors would like to give a special thank you to two non-author reviewers who were able to assist with peer reviews. Assistant Professor Dawn Owens from Nova Southeastern University Dr. Kiran C. Patel College of Allopathic Medicine, United States of America and Assistant Professor Anita Laloo from Nova Southeastern University Dr. Kiran C. Patel College of Allopathic Medicine, United States of America

Third, the editors wish to acknowledge the editorial contributions of Dr. Gabriella Dauer, MD from Nova Southeastern University Dr. Kiran C. Patel College of Allopathic Medicine, United States of America. Dr. Dauer assisted with the envisioning of the book and in providing a sample chapter for the editors. Her early contributions were invaluable.

Chapter 1
Mental Health Stigma

Omair Habib Abbasi
Memorial Health System, USA

Cory D. Horowitz
Memorial Health System, USA

Gabriella Dauer
Nova Southeastern University Dr. Kiran C. Patel College of Allopathic Medicine, USA

EXECUTIVE SUMMARY

This chapter discusses the ways in which stigma associated with mental health can impact access to appropriate care, not only for patients but also for healthcare providers themselves. Through these cases the authors will examine the ways in which implicit biases about mental health can impact the quality-of-care patients receive. In the first case, the authors look at the impact of mental illness on a medical student's career path in medicine. In the second case, they analyze the ways in which a person with a substance use disorder is scrutinized and judged in the emergency room setting. In the third case, an individual with a known history of autism and anxiety has their physical medical condition minimized which almost leads to a potentially poor outcome. Each case is unique in its presentation and only scratches the surface at the many different ways mental health and the stigma surrounding it continues to have an impact on the people alongside whom healthcare workers treat and work.

INTRODUCTION

The American Psychiatric Association defines mental illness as health condition involving changes in emotion, thinking, and/or behavior leading to distress or problems with functioning (or both). According to the World Health Organization, 1 in 8 people will be affected by mental illness at some point in their lifetime with the most common forms of mental illness being anxiety, depression, and post-traumatic stress disorder (Mental Disorders, 2022). Individuals who practice in the healthcare field are not excluded from this statistic. While medical students typically have lower pre-matriculation rates of burnout and depression than their college-graduating peers, approximately 1 out of 4 medical students

DOI: 10.4018/978-1-6684-5493-0.ch001

will meet criteria for depression during medical school (Rotenstein et al, 2016). A similar prevalence rate is seen amongst resident physicians and is linked to increases in medical errors and poor patient care (Mata et al, 2015). This high rate is also seen amongst students in other health professions including nursing (34%) (Yi-Jung et al, 2018), pharmacy (52.4%) (Al Faris et al, 2016), and physical therapy/occupational therapy (20%) (McDermott, 2018). This is in contrast to the prevalence of depression in the general population of 18- to 29-year-olds which is 21% (Villaroel & Terlizzi, 2020). Yet individuals with mental illness find themselves often being marginalized or discriminated for their diagnosis. Their illness is often considered to be less important or in need of attention than equally debilitating physical ailments. This is of major concern in an especially vulnerable population given the impact of mental illness on a person's ability to communicate and make decisions regarding their care. The stigma is also felt amongst healthcare workers themselves with members of the medical community being reluctant to seek out mental health treatment due to fear of judgement and effect on career trajectory (Knaak et al, 2017). The fact that stigmatization is not only felt amongst those we treat but also our colleagues lend to the endemic and systemic nature of the problem. Under the umbrella of mental illness there are also substance use disorders. In recent years the percentage of both emergency room visits and inpatient medical hospitalizations that are compounded by substance and alcohol use have been on the rise. From 2014 to 2018 alcohol use or substance use disorder in emergency room visits made up 9.4% and 11.9% of hospitalizations respectively, which showed a 30% and 57% relative increase from 2014 to 2018 (Suen et al, 2018). Despite the increasing prevalence of substance use disorders, they remain seriously undertreated (Yang et al, 2017). This stigmatization pervades not only how society perceives the person with substance use disorder, but also how that person perceives themselves and their illness. As such it can impact a person's willingness to engage in the healthcare system for preventative care and can also lead to other diagnoses of mental illness in addition to their substance use disorder. Studies have shown that the stigma associated with substance use as an independent factor can lead to worsening health outcomes even following completion of substance use treatment (Link et al, 1997).

CASE 1: SADAF'S SADNESS

Goal

This case exemplifies the barriers and stigma towards mental health treatment faced by medical professionals (in this particular case, a physician).

Learning Outcomes

1. Review the prevalence of mental illness amongst health professionals.
2. Identify barriers that prevent health care providers from seeking mental health treatment.
3. Examine the impact of health education curricula on the mental health of its learners.
4. Discuss changes that could be made in medical education and faculty development that may help decrease stigma towards mental health issues amongst healthcare providers.

Case

When Sadaf received her acceptance letter to medical school, she was ecstatic. As someone who had started her college journey with an interest in anthropology, she had never imagined she would find herself deciding to pursue medicine. However, after completing a paper on the history of medicine, she found herself deeply interested in the field and decided to take additional coursework in order to meet pre-matriculation requirements for medical school. She shared the news with her parents who congratulated her on her accomplishment and expressed pride in having their child be the first in the family to become a physician.

The reality of Sadaf's chosen path quickly came to realization when she began her first semester that summer. She noticed that she was somewhat behind in her knowledge when compared to her peers, especially those who had majored in basic sciences during their undergraduate studies. She struggled with feelings of shame when needing more time to grasp concepts and chose to study on her own so peers would not be aware of her knowledge deficits. She found herself utilizing large amounts of caffeine in order to keep herself awake in the evening so she could squeeze in a few extra hours of studying. This led to poor sleep, and she often felt tired the next morning during lab practicals. Although she was able to pass her first set of exams, she was approached by one of her professors who mentioned to her that she was "just barely passing" and expressed concern that she may have trouble obtaining residency placement in the future if she did not "try to make more of an effort." The professor suggested Sadaf seek help through a peer tutoring program, however Sadaf felt concerned that a peer might notice her struggles with the material and share the information with her classmates or professors. Sadaf continued to push herself, spending extra hours in the library, cutting down on her other hobbies, and reducing time with friends. She expressed concern to her family and friends who would often respond with "Isn't that typical for medical school?" often attempting to console her by telling her that things would get easier and congratulating her on choosing "such a noble profession".

During her second semester, Sadaf learned that her mother had been diagnosed with myasthenia gravis which was affecting her muscle tone and making it hard to breathe. Sadaf decided that she would try to provide support to her family over the phone – she did not feel she could take time off as she would most likely fall behind in her studies and not be able to maintain competitive grades. Knowing her mother was medically ill also drove Sadaf to work harder as she wanted to make sure she could one day help in her mother's treatment. Despite the increased conviction, Sadaf found herself having increasing difficulty in staying focused on her studies. She began to have insomnia even when she was not consuming caffeine. Her grades began to drop which made Sadaf feel that she was failing herself and her family. She frequently felt overwhelmed and would take breaks in between classes to go to the bathroom and cry. She began to dread calling her family as she didn't want to disappoint her mother who was already feeling unwell. Sadaf began to feel stuck. She kept pushing herself but felt she was only going through the motions in order to avoid disappointing others. Sometimes she would think to herself that it would be better if something were to happen to her so she could just pass away. She had experienced a similar thought while in college, but now the thought seemed to be crossing her mind more frequently. In some ways it brought her comfort, that perhaps there was a way out of all of this if she didn't feel she could keep going.

At a class-wide wellness session, Sadaf listened to a speaker discuss the symptoms of clinical depression and its prevalence amongst medical students. She could relate to the description provided by the presenter and wondered if she was indeed struggling with the condition. She checked in with some of her peers after the session. While many of her peers agreed with the presentation content and the importance of seeking mental health treatment, she didn't really hear anyone else mention a personal connection with the material. Sadaf again felt a sense of shame and decided not to mention anything to anyone.

As the year progressed, Sadaf started to fail coursework and was asked to meet with her faculty advisor. When the assistant dean went over Sadaf's grades and expressed concern over the decline in performance, Sadaf began to cry. She informed the dean about her struggles with medical knowledge, the medical issues with her mother, and feeling overwhelmed on a daily basis. The assistant dean encouraged Sadaf to take time off of school, to visit with family, and to work with a counselor. Sadaf agreed to do so. She started to reach out to friends and family but couldn't help but feel that she had somehow failed. She began to work with a therapist who eventually recommended Sadaf seek out a psychiatrist. When she mentioned the psychiatry appointment to her brother, he told her that he had heard from their mother that depression runs in the family and that there even was a cousin who committed suicide many years ago. He disclosed his own recent experience with depression and how medication was helpful which provided Sadaf with some comfort. Sadaf met with a psychiatrist and started an antidepressant. Combined with therapy, Sadaf noticed an improvement in her self-image and her outlook for the future. She returned to medical school 6 months later and successfully completed her pre-clinical course work.

During her clinical rotations, Sadaf came across patients who were struggling with mental illness on every service. She witnessed preceptors who would acknowledge mental illness and refer patients to psychiatric care, but she also noted physicians, nursing staff, and social workers making curt comments about such patients, often referring to them as "difficult" or "annoying." She encountered a patient who was having refractory pain and told her that he sometimes wondered if suicide would be the only way to get out of chronic pain. Sadaf felt she could relate to the sentiment. When she discussed it with her preceptor, he responded, "On top of everything else he now has to tell us he is suicidal? Now I'm going to be late for the next patient." Sadaf felt a tinge of shame in that moment, remembering that she had told her psychiatrist about similar thoughts and wondering if he had secretly had the same reaction.

Sadaf eventually went on to seek a residency in internal medicine with a desire to eventually specialize in rheumatology. The application and interviewing process was difficult for Sadaf as she often felt she could not disclose the exact reason she took time off from her coursework. She eventually ended up matching into a less competitive, but strong residency program and was happy to be starting the next phase of her career. Residency consisted of long hours, multiple demands on her time, and complex, frequently novel cases that Sadaf had not seen during her time in medical school. Despite it all, she did very well during her first 2 years. During her third year of training, Sadaf started to feel a sense of apathy. She was unsure why it was occurring as she had acclimated to the stress of residency, however a sense of lacking purpose continued to creep in. She began to struggle to listen to her patients, felt a lack of motivation, and had difficulty sleeping at night. She wondered if she was starting to "burn out," a term that had been presented to her as common amongst physicians. As time went on, the symptoms worsened. Her program director noted a change in her performance, "I know you can do better than this. You used to be so detailed in your assessments and now it feels like you're mailing it in." This only worsened Sadaf's experience. She began to have strong feelings of guilt and shame that she was not providing good care to her patients. Slowly, she began to re-experience a feeling of being trapped. That the only way out would be to end her life. She talked to a close friend and colleague about her history of depression. He expressed concern for her and told her that she should probably get help "you don't want to end up in a psych ward, they'll take away your license once you get to that point." Sadaf reconnected with the psychiatrist she had seen while in medical school. The psychiatrist encouraged her to speak with her program director to take time off, however Sadaf felt that it would impact her negatively. She had done so in medical school, and it had led to difficulty with candor during residency interviews, she did not want to have the same struggle with obtaining a fellowship. She took the prescription and began antidepressant treatment. She continued to struggle but noticed gradual improvements in her symptoms as the medication took effect. She continued to keep her struggles with mental illness to herself throughout the rest of her time in residency, worried that it might affect her chances at obtaining a competitive fellowship.

QUESTIONS AND ANSWERS

1. Discuss factors that may have increased Sadaf's risk of developing mental illness?

When reviewing risk factors for mental illness, one should take into consideration modifiable versus non-modifiable risk factors. That is, some individuals will enter health education with risk factors that cannot be directly changed (non-modifiable risk factors). For Sadaf such risk factors include a personal and family history of depression, age, and sex. It is important to note that having risk factors for mental illness does not guarantee that one will develop mental illness in their lifetime, however, compounding risk factors increase the overall likelihood. The health care educator should take into consideration modifiable risk factors that may respond to early intervention and prevention. Amongst the modifiable risk factors are interpersonal trauma, loss/grief, life stress, substance use, and poor nutrition. Lastly, neuroticism, a form of temperament in which an individual frequently perceives their surroundings as negative, threatening, or dangerous, can lead to poor resilience and difficulty coping with life stressors. Sadaf's perception of adjusting to the rigorous curriculum of medical school as a personal deficit led to a reaction of shame and guilt causing her to hide her struggles. Neurotic personality traits are responsive to psychotherapy and individuals who have these traits can benefits from seeking help early, before challenges and stress start to accumulate.

2. What barriers did Sadaf experience in seeking mental health treatment?

Sadaf faced many of the obstacles that students and trainees in health education encounter throughout the United States. High levels of stress and perfectionism are normalized in health education which causes struggling students and trainees to be less likely to seek out resources. The stigma associated with mental illness also imbues a feeling of shame and fear in individuals who could otherwise receive benefits from timely interventions. On a structural level, funding for mental health resources and particularly treatment is often limited in health education programs which leads to the cost of such interventions being prohibitive for students. If resources are available, there is often unclear guidance on how to access resources and what to expect during an appointment. There are also issues with confidentiality and whether seeking out such resources will be reported to governing bodies or documented in a student's records. Sadaf experienced a sense of internalized shame about her adjustment to the rigors of medical school. She avoided seeking out general resources due to concerns of confidentiality. She later had the opportunity to attend a seminar on depression in medical students, but it was unclear if resources were highlighted or encouraged during the session. She was encouraged to take a temporary leave of absence by her assistant dean, however due to stigma associated with mental health, Sadaf was hesitant to explain the exact cause of her leave of absence during residency interviews. This led her to question seeking help again when she experienced another bout of depression during residency. Her concerns about having to disclose a mental health diagnosis to state licensing agencies is valid as several state medical licensure boards require disclosure of mental health treatment even if it has never impacted a physician's ability to care for their patients.

3. How did the health education environment perpetuate Sadaf's depression and levels of stress.

As mentioned previously, high levels of stress are normalized in health care education. Perfectionism is often lauded as an asset and at times can be used recklessly to justify a need for constant achievement. High stakes performance measures such as clerkship grades, class rank, or exam scores cause students to feel pressured to over-study so to not risk losing out on competitive residency placement. Sadaf encountered these pressures, externally placed upon her by her professors but also internalized as she proceeded through medical school. When facing another episode of depression as a resident, Sadaf is reprimanded by her program director as not performing up to her typical standards. In this way, perfectionism is demanded as the standard from physicians who are only human and need to balance their efforts towards work with other aspects of their lives. Sadaf also witnessed stigma associated with mental illness during her clerkships. Frustration with mental health issues modeled by her preceptor not only caused a feeling of moral distress in Sadaf, but also imprinted social stigma that caused her to question her personal experiences with mental health care.

4. How could the wellness session that Sadaf attended be improved to make Sadaf more comfortable to seek help?

While educational sessions about mental health and wellness are becoming more common place in health care education, they are often marred by being impersonal and often utilizing an intellectual approach of didactic learning. Sadaf found herself relating to the topic and found it educational, but the session did not address barriers preventing Sadaf from disclosing her own struggles. An adjunctive session in which select faculty or students discuss their personal journeys through mental illness can help normalize the experience and empower students to seek out mental health care. Sadaf attended the session after she had already completed her first semester of medical school, by that time she was already experiencing symptoms of depression and had developed unhelpful methods of coping with her thoughts and feelings. Wellness sessions addressing mental illness, especially identification and resources for treatment, could have been presented in the curriculum sooner. This would have allowed Sadaf to catch the symptoms as they started to occur rather than attempting to treat them when they had become quite severe.

5. How could Sadaf's faculty and supervisors have been more helpful in their statements of concern?

Sadaf's faculty and supervisors often approached her out of concern. However, the concern was structured around Sadaf's academic or professional performance. Much of the commentary was prescriptive in nature, identifying a change in level of performance combined with a suggestion that Sadaf improve. The incentive for change was often related to concern for Sadaf's future or patient care as if these alone should be sufficient driving factors to motivate any individual. Attribution for the change or lack of performance was never explored. Health care careers often demand a constant level of high performance, not only during education and training, but for the remainder of a person's life. This type of pressure does not take into consideration that health care professionals are human and will have other aspects of their lives that need attention. Supervisors and instructors can change this by taking a more inquisitive stance when approaching a struggling student or trainee. The faculty or supervisor could have opened the conversation with an observation "I've noticed a decrease in the level of detail in your notes." This could be followed by a question that elicits reflection, "Have you noticed this yourself?" followed by a non-presumptive inquiry of what may be causing the change in performance and a collaborative stance on the approach to the problem. "Do you know what might be causing the change?" This is an un-intrusive, yet inquisitive approach to feedback and can allow for a bi-directional exchange of information to help the learner discuss concerns without being prescriptive in nature.

Epilogue

Mental health stigma not only plagues the patients who health care providers treat, but also health care providers themselves. Sadaf's journey is not uncommon amongst students and trainees in health education. While students will matriculate with their individualized pre-disposing factors for mental illness, it is important to address institutional factors that precipitate and perpetuate mental illness along with the barriers that prevent individuals from seeking care. Sadaf encountered many of these factors including a continuous pursuit of perfectionism encouraged by her instructors and supervisors that caused her to neglect her relationships, self-care, and values. Once she recognized that she needed help, she found herself at a loss of where to turn or whom to speak to leading to an increased sense of isolation. Even after she takes a leave from her medical education to seek out appropriate care, she continues to find herself facing obstacles in her career including having to explain the leave during residency interviews and wondering how a history of mental illness might impact her licensure and job prospects. Mental illness amongst health care providers is being increasingly discussed in the literature with emphasis on early identification, ease of access to resources, and modifications to the education curriculum to decrease stress on students. Mental health stigma remains a prominent obstacle and will take time to deconstruct. Most unfortunately, Sadaf's story is not uncommon with high rates of depression and anxiety being experienced by learners in all fields of health care education. Yet, the tendency to hide our stories as a source of shame rather than share them as examples of empowerment and overcoming adversity continues to drive a system that tends to avoid acknowledging the obvious, we are all human, we all struggle, we all need help. Health care educators can do their part by modeling positive approaches to mental health issues.

CASE 2: DR. LANGLEY'S LAPSE

Goal

This case exemplifies how individuals struggling with substance use disorders are often misperceived in the hospital which can impact quality of care.

Learning Outcomes

1. Discuss how the stigma associated with substance use disorders can affect an individual's self-worth and dignity.
2. Discuss how the provider's stigma toward substance use can impact patient outcomes with obtaining and maintaining sobriety.
3. Identify appropriate patient-centered language when speaking to or about persons with substance use disorders.
4. Explore how stigma towards substance use disorders can be addressed amongst medical professionals and healthcare workers.

Case

Brandi, a 29-year-old female, was found down outside a gas station. A call to the police had been made 15 minutes prior as Brandi was arguing very loudly with another person at the gas station. When the police arrived, Brandi was found slumped over on the curb, breathing very slowly. Law enforcement administered intranasal naloxone causing the Brandi to become responsive but agitated, cursing at the police officers. She was placed in handcuffs and brought to the emergency department by law enforcement for further treatment after an opioid overdose. On arrival, Brandi is received by an ER nurse who notes that Brandi's clothes are soiled. Law enforcement removes the handcuffs, and she is changed into a clean hospital gown, however she is not given the opportunity to wash her face or clean up before being placed in a hospital bed in a busy hallway of the emergency room.

She is assigned to be cared for by a resident ER physician, Dr. Langley. As Dr. Langley is approaching the patient to perform his initial evaluation, one of his supervising physicians, Dr. Howard, walks by and says, "Oh hello Brandi, I haven't seen you in a while, but it looks like you're back. Hopefully you won't give Dr. Langley too much trouble. We've got a lot of sick people in the ER tonight." Dr. Howard then turns to Dr. Langley and speaks softly, "Her urine drug screen came back dirty for marijuana, heroin, and fentanyl. She's somewhat of a lost cause but we try to help her when we can. She's definitely one of the less angry addicts we get here." Dr. Howard then walks away to go take care of his own patients. Brandi is guarded and answers Dr. Langley's questions with short, curt responses, taking brief breaks from the interview to vomit. Dr. Langley notices that Brandi has some cellulitis on her left hand. He points it out to Brandi who replies, "Oh now you care all of a sudden?" Dr. Langley finds himself irritated by Brandi's demeanor and cuts the interview short, "let's just get you in shape to leave. No one is forcing you to stay." Dr. Langley continues his assessment and finds that the patient appears to be in withdrawal from opioids with tachycardia, elevated blood pressure, rhinorrhea, nausea, hot and cold sweats, loose bowel movements, and muscle cramps. Brandi is offered oral antibiotics for her skin infection. She takes the medication. She requests help with her pain in her hand, but Dr. Langley responds that she is not allowed to have narcotic pain medications, "we can't give you anything like that because of your drug problem." Brandi becomes irritated that Dr. Langley is assuming she wants opiate pain medication and decides to sign out against medical advice.

Later in the night, a hospital dispatcher receives a call from rescue services that they are on route with a patient who was found down on the street and responded to naloxone administration. The patient arrives to the hospital in an ambulance on a stretcher and is placed under Dr. Langley's care. Dr. Langley enters the room to see that it is Brandi who has returned after being discharged several hours ago.

However, at the bedside is the ER nurse, Hannah, who is sitting next to the patient speaking with her. Nurse Hannah asks to speak with Dr. Langley in the hallway. She tells Dr. Langley that she has known Brandi for several years and that until recently Brandi had been in recovery for over a year. The nurse shares with Dr. Langley that Brandi's younger brother had unexpectedly passed away three months ago. Brandi subsequently relapsed on heroin. She subsequently lost her job and was evicted from her home and has been living on the streets for the last few weeks. Brandi told nurse Hannah that she had left the hospital against medical advice as she was not getting help with her pain and felt that she was being judged by the doctors. Hannah tells Dr. Langley, "She trusts me so I told her you're actually a nice guy and that I would talk to you about what's going on; that this visit would be better and we'd be able to take care of her." Dr. Langley appreciates Nurse Hannah's help and visits with Brandi. He expresses his remorse to Brandi about her loss and begins his interview. The patient appears quite uncomfortable and snaps at the physician, "Don't pretend like you care! I'm just an addict and that's all I'm ever going to be". Dr. Langley apologizes to Brandi and recognizes that his demeanor towards her may have made her feel that way. He asks her to work with him so he may be able to get her hand feeling better. Nurse Hannah stands next to Dr. Langley and states, "Give him another chance, Brandi. He's still learning!" Brandi begrudgingly agrees. He screens Brandi for symptoms of depression and finds that she does meet criteria for major depressive disorder. He requests a consult with psychiatry and social work to help Brandi obtain resources for housing and addiction treatment. Brandi is started on an opioid withdrawal protocol and provided with non-narcotic pain medication. She agrees to stay at the hospital to get her care.

Months later Dr. Langely meets Brandi in the ER for another visit. This time it's for a fractured toe. He notices a major change in Brandi's appearance as she is well dressed, groomed, and very pleasant. She greets Dr. Langley and says she remembers him. She updates Dr. Langley that she was able to get into a residential recovery program and is now on buprenorphine which has been helping her greatly with her opioid use. She is working full time and has found some stable housing. She apologizes to Dr. Langley about her cursing and being curt with him during her previous visit, "When they give you that naloxone, it throws you into withdrawal and you are just angry with anyone and everyone." Dr. Langley thanks her for giving him a second chance and proceeds to examine and treat her toe. After Brandi leaves, he runs into Dr. Howard and tells him about the good news. He shakes his head and responds, "She couldn't get totally sober, huh? Had to get on that replacement therapy. Well, at least she's off the streets." Dr. Langley is surprised by his supervisor's response. He wonders how often Dr. Howard runs across individuals with substance use issues and what Dr. Howard's trainees may have learned from watching him.

QUESTIONS AND ANSWERS

1. Discuss how the manner in which Brandi arrives and is stationed in the emergency room during her first visit can affect her dignity and self-worth.

Unfortunately, Brandi's initial experience in the emergency room is not uncommon for individuals with substance use disorders. Often individuals may be brought in under custody dawning handcuffs. This form of presentation to the emergency room relays a message of criminality which can activate unconscious biases in her healthcare providers. Consequently, Brandi may be approached in a guarded manner by those taking care of her or worse, she may not be provided with cares or resources that others would receive. The criminalization of substance use, although slowly being reformed, has caused a societal view of substance use disorders as a deficit in morality rather than a specific disease process. While society at large needs ongoing education about the biological underpinnings of addiction, health education fields have been incorporating biological determination, precipitation, and perpetuation of addiction into their curriculum. Healthcare providers must keep in mind that this is a disease process like any other. When Brandi arrives to the ER, she is asked by Dr. Howard to not cause too much trouble as there are a lot of "sick" people in the emergency. Such a statement does damage to Brandi's dignity and self-worth in two ways, it labels Brandi as a troublemaker insinuating that she may have a poor understanding of moral or societal norms. It also deems Brandi's substance use disorder as less deserving of prioritization or understanding compared to other illnesses. This may explain Brandi's angry response when Dr. Langley points out the cellulitis on her hand, as if the presence of an observable ailment now makes Brandi more deserving of care. This can also be an unconscious process for Dr. Langley who may have switched to observations of objective signs rather than further exploring Brandi's social history and substance use as a response to Brandi appearing frustrated. This can also be due to a lack of confidence in speaking about substance use or difficulty empathizing with someone who struggles with a substance use disorder. Training on approaching substance use disorders through simulation or case discussion can be helpful for health education learners as they will encounter individuals with the disorder regardless of what field they enter. Lastly, while Brandi is provided with a gown, she is not given an opportunity to clean herself up. She is in opioid withdrawal which while not fatal, can cause significant distress and discomfort for individuals. Even then, she is left in the emergency room hallway to eventually be seen. Some of these factors cannot be controlled in a busy emergency room setting, but even a simple gesture of handing Brandi a wet towel could be beneficial and help her preserve some level of dignity.

2. Compare Dr. Howard and Nurse Hannah's approach to Brandi and how it impacts Dr. Langley's care of Brandi?

Addiction is a chronic disease with remissions and relapses. While the goal is to hopefully prevent a relapse from occurring in the future, it should be considered that relapse is part of the disease process. Yet individuals with substance use disorders are often judged for their relapses compared to other disease models (e.g., multiple sclerosis). Dr. Howard mentioned that he had not seen Brandi for a period of time but did not attempt to learn why that may have been. As discussed previously, his greeting to Brandi contains comments that are demeaning of her illness and signal to Dr. Langley that he should deprioritize her symptoms and possibly constrict the interview. In turn, Dr. Langley finds himself becoming quickly irritated with Brandi and cuts the interview short. When Brandi returns for a second time, nurse Hannah, who is also familiar with Brandi, speaks with her. However, nurse Hannah does not identify Brandi by her addiction and instead learns more about Brandi's personal situation. Hannah then provides Dr. Langley with some background about Brandi which humanizes her. Additionally, Hannah plays a powerful role as the liaison between Dr. Langley and Brandi, helping both parties communicate with one another and helping rebuild a ruptured rapport. Dr. Langley follows suit and apologizes to Brandi which helps relieve the tension in the situation. Learners in health education are often impacted by the "hidden curriculum." This refers to the unstructured, sometimes unspoken lessons learned from students and trainees by observing others in the healthcare environment. In many cases, the hidden curriculum can leave more of a lasting effect on a learner than a didactic lecture or curricular activity. Both Dr.

Howard and nurse Hannah modeled different approaches to the care of Brandi which caused a change in Dr. Langley's interaction with the patient.

3. Dr. Howard uses several stigmatizing words when referring to Brandi and her care. Identify the words used and how they could be changed to be more patient centered.

Language matters when taking care of frequently stigmatized individuals. Using the appropriate words when speaking about and to patients can reduce feelings of judgement and discrimination amongst patients and healthcare providers alike. In this case Dr. Howard uses several words that could be replaced with alternatives that are more patient centered. In his comment to Dr. Langley, he reports that Brandi's urine drug screen was "dirty". Alternatively, he could say that the urine drug screen returned positive for substances. He also refers to Brandi as an "addict". He could alternatively refer to Brandi as a person with a substance use disorder. This allows Brandi to be identified as a person who can be separated from the disorder, not defined by it. Dr. Howard's response to Dr. Langley months later is also problematic. Often there is a misconception that a person with substance use disorders is only doing well when he or she is "sober." The term sober or sobriety is problematic as it implies that the primary purpose of treatment is for the individual to stop using substances – this again defines the person by their diagnosis rather than taking the individual in their entirety and engaging them in ways to move forward in their life. The term "recovery" is a more suitable term. It entails not only addressing a person's substance use, but also considering the individual's overall goals and values. The term sobriety has also caused healthcare providers to misconceive success as complete abstinence from all substances, rather than improved overall functioning. Lastly, Dr. Howard refers to Brandi's treatment with buprenorphine as "replacement therapy." Terms such as replacement therapy or substitution therapy should be replaced with medication-assisted treatment. Due to long term effects of chronic substance use on a person's neurobiology, some individuals do best with medication-assisted treatment to maintain recovery and move forward in their lives. Labeling this life changing treatment as simply "replacement therapy" degrades its value and purpose. It again makes the focus on solely abstinence from a substance rather than rebuilding one's life and purpose.

4. How could Dr. Langley approach Dr. Howard about his conscious or unconscious biases towards individuals with substance use disorders?

Addressing biases in colleagues can be difficult. This can be especially complicated in health education due to the hierarchical nature of many institutions. As a resident, Dr. Langley may be hesitant to speak with Dr. Howard about such matters. If Dr. Langley does not feel he has the rapport with Dr. Howard to bring up the topic, a first step may be to share the concern with another supervisor or trusted ally in his organization. That individual may be able to provide support, raise the issue on Dr. Langley's behalf, or may be able to identify the right person to contact. Whether addressing Dr. Howard directly or indirectly, Dr. Langley will want to make sure to avoid using accusatory language. Unless there is clear evidence to the contrary, it is best to assume that Dr. Howard's bias is unconscious, and that Dr. Howard is not purposely attempting to harm patients. When speaking to Dr. Howard, using "we" statements can help reduce a feeling of blame as in, "I think we can work on our approach to people with substance use disorders." This includes Dr. Langley in the process and makes the effort feel more collaborative. Dr. Langley can provide suggestions to Dr. Howard for using alternative language to improve patient care.

He could also offer to provide a brief presentation on updates in substance use disorder treatment and explain how sobriety in and of itself may not be the sole solution. He may demonstrate more empathic behaviors towards patients with substance use disorder. Lastly, individuals with unconscious biases tend to focus on events that confirm their bias and often fail to recognize instances that counteract their assumptions. Highlighting instances in which patients do well or respond better to an alternative approach may also help Dr. Howard recognize his blind spots and foster change.

5. How can stigma towards substance use disorders be addressed amongst medical professionals and healthcare workers?

The stigma associated with substance use disorders and addiction is prevalent in both the healthcare profession and in society. This stigma serves to marginalize these persons and make them be perceived as the “other”. So, we can tackle this stigma by humanizing our patients who struggle with substance use and viewing them as people with a substance use disorder as opposed to “just an addict”. The case above exemplifies the importance of humanizing the patient and treating them with dignity and respect. In Brandi’s first encounter we see that the only background information provided is from Dr. Howard’s description of her and otherwise she is described by symptoms and vital signs. In her second encounter we see that Brandi is a person with a story and experiences that have led her to this moment. It does not diminish her illness, but rather provides context and understanding to it. So should this be our goal as healthcare professionals in addressing the stigma associated with substance use disorders. We should be striving to get to know the person as a whole, including their illness, so that we can see them as a person first and foremost.

Epilogue

The stigma associated with mental health problems, notably addiction, can have far reaching consequences in the healthcare profession. In this case we see how the stigma associated with persons struggling with addiction impacts the care Brandi initially receives by Dr. Langley in the emergency room. Everything from the manner in which Brandi is brought into the emergency room to Dr. Langley’s interaction with Dr. Howard colors the entire emergency room encounter before Brandi has even spoken a word to Dr. Langley. This leads to Brandi feeling ashamed and embarrassed, responding to Dr. Langley’s questions with one-word answers, and being discharged a few hours later only to have another accidental overdose shortly thereafter. On her subsequent visit just a few short hours later the tone is different from the very beginning. Brandi is brought in by an ambulance, has a positive experience with her nurse, and she is humanized by being given space to describe the events surrounding her situation. This allows Brandi to receive care from a biopsychosocial approach which addresses her needs not only as a person with addiction, but as a person as a whole. Our innate biases and the stigma associated with those struggling with addiction can often color not only our perception, but also our interactions, with this population. It is important that we as healthcare professionals are aware of our innate biases and the stigma associated with addiction so that we can provide the highest quality of care that all of our patients deserve.

CASE 3: DR. R'S OVERSIGHT

Goal

This case demonstrates how the stigma associated with mental health can have repercussions on the care of a patient with mental illness.

Learning Outcomes

1. Discuss and analyze how the stigma associated with mental illness, particularly in the healthcare profession, can impact the care of a patients.
2. Discuss how healthcare providers can approach an individual with mental illness in the context of a co-occurring physical condition.
3. Evaluate how the stigma toward mental illness can be addressed in the healthcare profession to improve quality of care.

Case

The emergency room was staffed by a rotating resident when Orlando came in. He had been brought in by his mother, Mrs. S, for fever and difficulty breathing. He appeared short of breath and very anxious. Mrs. S explained to the ER nurse that Orlando is a 19-year-old male with autism, he is minimally verbal, and has a diagnosis of anxiety for which he takes nightly medication. Nurse documented "Autism with anxiety having SOB" in notes. His anxiety is well managed, and he has only had one prior episode of severe anxiety with panic attack requiring a visit to the emergency room for acute medical management. When Orlando came into the emergency room this time, a familiar face- Dr. R-an emergency room resident greeted them.

Dr. R recognized Orlando and his mother from a previous visit to the emergency room during an acute panic attack. Dr. R pulled Orlando's chart, reviewed his vitals, and proceeded to review the triage nurse notes, which read "19-year-old male, anxious, short of breath." Dr. R noted that Orlando was tachycardic and hypertensive on review of initial triage vitals. Dr. R looks over to the covering attending physician and says, "I know this guy. He has autism and a strong history of anxiety. I took care of him recently when he was brought in by his mom for a panic attack. Looks like he's here for the same thing. He will probably need some lorazepam like he did last time."

Dr. R enters into the patient's room to take a history and complete a physical exam. "Orlando and Mrs. S, I see that you are back, do you remember me?" Orlando is visibly uncomfortable and unable to respond. His mother is clearly worried. Mrs. S notes that they presented to their usual hospital a few days ago for fever and muscle aches. They were told by the physician team that Orlando likely had a viral infection and discharged him home without further investigation. They are returning to this larger academic center for a second opinion as over the last 24 hours Orlando has developed worsening muscle aches, specifically on his chest and back, and has been having difficulty breathing. Dr. R attempts to perform a physical examination however Orlando is irritable and will hold still only momentarily before attempting to swat Dr. R's stethoscope away, making the examination difficult. Mrs. S notes Dr. R's difficulty and attempts to explain that Orlando is in distress because of his breathing. Dr. R interrupts and quickly responds, "Oh poor guy, he must be very anxious, and the virus is probably worsening his anxiety, let me get him some lorazepam to help him out." Dr. R exits the room and Mrs. S is confused as she believes there is an underlying medical etiology beyond Orlando's anxiety that are causing the symptoms. Mrs. S attempts to explain this, however Dr. R dismisses this and tells her that "I'm sure it's just anxiety so we will give him some anxiety medicine and he should calm down". Feeling uncomfortable with this Mrs. S requests to see the attending immediately as Orlando is beginning to look worse. Dr. R obliged and called the attending Dr. P over to examine Orlando per the mother's request.

Dr. P enters the room, listens to the history of the patient having fever and muscle aches with now worsening shortness of breath. "Let's do some labs to see what is going on, I see that you are concerned. In the meantime, we can give Orlando some lorazepam to help him relax." The mother agrees to the labs and the anxiolytic medication. A full lab panel is sent, and 1 milligram of Lorazepam given to the patient. Orlando is given the lorazepam and labs are waiting to result, but Orlando continues to have increased work of breathing, tachycardia now to 160, and seems restless sitting upright and bending forward in the patient bed.

The nurse enters the room again and alerts both Dr. R and Dr. P of Orlando's worsening condition. Dr. P reviews the labs and notes an elevated creatine kinase. He diagnoses Orlando with an infection, starts intravenous fluids, and calls the hospitalist team for admission for rehydration and antibiotics. Orlando now receives a second dose of lorazepam for worsening agitation, and his oxygen saturation slips down to 93% without notice.

The hospitalist is called for admission and review Orlando's vitals and labs. Vitals are notable for persistent and worsening tachycardia; labs are notable for derangements throughout. Alongside an elevated creatine kinase, Orlando has severely abnormal labs notable for leukocytosis, thrombocytosis, coagulopathy, transaminitis, and elevated creatinine consistent with severe infection or inflammation and possible multi-organ failure. The hospitalist goes down with her resident team to evaluate Orlando who is now in a tripod position on his bed, visibly short of breath, febrile, and severely anxious despite 2 mg of lorazepam. Orlando is started on supplemental oxygen; blood cultures are obtained, and he then receives empiric broad spectrum antibiotics. His blood cultures return positive for Methicillin Resistant Staph Aureus (MRSA) which is sensitive to the antibiotics he was started on and over the course of several days his symptoms improve and he is able to be discharged home.

QUESTIONS AND ANSWERS

1. How does the stigma associated with mental illness impact the care Orlando receives in a medical setting?

In the case above we see a patient with autism spectrum disorder who is minimally verbal with a known history of anxiety presents with a chief complaint of shortness of breath. At the beginning of the case we see that Dr. R has assumed a diagnosis and treatment plan before he has even seen the patient. He then proceeds to hold to his diagnosis despite Orlando's mother voicing her concerns that the presentation is not typical for Orlando's anxiety. What Dr. R is demonstrating is known as an anchoring bias. An anchoring bias is the tendency to prioritize information and data that confirms an initial diagnosis, even if the diagnosis may be incorrect. Individuals with mental illness are often vulnerable to marginalization and misinterpretation of symptoms as are the family members who may attempt to advocate for them. The minimization of Orlando's mother's concerns, while not conscious on Dr. R's behalf, could have led to a poor outcome. It is important for healthcare providers to keep in mind that physical symptoms, whether benign or dangerous, may often elicit an emotional response from patients. Psychiatric symptoms are not always indicative of onset or exacerbation of an underlying psychiatric disorder and therefore healthcare providers need to be cautious of misattribution. In the same vein, it is appropriate for healthcare providers to acknowledge, validate, and manage co-occurring psychiatric or emotional symptoms, but they must be cautious not to do so at the cost of leaving other potential differential diagnoses unexplored.

2. Discuss how Orlando's mental health diagnosis may have impacted Dr. R's ability to elicit a history from his patient?

There may be times when a healthcare worker enters a room, and the most prominent symptoms is the patients affect (their outward expression of emotion). When this occurs, one should always be mindful of one's internal response to the affect – does it cause a desire to shorten the interview or reduce engagement with the patient or family, does it cause avoidance of performing certain exam maneuvers? Being mindful of these feelings can help healthcare providers to ensure they are maintaining their due diligence in the treatment of patients. It is also important to remember that patients are not always going to present in a classic textbook manner. Our minds and bodies are linked and therefore our physical and mental health can impact each other. For example, when a person is experiencing flu-like symptoms they are unlikely to be as upbeat and outgoing as they might normally be because they do not feel well. By that same token when a person is experiencing anxiety it can often lead to a difficulty in obtaining an appropriate and distinct assessment of their physical health. For example, is their tachycardia due to a physical illness or is it a physiologic response to their anxiety? In the case above we see that Orlando has a known history of anxiety in addition to being minimally verbal at baseline. Dr. R was not necessarily wrong in her line of thinking that Orlando's physical illness of the suspected virus was leading to a worsening of his anxiety. However, is it important for healthcare providers to obtain and integrate collateral information into their assessment whenever possible. Had Dr. R considered the collateral information from Orlando's mother then she may have been able to accurately diagnose Orlando's physical illness as opposed to misattributing his symptoms to his co-occurring anxiety.

3. How does Dr. R's initial interaction with Orlando and his mother during this visit lead to Dr. R missing the actual diagnoses of MRSA bacteremia?

When Dr. R first interacts with Mrs. S, Dr. R assumes that Orlando is presenting because his previously diagnosed virus at the previous hospital is causing the patient to be more anxious. It is valuable to recognize that a patient who is physically unwell is prone to have heightened anxiety and to try and help minimize the patient's discomfort, it is equally important to not let the belief that a patient's anxiety or other mental illness is the sole contributor to a patient's presentation. For example, Orlando is having physical complaints of worsening muscle aches and fever that are concerning enough to Mrs. S that she has taken him to another hospital for a second opinion. When Dr. R tells her that they believe that "the virus is probably worsening his anxiety" and Mrs. S communicates her further concern, Dr. R is dismissive of her. This is where Dr. R's bias towards mental health becomes apparent because Mrs. S is trying to communicate that this time is different than Orlando's previous panic attack, but Dr. R continues to insist that it is anxiety again and thus does not need further workup. This is why having a new pair of eyes, notably Dr. P, evaluate Orlando and order further lab workup is important. Keeping a broad differential at the beginning of an encounter, listening to the patient's concerns, and assimilating the entirety of the data to treat the patient is important to provide high quality care to our patients.

4. How could. Dr. P have a debrief with Dr. R following this case to discuss his bias in a way that would allow for Dr. R to provide a more informed and higher quality of care with his patients moving forward? Try roleplaying this scenario with a peer or in small groups to see how you would handle it.

When having conversations about bias and stigma it is important address the learner/trainee in an open, understanding and educational manner without judgment. It is clear that Dr. R cares about her patients as she remembers Orlando from a previous visit and is prompt in getting the patient the treatment, she believes he needs. One potential way to approach this would be for Dr. P to sit with Dr. R privately and ask them what they learned from the case and how it can be used as an example to improve their care. It is also important to normalize that everyone has innate biases and stigma and therefore it is necessary to be vigilant to make sure they do not dictate care. One can do this by making sure to assimilate new information into an evaluation and keep a broad differential. It is also important to recognize ways that Dr. R was trying to provide a higher quality of care by attempting to treat the patient's anxiety as opposed to dismissing the possibility for mental health concerns outright. It may be helpful to explore the etiology of psychiatric symptoms and correlate onset with the use of a new medication or underlying medical diagnosis. It would also be beneficial to discuss with Dr. R that they are a trainee and that it is for this reason there is the oversight of an attending provider. However even if in the future this happens and Dr. R is an attending or you are having this conversation with a peer, this can be approached from the perspective that we in the healthcare profession are lifelong learners (which is why we have continuing medical education) and so we have something new to learn from every patient encounter.

5. How would this case have been different if Orlando had truly been presenting for a mental health reason as opposed to a physical illness?

Had Orlando truly been presenting for a panic attack and anxiety then a further medical workup would have been technically unnecessary. However, it is important to keep in mind that we treat the whole person, which includes their family and the reason for them showing up to see us. In this case Orlando was brought by his mother for a second opinion because she was concerned that he had not had an appropriate medical workup, which does include working up his mental health. While we want to assume the best of others, if a patient or their parent is worried that something may have been missed, especially if they are noting the symptoms are not resolving or worsening, it is important for health care providers to perform their due diligence in ruling out underlying causes for psychiatric symptoms. If Orlando's symptoms were solely caused by anxiety, then the appropriate treatment for those symptoms would have been the anxiolytic, however Dr. R would still have not been treating the other reason for his presentation which was his mother's concern of wanting a further workup. In this case the further workup required was minimal and with low risk in that it was blood work. Mrs. S was looking for peace of mind that her son's health and well-being was not at risk, so even if the sole reason for his physical presentation was anxiety, it is important to take into account that we are treating the whole person in healthcare. We still need to be stewards of medicine and not order extraneous tests that patients do not need, but it is important to always have informed and thorough conversations with our patients about why we are performing each specific treatment plan and what is leading to our decisions.

Epilogue

The stigma associated with mental health and mental illness can have far reaching consequences in the healthcare profession. In the case above we see how the stigma associated with mental health, notably persons with anxiety, can impact the care these patients receive. At the beginning of the case Dr. R decides on his diagnosis and treatment for Orlando before he has even laid eyes on him all based on the premise that Orlando has a history of panic attacks and anxiety. Rather than take a thorough history and thoughtfully listen to what Mrs. S has to say, Dr. R instead dismisses her and rushes off to order anxiolytic medication. While on one hand this is beneficial as Dr. R is wanting to quickly and efficiently treat what they believe is causing Orlando's presentation, it ends up leading them to miss the actual diagnosis. Fortunately, Mrs. S is an advocate for her son and asks for another physician to evaluate Orlando, however patients may not always voice these concerns after being dismissed by the physician. As such it is important for healthcare providers to be cognizant of the bias and stigma associated with mental illness so that we continue to keep a broad differential without becoming anchored into our preconceived diagnosis and to provide the highest quality of care to our patients that we possibly can.

REFERENCES

AlFaris, E., Irfan, F., Qureshi, R., Naeem, N., Alshomrani, A., Ponnamperuma, G., Al Yousufi, N., Al Maflehi, N., Al Naami, M., Jamal, A., & van der Vleuten, C. (2016). Health professions' students have an alarming prevalence of depressive symptoms: Exploration of the associated factors. *BMC Medical Education, 16*(1), 279. doi:10.118612909-016-0794-y PMID:27769235

Knaak, S., Mantler, E., & Szeto, A. (2017). Mental illness-related stigma in healthcare: Barriers to access and care and evidence-based solutions. *Healthcare Management Forum / Canadian College of Health Service Executives = Forum Gestion Des Soins de Sante / College Canadien Des Directeurs de Services de Sante, 30*(2), 111–116.

Link, B. G., Struening, E. L., Rahav, M., Phelan, J. C., & Nuttbrock, L. (1997). On stigma and its consequences: Evidence from a longitudinal study of men with dual diagnoses of mental illness and substance abuse. *Journal of Health and Social Behavior, 38*(2), 177–190. doi:10.2307/2955424 PMID:9212538

Mata, D. A., Ramos, M. A., Bansal, N., Khan, R., Guille, C., Di Angelantonio, E., & Sen, S. (2015). Prevalence of Depression and Depressive Symptoms Among Resident Physicians: A Systematic Review and Meta-analysis. *Journal of the American Medical Association, 314*(22), 2373–2383. doi:10.1001/jama.2015.15845 PMID:26647259

McDermott, R. C. (2018). *Rates of Depression and Anxiety in Physical Therapy and Occupational Therapy Students: A Cross-Profession Comparison study*. Educatationa; Leadership Conference. Jacksonville, Florida. https://aptaeducation.org/abstract-archive/view.cfm?id=2996450

Rotenstein, L. S., Ramos, M. A., Torre, M., Segal, J. B., Peluso, M. J., Guille, C., Sen, S., & Mata, D. A. (2016). Prevalence of Depression, Depressive Symptoms, and Suicidal Ideation Among Medical Students: A Systematic Review and Meta-Analysis. *Journal of the American Medical Association*, *316*(21), 2214–2236. doi:10.1001/jama.2016.17324 PMID:27923088

Suen, L. W., Makam, A. N., Snyder, H. R., Repplinger, D., Kushel, M. B., Martin, M., & Nguyen, O. K. (2022). National Prevalence of Alcohol and Other Substance Use Disorders Among Emergency Department Visits and Hospitalizations: NHAMCS 2014-2018. *Journal of General Internal Medicine*, *37*(10), 2420–2428. doi:10.100711606-021-07069-w PMID:34518978

Tung, Y.-J., Lo, K. K. H., Ho, R. C. M., & Tam, W. S. W. (2018). Prevalence of depression among nursing students: A systematic review and meta-analysis. *Nurse Education Today*, *63*, 119–129. doi:10.1016/j.nedt.2018.01.009 PMID:29432998

Villarroel, M. A., & Terlizzi, E. P. (2020). Symptoms of Depression Among Adults: United States, 2019. *NCHS Data Brief*, *379*, 1–8. PMID:33054920

WHO. (n.d.). *Mental disorders*. WHO. https://www.who.int/news-room/fact-sheets/detail/mental-disorders

Yang, L. H., Wong, L. Y., Grivel, M. M., & Hasin, D. S. (2017). Stigma and substance use disorders: An international phenomenon. *Current Opinion in Psychiatry*, *30*(5), 378–388. doi:10.1097/YCO.0000000000000351 PMID:28700360

Chapter 2
Ableism in Medicine:
Disability-Related Barriers to Healthcare Access

Kristina H. Petersen
New York Medical College, USA

Amanda J. Chase
https://orcid.org/0000-0003-0761-3769
Nova Southeastern University Dr. Kiran C. Patel College of Allopathic Medicine, USA

EXECUTIVE SUMMARY

As defined by the U.S. Surgeon General's Call to Action in 2005, disabilities are characteristics of the body, mind, or senses that, to a greater or lesser extent, affect a person's ability to engage in some or all aspects of day-to-day life. Approximately one in four individuals in the U.S. self-identify as having a disability. As such, healthcare providers, educators, policymakers, and the population at large have a responsibility to promote accessible and comprehensive healthcare and wellness promotion services that support persons with disabilities. Furthermore, to ensure that persons with disabilities receive appropriate and culturally competent healthcare, it is imperative that healthcare educators teach about disability and future healthcare providers learn to treat the whole person, not just the disability. This chapter highlights a few of the many barriers that are experienced by persons with disabilities and the impact of insufficient knowledge and awareness on the delivery of quality care.

INTRODUCTION

Approximately 15% of the world's population lives with some form of disability (World Health Organization, 2021), and 1 out of 4 Americans self-identify as having a disability (Okoro et al., 2018). The Americans with Disabilities Act (ADA), a U.S. federal law passed in 1990, defines a person with a disability as one who has a physical or mental impairment that substantially limits one or more major life activities. This includes people who have a record of such an impairment, even if they do not currently have a disability (Americans with Disabilities Act, 1990). Congress later passed the ADA Amendment

DOI: 10.4018/978-1-6684-5493-0.ch002

Act (ADAAA) of 2008 to expand the definition of disability, thereby rejecting the inappropriately high standards applied by courts to the term "substantially limits" and increasing the number of "major life activities" covered by the ADA (ADA Amendments Act, 2008). Disabilities can be categorized into non-apparent (e.g., psychiatric or learning disability, attention deficit disorder, chronic health conditions, traumatic brain injuries, etc.) and apparent disabilities (e.g., physical or mobility disabilities, deaf or hard of hearing, blind or low vision, intellectual or developmental disabilities, etc.). Persons who are protected by the ADA and ADAAA may not be discriminated against on the basis of their disability (Americans with Disabilities Act, 1990; ADA Amendments Act, 2008).

Persons with disabilities receive fewer preventative screenings, less health education, and inadequate emergency care (Carmona & McCabe, 2005; *Healthy People 2010 Final Review*, 2012; Iezzoni & Agaronnik, 2020; *The Surgeon General's Call to Action to Improve the Health and Wellness of Persons with Disabilities*, 2005). Furthermore, studies have cited health disparities in areas that include Pap testing (Iezzoni et al., 2016), mammograms (Andresen et al., 2013; Iezzoni et al., 2015), and treatments for colorectal cancer (Gofine et al., 2018) and lung cancer (Iezzoni et al., 2008), among others (Agaronnik et al., 2022; Iezzoni, 2022; Iezzoni et al., 2022). In one study, most of the practicing physician participants had superficial or incorrect knowledge of their legal obligations when treating patients with disabilities (Agaronnik et al., 2019). Iezzoni and colleagues subsequently surveyed physicians and found that 35.8% of those surveyed knew little or nothing of their legal obligations under the ADA, 71.2% did not know who determines reasonable accommodations, and 68.4% felt they were at risk for ADA lawsuits. These physicians reportedly felt that a lack of formal training or medical education dedicated to these topics was a barrier to their understanding of the needs of persons with disabilities (Iezzoni, Rao, Ressalam, Bolcic-Jankovic, Agaronnik, et al., 2022).

Within medical education, the proportions of physicians and medical students with disabilities are considerably lower than in the general population. Disability prevalence among U.S. medical students in 2019 was reported to be 4.52%, with allopathic (MD) schools reporting 4.62% and osteopathic (DO) schools reporting 4.27% (Meeks et al., 2019; Meeks et al., 2020). Disability prevalence among practicing physicians in 2021 was reported to be 3.1% (Nouri et al., 2021). In conjunction with the amplification of barriers when we consider the intersectionality of race, ethnicity, poverty, and disability, the low prevalence of physicians with disabilities likely contributes to health inequities experienced by patients with disabilities.

Recently, leading organizations in medical education have expressed a commitment to supporting the inclusion of clinicians with disabilities (American Medical Association, 2021; Association of American Medical Colleges, 2015, 2019; Meeks & Jain, 2018), and calls to action have been made to amend the Liaison Committee on Medical Education standards to better ensure support of medical students with disabilities (Meeks et al., 2022). Cultural concordance, or a shared identity between clinician and patient, has been shown to support patient outcomes (Battalova et al., 2020; Miller et al., 2022; Shapiro, 2008). A study that examined perceptions of 714 practicing U.S. physicians nationwide reported that 82.4% believed that people with a significant disability have a worse quality of life than those without a disability, and only 40.7% felt "very confident" in their ability to provide equal care to individuals with a disability (Iezzoni et al., 2021). It is unclear how these negative perceptions may influence the choices made by physicians when caring for a patient with a disability. However, studies suggest that the experience of a physician with a disability allows for a unique patient-centered, rather than a "one size fits all," approach when treating a patient with a disability (Battalova et al., 2020; Bulk et al., 2017).

An analysis of a nationwide survey of patients with and without disabilities revealed that persons with disabilities are at increased risk of experiencing ineffective patient-physician communication (Smith, 2009). Specifically, persons with a disability were more likely than persons without a disability to perceive that the physician did not: listen to what they had to say, treat them with respect, spend enough time with them, and/or involve them in treatment decisions. Suggestions to work toward mitigating these gaps include the promotion of disability awareness among healthcare providers and assessments of the accessibility of health facilities (DeJong et al., 2002; Smith, 2009). In the U.S., few nationwide guidelines and resources have been compiled to educate healthcare providers on care of persons with disabilities, and those that are available are limited in scope (American Association of Medical Colleges, 2022; American Medical Association, 2022; Centers for Disease Control and Prevention, 2020). In contrast, in 2018 Canada updated their 2011 clinical practice guidelines for treatment of patients with intellectual and developmental disabilities (Sullivan et al., 2018), which provides a detailed guide to support this patient population. Further work is needed to increase clinicians' access to comprehensive information on best practices for treating patients with all types of disabilities.

The goal of this chapter is to highlight and review important considerations to help inform healthcare providers and educators as they take care of, interact with, and educate their patients, colleagues, or learners with disabilities. Cases created for this chapter include individuals with diabetes, a visual impairment, an orthopedic impairment, and autism spectrum disorder. We must acknowledge, however, that disability identities are inherently heterogeneous and often intersectional, with varying barriers and needs. We attempt to present a sampling of patients with apparent and non-apparent disabilities, but not every disability is represented, and it is impossible to present the nuances of every case.

CASE 1: BLINDSIDED

Goal

This case portrays barriers to culturally competent and accessible services at multiple points of contact during a health visit by a patient with more than one disability.

Learning Outcomes

1. Review ADA (1990) and ADAAA 2008, and what clinician's offices are legally required to provide as accommodations for persons with disabilities.
2. Describe barriers to effective health care for individuals who are blind or visually impaired.
3. Discuss techniques to enhance communication, convey trust, and build an atmosphere of caring between a provider and persons with disabilities.
4. Review principles of inclusive language when obtaining informed consent to ensure the patient comprehends and consents to care and procedures.
5. Describe standards for ethical and professional communication when discussing patients with the interprofessional healthcare team.

Case

Ms. K is a 51-year-old female who is visually impaired due to diabetic retinopathy from Type 1 Diabetes. Today, she has a colonoscopy scheduled at an outpatient surgery center. Ms. K wears tinted glasses that are not vision-correcting, and she uses a long cane. After being dropped off by her neighbor, she maneuvers through the waiting room and heads toward what appears to be the check-in desk. She starts by saying, "Good morning, I'm here for…" but is immediately cut off by a man behind the desk who barks at her, "Check in at the kiosk and we'll call you when we're ready!" Ms. K calmly asks which direction the kiosk is located. The man behind the desk responds, "Over there!"

Someone in the waiting room says, "It's to your right." Ms. K makes her way over to the kiosk, touches the screen a few times, but doesn't hear anything. She goes back to the front desk and says, "My vision is not great, and I can't see the screen. Does your kiosk have screen-reading software or a headphone connection?" The person at the front desk sighs heavily, asks for her name, and says, "I'll check you in manually and our medical assistant will complete the patient forms with you."

After about 20 minutes, a medical assistant leads Ms. K into the hallway and says, "I'm taking you to a room to finish filling out these forms." The medical assistant grabs Ms. K's cane and proceeds to pull her down the hallway. Startled and about to lose her balance, Ms. K pulls back on the cane and says, "I'm perfectly fine walking on my own. Can you please use verbal cues to let me know where I'm going?" Ms. K follows the medical assistant to a patient room where the medical assistant proceeds to read through the intake and patient history forms hurriedly and transcribes Ms. K's responses. The medical assistant points to a gown laying on the bed and instructs Ms. K to change.

Ms. K hears the medical assistant shut the door. She undresses, puts on the gown, and lies down on the exam bed. About 30 minutes later, Nurse J walks in and says, "My name is Nurse J. I'm here to take your vital signs and establish an IV." Nurse J provides some information about the upcoming colonoscopy and confirms that Ms. K has complied with the bowel preparation. Nurse J finds it odd that the patient is wearing dark glasses. The last piece of information that Nurse J provides is that Ms. K can use the call button to contact the nurse's station. Ms. K looks around and asks Nurse J where the call button is. Nurse J points at the call button on the exam bed rail and says, "Right there!" and walks out of the room.

Nurse J heads down the hallway, pulls aside the floor nurse, and says, "The patient in room 106 is disoriented. Can you interview her to make sure she's sane enough to consent to the procedure?"

The floor nurse, Nurse CA, walks into Ms. K's room, shuts the door, and says, "Good Morning Ms. K, my name is Nurse CA. Is it okay if I ask you some questions about your medical history so that Nurse J can get your consent?" Ms. K nods her head in approval. Nurse CA sits down next to Ms. K's bed and puts down the bedside rail so that her view of Ms. K is unimpeded. Nurse CA asks, "What medical conditions do you have, or have been told you have?"

Ms. K thinks for a minute and then says, "Well, I have Type 1 Diabetes. I can't see anything out of my left eye and can only see light and dark through my right eye."

Nurse CA says, "Let me know how I can help to make you comfortable during your visit." Ms. K then asks her to dim the lights a little. Next, Nurse CA asks her if she takes any medications, and Ms. K tells her that she takes insulin.

After answering some of Ms. K's questions, Nurse CA raises the bedside rail and says, "I'm leaving now. Nurse J will be in soon to run through the consent with you." After leaving, she checks through Ms. K's chart and notes that Ms. K's disabilities were, in fact, included in her medical history. Back at the nurses' station, Nurse CA speaks to Nurse J about Ms. K's disability, some of the signs that Nurse J could have noticed, and the importance of conducting a chart review prior to caring for each patient.

Nurse J enters Ms. K's room and sits down in the chair by Ms. K's bed. Startled, Ms. K asks, "Who's here?"

"Oh, it's Nurse J. I'm here to get your consent." The surgery center does not have the consent form in electronic format, so Nurse J must read the consent form aloud to Ms. K. Nurse J does not lower the side rail of the bed and keeps her head down as she reads through the consent form hurriedly, without checking for understanding.

When Nurse J is finished, she puts a pen in Ms. K's hand, points to the signature line, and says, "If you consent to everything that I've read, sign here." As Ms. K is slowly moving her hand towards the page, Nurse J grabs her hand, moves it to where the pen is above the signature line, and says, "Here, sign here." After Ms. K signs, Nurse J leaves the room and says to Dr. B, the gastroenterologist, "The blind woman in room 106 has consented and is ready for the colonoscopy."

Ms. K is startled when she wakes up. She is in a different room and doesn't remember how she got here. She presses the call button frantically. Nurse J comes in, checks Ms. K's blood pressure and pulse, removes her IV, and tells her that Dr. B will be in soon to explain the results of the colonoscopy. As Nurse J is finishing up, Dr. B arrives and talks with Nurse J about Ms. K's vitals, then they talk about the schedule for the rest of the day. Finally, Dr. B sits next to Ms. K, looks down at the iPad, and says in a very loud voice, "Everything looked great. We found only two polyps, likely benign, and we biopsied one to send to the lab."

Ms. K notices that Dr. B is using a much louder voice than what was used in the conversation with Nurse J. Ms. K says to Dr. B, "I'm blind, not hard of hearing."

In a normal tone, Dr. B then asks Ms. K, "Well, did you bring someone with you that I can talk to?"

Ms. K responds, "Why would I need somebody with me?"

Dr. B asks, "How are you getting home?"

Ms. K responds, "My neighbor dropped me off, and she will drive me home."

Dr. B looks back down at the iPad and tells Ms. K that she can resume her medication and regular diet by noon but needs to avoid activity that takes a lot of energy for the rest of the day. Dr. B then asks Ms. K if she has any questions. Ms. K thinks for a minute and says, "Lately, the vision in my right eye has been getting blurrier, and I'm having trouble guiding the syringe needle into the bottle."

Dr. B sighs and says, "That's a question for your family physician." Dr. B stands abruptly and turns toward the door, saying, "I'll let the front desk know that they can call your ride." Dr. B walks out of the room.

Not realizing that Dr. B has left, Ms. K says "Wait, what is a polyp?"

Again, Ms. K presses on the call button. Nurse CA arrives, knocks on the door, verbally announces her arrival, sits down next to Ms. K, and asks her what she needs. Ms. K recollects the events of the morning, explaining her disappointment at just how uncomfortable and uninformed everyone seemed around her, except for Nurse CA. Nurse CA apologizes for her entire team.

After leaving the room, Nurse CA pulls Dr. B aside and says, "We need to have a team debrief about the patient in room 106 who is visually impaired, and I believe some disability training is in order."

QUESTIONS AND ANSWERS

1. In this case, which diagnoses fall under the category of a disability, as defined by the ADA?

Some disabilities are visible (apparent) while others are not (non-apparent). They can be physical, visual, auditory, developmental, cognitive, or behavioral, and impact a person's ability to engage in one or more major life activities. Two disabilities were disclosed by Ms. K: type 1 diabetes and a vision impairment. When people think of disabilities, non-apparent conditions such as diabetes are often overlooked or not recognized as disabilities. A person with diabetes or another chronic health condition is entitled to protection under the ADA.

2. What are some accessibility recommendations for persons with a vision impairment in the healthcare setting?

Hospitals, nursing homes, surgery centers, or any other healthcare facility must ensure that patients who are blind, deaf-blind, or visually impaired have an equal opportunity to participate in and benefit from all of the services provided by the facility. Effective communication in healthcare settings may require the provision of auxiliary aids and services, such as materials provided in braille, text-to-speech software, large print, magnifiers, and/or accessible electronic formats. Federal law stipulates that all patient forms, documents, and communication be available in accessible formats for patients who are blind or have visual disabilities (Americans with Disabilities Act, 1990). The American Foundation for the Blind provides a checklist for providers and all healthcare facility staff that includes communication guidelines, such as verbalizing directions, using disability-sensitive language, verbalizing procedures before they are performed, and providing written materials in auditory, tactile, or electronic format (American Foundation for the Blind, 2006).

3. What missteps occurred during Ms. K's visit to the surgery center?

There were several missteps in the way Ms. K was cared for during her visit to the surgery center. Admitting staff should initiate an introduction to a patient. Even after Ms. K alerted the reception desk staff to her low vision, they did not apologize, nor did they adapt their communication to better meet Ms. K's needs. In addition, the surgical facility was not in compliance with the ADA, as they did not provide access to an ADA-compliant kiosk or medical forms in braille, large print, or in an auditory format.

The medical assistant grabbed Ms. K's long cane, which Ms. K relies on to orient herself and walk independently. Healthcare professionals should always ask a patient's permission before touching them, guiding them, or handling their assistive devices. They should ask how patients would like to be assisted and not touch or remove mobility canes unless requested to do so, unless there is an emergent situation that requires it. Persons with disabilities experience specific functional limitations, but they are capable of functioning on their own, and assistance should be given only if an offer of assistance is accepted. Training of health professionals should include verbalizing directions; even the layout of a patient's room can be verbalized. In addition, the intake staff did not alert the healthcare team of Ms. K's visual impairment. This should be done in a dignified manner and in a way that communicates the patient's functional limitations and informs necessary accommodations.

Neither Nurse J or Dr. B announced their arrival into or exit from Ms. K's room. It is important for providers to verbally identify themselves when they approach and to introduce other people who enter the room. When orienting the patient to locations of devices such as the call button, providers should specify verbally where it is located in space (e.g., "to your right, at shoulder level"). Nurse J failed to read the patient's medical history and mistakenly assumed that Ms. K was not mentally competent to consent to the procedure. In addition, Nurse J was short with Ms. K, did not make eye contact, and failed to follow appropriate consent procedures like checking for understanding or asking if the patient has any questions. When Ms. K was signing the consent form, Nurse J grabbed her hand instead of asking permission to do so. Randomly touching a person with a visual impairment can be disconcerting and scary.

Healthcare organizations can ensure that they provide equitable care for the blind or visually impaired by training the healthcare team, planning how they will provide effective communication, and documenting their approaches in a comprehensive communication access plan (Centers for Medicare and Medicaid Services, 2022).

4. How did the communication strategies used by Nurse CA differ from those of Nurse J?

To ensure equitable quality of care, the ADA stipulates that communication with persons with disabilities should be equally effective as communication with persons without disabilities. The actions taken by the floor nurse upon entering the room enhanced the notion that she was completely focused on the patient. Nurse CA's simple maneuvers that put the patient at ease included announcing herself upon entering the room and lowering the bedside rail to put Nurse CA and the patient on equal footing while also giving Nurse CA a clear view of Ms. K. Even after Nurse CA alerted Nurse J to Ms. K's disability, Nurse J did not improve in her interpersonal interactions with Ms. K, suggesting a need for disability training. Nurse CA used disability-inclusive language when discussing Ms. K with the care team. In contrast, Nurse J referred to Ms. K as "the blind woman in room 106." When referring to patients with disabilities, the person should be referred to first, then the disability.

5. Discuss Dr. B's blunders. How could Dr. B have communicated better with Ms. K?

Instead of speaking in a normal conversational tone, Dr. B raised his voice, perhaps out of discomfort or an incorrect assumption that Ms. K was also hard of hearing. Dr. B did not make eye contact with Ms. K when speaking to her. Visual impairments exist in varying degrees and it is likely that Ms. K recognized that she was not being looked at when Dr. B was speaking to her. Dr. B offered standard advice post-colonoscopy without considering the barriers Ms. K may encounter due to her specific disability. Instead of finding an answer to Ms. K's question about insulin administration, Dr. B disregarded it as something that didn't pertain to his medical specialty. Dr. B does not take the time to respond to Ms. K's concerns. Finally, Dr. B exits the room without informing the patient.

Epilogue

This case provides an examination of multiple failures in communication that can be experienced by persons who are blind or visually impaired when visiting healthcare facilities. Many of the missteps in care, committed by healthcare staff and clinicians, can be addressed through disability awareness training. Of note, only one member of the healthcare team used language and behavior that demonstrated disability awareness when caring for Ms. K. Many members of the healthcare team treated Ms. K through an ableist lens and presumed that a patient with a disability is not competent enough to care for themselves. They did not wait for an offer of assistance to be accepted by the patient before providing it and underutilized verbal instructions. An equitable health system engages fairly and respectfully with everyone who seeks care. Negative perceptions of healthcare experiences by persons with disabilities can influence subsequent health care-seeking behaviors and poorly impact future wellness and health outcomes (Krahn et al., 2015). Increasing disabilities awareness training at all levels of health sciences education can contribute to a more positive patient experience for patients with disabilities, therefore hopefully impacting health outcomes.

CASE 2: TRANSITION LIMBO

Goal

This case highlights the barriers faced by patients with intellectual disabilities as they transition from the care of a pediatrician to an internal medicine physician, while simultaneously losing some of the supportive services provided by the K-12 educational system.

Learning Outcomes

1. Recognize the broader issue of gaps in care when children with disabilities require a transition from pediatric to adult-centered care.
2. Outline best practices associated with a successful transition of care for a patient with an intellectual disability.
3. Propose how assistive technology can be incorporated into the medical visit to improve collaborative care for patients with autism spectrum disorder.
4. Discuss strategies to enhance communication, convey sensitivity, and build trust between a provider and a patient with autism spectrum disorder.
5. Describe programs and supports for families and caregivers of children with autism spectrum disorder.

Case

CJ is a 22-year-old male with autism spectrum disorder. It's time for CJ's annual influenza shot, and CJ's mother also wants to speak with his pediatrician about getting him back on medication for his anxiety, which has worsened over the past few months. When she calls to make an appointment, the receptionist informs her that their pediatrician stops seeing patients at age 21. The receptionist offers to make one last appointment, but CJ's mother doesn't think this is a good idea. She declines, ends the call, and goes to her computer to start searching for a doctor who accepts CJ's health insurance. She finds an internal medicine practice located nearby and thinks that it will be good to go to a small community practice where CJ can get to know his new physician. She calls the office and makes an appointment for the following week. She lets them know that CJ is on the autism spectrum and tells them that injections trigger

CJ's anxiety. She then calls the pediatrician's office to let them know that she has found a new doctor for CJ - and finds it odd that the receptionist doesn't ask for the new doctor's information.

A few weeks later, CJ and his mother enter the new doctor's office and the front desk attendant looks at CJ, then back at his mother and says, "Is he competent?" CJ says, "I'm CJ." CJ's mom looks pointedly at the attendant and says, "I am CJ's mother and make his medical decisions for him, but we appreciate when staff communicate with CJ before involving me." The attendant shrugged and replied, "I have to ask."

CJ takes out his iPad and plays a game while they wait for his name to be called. After 45 minutes, Nurse F calls his name and CJ refuses to get out of his seat and starts grunting. CJ's mom tells Nurse F that she will need a minute to get CJ to the exam room. Nurse F is visibly annoyed and sighs loudly. After CJ's mom talks to him for a few minutes, he stands up and walks toward the exam room. CJ's mom explains to Nurse F, "It's difficult for him to adjust to new places, and the long wait makes it worse."

As they approach the exam room, CJ starts grunting and screaming. His mom gets him into the exam room and pulls out a photo book that she created to help keep him calm. Nurse F says, "He's here for a flu shot? I'll get it ready and do his vitals in a minute."

Nurse F returns to the exam room with a syringe. CJ is calm, so Nurse F approaches him and tries to get his vitals. When the nurse touches CJ, he pulls his hand away and screams. CJ's mom says, "You need to tell him what you are going to do before you do it. He doesn't like to be touched, but if you prepare him, he won't scream." Nurse F rolls her eyes and exits the room in frustration. She can be heard saying to a colleague, "I don't have time for this difficult patient. You're up. He needs vitals and a flu shot."

Nurse A enters the room. CJ's mom says, "He's ready for you to take his temperature and blood pressure. I explained to him what to expect." Without saying anything, Nurse A takes CJ's temperature and vitals, then picks up the alcohol swabs and starts to prepare his arm for the flu shot. When she picks up the syringe, CJ jumps off the table, screams, sits on the floor, and bangs his head against the wall. CJ's mom tries to comfort CJ and tells the nurse, "Our pediatrician always used a procedure photobook before giving CJ a shot."

Nurse A says, "I don't believe we have that, Ma'am. I'll come back in a few minutes and see if Dr. T is ready to see you. Then we can try again."

About 15 minutes later, Dr. T enters the room. He looks at CJ, who is sitting on the ground, then at CJ's mom. Dr. T addresses all his questions about CJ's medical history to CJ's mom. The doctor hears what CJ's mom is saying about anxiety, interrupts her, and writes a prescription. "Yes, I see he has elevated anxiety in new situations," Dr. T says. "Let's try this and see how he does with it."

CJ's mom doesn't take the prescription. Instead, she says, "This office isn't going to be a good fit for us. We'll take his pediatrician up on the offer to see him one last time to do the flu shot and go from there. Thanks for your time." CJ's mom helps CJ pack his iPad and leads him down the hallway. She tells herself that she will call the pediatrician and beg them to continue caring for her adult child.

QUESTIONS AND ANSWERS

1. What proactive strategies could CJ's pediatrician have implemented to ensure a smooth transition to CJ's new physician?

CJ's pediatrician did not take proactive steps to prepare CJ and his caregiver for a transition to adult care. Clinicians should provide anticipatory guidance to patients with intellectual disabilities for transition to adulthood, including healthcare transition planning. Strategies that could enhance communication include using a templated medical summary prepared by the pediatric team and facilitating a warm handoff between the pediatric and adult care teams (White et al., 2018).

According to data collected by the Centers for Disease Control and Prevention between July 2018 to December 2020, only 1 in 13 adolescents with autism spectrum disorder (ASD) received the recommended guidance to move from pediatric to adult health care (Powell et al., 2021). In addition, communication between the pediatric and adult providers occurred inconsistently, with few systems in place to connect families with adult providers specializing in health care for persons with intellectual disabilities. Greater coordination among healthcare programs and interdisciplinary training for clinicians could expand access to services, increase provider comfort in treating the unique healthcare needs of adolescents with ASD, and support healthcare planning as they transition from pediatric to adult care.

Pediatricians' offices should have health care transition plans in place to foster a proactive, planned transition from pediatric to adult health care. The Six Core Elements, established by the American Academy of Pediatrics, include three phases of transition support: preparation, transfer, and integration into adult health care (White et al., 2018). In CJ's case, all three phases of the health care transition were absent, leading to an anxiety-filled, abrupt transition that may have an adverse psychiatric impact on CJ.

2. What strategies could the healthcare professionals have implemented to improve CJ and his mother's experience?

Bearing in mind CJ's functional limitations and the associated barriers, the clinical staff could have better accommodated CJ's needs. Patients who require extra time and/or have difficulty waiting may benefit from being scheduled as the first appointment of the day. This would allow CJ to wait for a shorter period of time with fewer people in the waiting room and would hopefully prevent his mom from having to use his iPad to keep him entertained (thereby preventing the problem when CJ doesn't want to stop using the iPad). Another possibility would be to book a double-appointment to allow for additional time and attention, especially the first time a person with a disability is seeing the new clinician team. This may have lowered the pressure on the clinical staff, who demonstrated their frustration inappropriately and referred to CJ as a "difficult patient." Of course, the entire healthcare team should be trained to be sensitive to disability-related issues and consider how their office can better serve patient needs. Every clinical office would be well served by a few basic procedure photo books (addressed below in question 3), which can support many different types of patients. In fact, these photobooks may even help some patients who do not have a disability by giving them an opportunity to understand a procedure visually while the clinician talks them through it.

3. What specific assistive technology may have helped to mitigate CJ's disability-related barriers to communication?

CJ would have benefited from the use of a procedure photobook, which demonstrates the step-by-step process of various procedures using pictures. Ideally, this would be done on an iPad (since he already uses one and is comfortable with it, as are many patients on the autism spectrum), as a series of images or potentially as a cartoon video. Regardless of the format, any sort of pictorial tool to demonstrate the procedure step-by-step, along with a simple verbal description, could have aided CJ in feeling more comfortable and less anxious about the care he was about to receive.

4. How can clinicians partner with families and caregivers of children with ASD to improve psychosocial outcomes?

It is important to recognize that when a person with a disability turns 18 in the US, they are no longer eligible for the numerous services they easily accessed in their childhood years, many of which are associated with the K-12 educational system. Consequently, it is critical that clinicians understand the socioeconomic impact and financial barriers associated with adult patients with intellectual disabilities obtaining supportive services - particularly services they require to live independently. Additionally, healthcare providers should educate patients on resources that are available to support adult patients with disabilities in obtaining necessary assistive technology and devices, access to supportive services, etc. These programs differ by region and state, but most states have programs that support persons with disabilities (e.g., New York state has a program whereby persons with a mobility disability can apply for financial support to modify a car or van to render it accessible). This may involve partnering with a social worker trained to support patients in these areas.

It is critical for clinicians to recognize the personal and financial resources that families and caregivers invest in supporting their loved ones with intellectual disabilities. Many groups have formed to provide support to caregivers, who may encounter similar barriers, and opportunities to share resources and personal experiences. Clinicians should educate themselves on the groups that are available within their region and encourage patient families to participate.

5. What strategies can healthcare professionals use to facilitate effective and sensitive communication when treating patients with intellectual disabilities?

When clinicians are treating patients with disabilities, it is best to start by using person-first language (e.g. "person with autism"). However, it is important to recognize that some persons with disabilities are re-claiming their disability identity and prefer disability-first language, so clinicians should be prepared to be corrected. Alternatively, the clinician may ask the patient if they have a preference of person-first or identify-first language.

It is critical that clinicians direct their questions and attention to the patient, not the caregiver, for as much of the time in the clinical interaction as possible. Most persons with disabilities find it condescending when clinicians presume that they cannot make their own decisions and instead address their caregiver. That being said, information provided by a caregiver about how to best serve a patient should be considered in the treatment plan. Caregivers will often offer ideas about how to best meet their loved one's needs, and taking specific suggestions may allow the clinician to serve the patient effectively and create a positive experience that could encourage future access to care.

6. Why is it crucial for young adults with intellectual and developmental disabilities to receive adequate support during their transition to adulthood?

Intellectual and developmental disabilities encompass hundreds of diagnoses including autism, cerebral palsy, and Down syndrome which affects about 6.5 million people in the U.S. As these children reach adulthood, they face unique challenges navigating the healthcare system (Association of American Medical Colleges, 2022). These include the loss of supportive services that were available to them in the K-12 educational system, which often results in increased financial barriers. In addition, depending on the diagnosis, persons with intellectual and developmental disabilities face significant barriers to living independently.

Over the last 20 years, the prevalence of ASD in children in the U.S. has climbed from fewer than 10 per 1,000 to over 25 per 1,000 children, the prevalence ratio being 4 males for every 1 female diagnosed (Centers for Disease Control and Prevention, 2022). Research suggests that young people with ASD are more likely to continue living with family members, have higher rates of unemployment or under-employment, and have lower rates of participation in education beyond high school. In addition, individuals with ASD may experience changes in their ASD symptoms, behaviors, and co-occurring health conditions during young adulthood, which can affect their ability to function and participate in the community (Levy & Perry, 2011). For all these reasons, it is especially critical that this health care transition be approached proactively and with great attention to the well-being of the patient.

Epilogue

Patients with disabilities, particularly those with intellectual disabilities, encounter significant barriers when transitioning from pediatric to adult care. These barriers contribute to the overall health inequities experienced by patients with disabilities. It is critical that pediatricians follow the recommendations provided by the American Academy of Pediatrics for health care transition from adolescence to adulthood. As part of these recommendations, the family and internal medicine practices receiving patients play a role in interacting with pediatricians to ensure a smooth transition. Clinicians should consider providing accommodations to patients with intellectual disabilities, which may include: first appointment of the day, double appointments to allow extra time for new patients and/or complex procedures, and having procedural photobooks or cartoons available to facilitate communication with patients who may not be able to express themselves verbally (White et al., 2018). By addressing the disability-related barriers patients face in obtaining access to care, the health disparity gap can be lessened.

CASE 3: DR. G'S ABLEIST LENS

Goal

This case demonstrates some of the barriers to culturally competent and accessible services for a patient who is paraplegic and explores some of the stigma experienced by physicians with disabilities.

Learning Outcomes

1. Review the use of inclusive language in the context of persons with disabilities having the potential to be excellent physicians, including surgeons.
2. Consider disability-related barriers that a person who uses a wheelchair may encounter as a student in the clinical and gross anatomy lab settings.

3. Engage in a conversation about what types of accommodations would mitigate this patient's disability-related barriers.
4. Review ADA (1990) and ADAAA 2008, Section 504 of the Rehabilitation Act, and what educational institutions are legally required to provide as accommodations to persons with disabilities.

Case

Mr. J enters the health clinic's parking lot and all the ADA parking spots are taken. Mr. J is paraplegic and uses a wheelchair. He parks his car in the farthest part of the lot to ensure nobody parks next to him - so he will be able to access his car when the appointment is over - then makes the long journey to the front door. After entering the lobby, he sees a sign on the elevator "Out of order - use freight elevator - rear entrance." Mr. J exits and goes through the parking lot to the rear of the building, but cannot find any easily visible door. He asks a few people before finding the rear entrance. The doors are not equipped with an ADA-compliant push-button, and when he tries to open the doors, they are too heavy. Mr. J waits until someone opens the door and then finds the freight elevator. He traverses the extra distance to get to the clinic but is 15 minutes late for his appointment. Mr. J approaches the desk and tells the attendant his name. The attendant, on the phone, looks at him and rolls her eyes. "You're late."

Twenty minutes later, Nurse Z, who Mr. J is familiar with, greets him and asks how his application to medical school is going. Mr. J tells Nurse Z that he was admitted and is excited to begin his journey to becoming a surgeon. Nurse Z stops in her tracks, turns to Mr. J and says, "Have you thought about psychiatry? It would be so much easier. You can do that sitting down." Mr. J's heart drops and he can't muster the courage to say anything except, "I don't know. Maybe."

Nurse Z and Mr. J enter the exam room, and Nurse Z realizes the adjustable exam table isn't functioning properly. She turns to Mr. J with a stressed countenance and says, "It looks like I'll have to find some folks to transfer you to the table, but we are really short-staffed…" Mr. J informs Nurse Z that he is only there to ask the doctor a few questions related to accommodations and to get routine blood work, so he may not need to move to the exam table. Nurse Z looks at Mr. J with relief and leaves the room.

Dr. G and Mr. P, the physician assistant, enter the room. Dr. G says, "How are you doing, Mr. J?"

"Pretty good. Just here for my annual physical which I need to start medical school in a few weeks. Also, the campus disability office asked for a clinician letter recommending any educational accommodations that may support me in the anatomy lab."

Dr. G says "Well, I can take care of the physical. I don't know anything about accommodations. What field of medicine do you want to go into? Psychiatry?"

"No, surgery," replied Mr. J.

Dr. G smirks and says flippantly, "Not sure you can keep up with those hours. Psych may be better for someone like you." Dr. G flashes a big smile and slaps Mr. J on the shoulder playfully. Mr. J shrinks down in his chair and decides not to share his ambitions with others moving forward.

Mr. P chimes in, "I worked with a wonderful surgeon who used a standing wheelchair on one of my rotations. She was excellent and the patients loved her." Dr. G ignores Mr. P and conducts the physical exam.

Mr. J waits until the end of the meeting to remind the doctor: "I need a letter for disability services to get accommodations approved. They asked what accommodations I will need for the anatomy lab and I was hoping to get your recommendations."

"I can write you a letter telling them you have a mobility disability, but it's up to them to determine if they'll give you any accommodations. When I was in school, they didn't do that sort of thing - it was sink or swim."

"Sure thing, Dr. G. Thanks for writing the letter." Dr. G grabs Mr. P and they exit in a rush.

Mr. J, defeated, starts the long journey back to the parking lot via the freight elevator. Mr. P finds Mr. J in the hallway and says, "I learned about some accommodations in PA school; one of my lab partners was paraplegic and he used a standing wheelchair in combination with an adjustable dissection table. Maybe look into that."

Mr. J thanks Mr. P and tells him how much he appreciates the information.

Mr. J changes his evening plans so he can focus on googling accommodation options. He is starting to realize that he is going to have to educate himself to be able to advocate for what he needs in order to pursue his dream to become a surgeon.

QUESTIONS AND ANSWERS

1. How could the desk attendant have improved the interaction with Mr. J when he arrived late? How could the parking situation be improved for Mr. J?

The desk attendant should be aware that persons with disabilities may take longer to arrive for their appointments, particularly when the elevator is out of order. The desk attendant should have apologized for the inconvenience caused by the elevator being out of order, rather than focusing on the patient's late arrival. While the number of parking spots may be in compliance with the ADA, it would be wise for health care clinics to exceed the minimum requirement. Hospital outpatient facilities are required to provide 10%, while rehabilitation facilities are required to provide 20% of their total spaces as ADA parking. Since the prevalence of persons in the U.S. with disabilities ranges from 15-25%, and people with disabilities tend to have more health care appointments than those without disabilities, additional ADA parking spots should be included in parking structure plans. When there is not ample ADA parking available, often persons who really need the ADA parking must park at the furthest point away from the clinic to ensure they will be able to access their car after the appointment. Note the use of the term "ADA parking," which is more inclusive than the typically used term "handicapped parking."

2. When an elevator is out of order in a medical office building, what needs to be considered?

People often view a non-working elevator through an ableist perspective as simply inconvenient but not an urgent matter. This is where education and reflection may help people view this issue through the lens of someone who requires the use of the elevator to fully access a building. It is critical that medical offices, in particular, hire a repair company that ensures a quick turnaround when issues arise. In addition, it is important to have a back-up option whenever possible. In the case of Mr. J, he was directed to use a freight elevator at the rear entrance; this may have been appropriate if the rear entrance was clearly labeled and, most importantly, equipped with an ADA-compliant entrance.

Unfortunately, often buildings only install one ADA-compliant door, so it is critical to be aware if that is the case before redirecting persons with disabilities to a non-ADA-compliant entrance. Equipping the rear entrance with a compliant door would rectify this issue, but staff should be sensitive to the increased amount of time it will take patients with disabilities to physically navigate their way to the office. It would be courteous to call the patients ahead of time to let them know they may wish to allow extra time to get to the rear entrance - or, even better, to tell them to plan to park closer to the rear entrance to lessen the barriers to entering the building through the alternate entry point. It may also be prudent to designate additional ADA parking spots closer to the rear entrance until the elevator is fixed.

3. When an assistive device, such as the adjustable exam table, is not functioning properly what would be an appropriate response? How could Nurse Z have improved this interaction to prioritize Mr. J's needs?

Ideally, each clinic would have more than one adjustable exam table (and/or other necessary assistive technology/devices), and a simple move to another room would ensure the patient can be fully examined. If an adjustable exam table is not functional and there is no other option than to manually transfer the patient to the exam table, the staff member should make it clear that they apologize for the inconvenience of the table not being available and will get a team together to move the patient to the exam table. Staff should not imply through any part of their communication that this is inconvenient for the staff, as the non-functional adjustable exam table was not the fault of the patient. It is the legal responsibility of the clinical staff to ensure patients have full and equal access to care, regardless of disability status.

In this case, it is possible that Mr. J did not need to be examined on the table - but under no circumstances should he feel pressured to make the staff's day easier by forgoing transferring to the exam table if it will hinder his access to equitable care. Nurse Z should have clearly communicated that the staff is happy to transfer Mr. J to the exam table and make arrangements to do so in the event that Dr. G felt a full physical examination was necessary. It is also important to note that when a person is being transferred by medical staff, they are in a vulnerable position - and staff should pay close attention to the patient's safe transfer. Many persons with disabilities have relayed experiences wherein health professionals get distracted or chat with each other during the patient transfer - and an injury occurs. When a patient with a disability sustains an injury, it can set them back considerably and may even prevent them from living independently. Clinicians need to treat any patient transfer with the utmost care and respect, and consider it a critical part of the patient's medical treatment.

4. How could Nurse Z and Dr. G improve their communication with Mr. J regarding his entry to medical school and ambition to become a surgeon?

Persons with disabilities experience specific functional limitations, but with reasonable accommodations they can fully access opportunities to achieve the same goals as persons without disabilities. Of course, not every disability presents the same functional limitation - and not everyone with a disability, even with reasonable accommodations, could meet the academic and technical standards to perform the necessary duties of health care clinicians. With reasonable accommodations, many persons with disabilities are pursuing rewarding careers in the health professions and receiving positive patient feedback – including reports of strong levels of empathy and understanding, understanding of disability-related barriers, and approachability (Battalova et al., 2020; Bulk et al., 2020; Jarus et al., 2020).

5. Should the physician be able to recommend accommodations that may support a patient with a disability in their education or work setting?

In order to recommend an appropriate accommodation, first the functional limitation(s) must be identified, after which feedback should be sought from the patient regarding preferences and any experiences they have already had with accommodations. After this conversation is fully considered by the clinician, options can be recommended to mitigate the patient's specific functional limitation(s) (Magence et al., 2021; New York Medical College, 2022). Health professions education training programs should incorporate content to help future clinicians understand how a patient's diagnosis may result in specific functional limitations that affect major life activities.

In employment or educational settings, disability accommodations are only implemented after the patient provides medical documentation supporting their need for an accommodation. Hence, clinicians should understand how to identify functional limitations and recommend some potential accommodations (e.g., assistive technology or devices, alteration in environment or formatting of examinations, etc.) that would mitigate the disability-related barriers and facilitate equitable access. While many groups have done important work to support the inclusion of a disability curriculum in medical education (Doebrich et al., 2020; Juster & Edwards, 2001; Sarmiento et al., 2016; Symons et al., 2009), these efforts face many barriers and no explicit curricular mandates are in place for medical schools. To date no program has developed a fully integrated, universal design approach to teaching disabilities in medical education. One such program has been proposed and is currently under development (Magence et al., 2021; New York Medical College, 2022). In 2019, dental schools announced a stronger curricular mandate that "dental graduates must be competent in assessing and managing the treatment of patients with special needs," which is a step in the right direction, but this new mandate continues to face barriers to its implementation (Commission on Dental Accreditation, 2022).

6. What disability-related barriers might a person in a wheelchair encounter in a medical school anatomy lab and what types of accommodations would address these barriers?

Ideally, at least one adjustable table would be available in every gross anatomy laboratory, in the event that students with disabilities may require its use to ensure equitable access to the educational laboratory programs. In addition, a standing wheelchair would be optimal for a paraplegic who is performing a dissection. The standing wheelchair is utilized by surgeons in the operating room, allowing them to use the leverage necessary to conduct certain surgical maneuvers while standing (National Institutes of Health, 2018).

7. What additional accommodations might Mr. J seek in an educational or work setting?

Mr. J may require a specific type of desk, access to materials on lower shelves, ADA-compliant facilities and housing, and ADA parking, among other accommodations. In addition to the accommodations that are provided by the employer or educational institution, persons who use a wheelchair will also have to supply many of the following for themselves: a modified accessible vehicle to allow them to operate and enter/exit a vehicle safely (which also requires the purchase of additional auto insurance), leather gloves to avoid blisters when operating a manual wheelchair, and a pressure relief cushion to prevent pressure ulcer formation, among other items.

8. Are educational institutions legally required to provide accommodations to persons with disabilities? What laws govern these regulations?

U.S. educational institutions, including those in higher education, are mandated to provide equal access by the ADA of 1990 and the ADA Amendment Act of 2008. Most educational institutions receive federal funding (this includes financial aid) and, therefore, are also regulated by Section 504 of the Rehabilitation Act. Specifically, institutions must provide reasonable accommodations to persons who disclose their disability and demonstrate that a disability-related barrier impedes their access to the educational program. Students must go through an "interactive process" outlined by the institution that involves documenting one or more functional limitation(s) associated with their disability and identifying associated barriers to accessing the educational program. Once these barriers are identified, an accommodation plan can be created and may be updated as needs change. For example, the access barriers in a classroom curriculum would differ greatly from those in a clinical curriculum.

Epilogue

This case considers a patient who is paraplegic and just about to start medical school. When the patient approaches the health care team to seek recommendations for accommodations to allow for his equitable participation in the Gross Anatomy laboratory, he is met with commentary discouraging him from becoming a surgeon due to his use of a wheelchair and ignorance of accommodations that may mitigate disability-related barriers.

Physicians with disabilities are well received by patients, and increasing the number of physicians with disabilities would allow for increased opportunities for cultural concordance. Evidence suggests this would support amelioration of the health inequities seen in this population (Battalova et al., 2020; Miller et al., 2022; Shapiro, 2008). It is critical for health care professionals to be aware of the specific barriers that persons with disabilities face when seeking full access to health care, and to take measures within their practice to minimize these barriers from the outset. Health care professionals also need to increase awareness around their colleagues who have disabilities and encourage the next generation of clinicians to achieve their goals, regardless of disability identity.

REFERENCES

ADA Amendments Act of 2008. (2008). 42 U.S.C. § 12101 et seq. Retrieved July 22, 2022 from https://www.ada.gov/pubs/adastatute08.htm

Agaronnik, N. D., El-Jawahri, A., & Iezzoni, L. I. (2022). Implications of physical access barriers for breast cancer diagnosis and treatment in women with mobility disability. *Journal of Disability Policy Studies, 33*(1), 46–54. doi:10.1177/10442073211010124 PMID:35875606

Agaronnik, N. D., Pendo, E., Campbell, E. G., Ressalam, J., & Iezzoni, L. I. (2019). Knowledge of practicing physicians about their legal obligations when caring for patients with disability. *Health Affairs, 38*(4), 545–553. doi:10.1377/hlthaff.2018.05060 PMID:30933590

American Foundation for the Blind. (2006). *ADA Checklist: Health Care Facilities and Service Providers.* AFB. https://www.afb.org/blindness-and-low-vision/your-rights/advocacy-resources/ada-checklist-health-care-facilities-and#%5B1%5D

American Medical Association. (2021). *AMA seeks more help for medical students, residents with disabilities*. AMA. https://www.ama-assn.org/education/medical-school-diversity/ama-seeks-more-help-medical-students-residents-disabilities

American Medical Association. (2022). *AMA Guides to the Evaluation of Permanent Impairment*. AMA. https://ama-guides.ama-assn.org/books/book/8/AMA-Guides-to-the-Evaluation-of-Permanent

Americans with Disabilities Act of 1990. (1990). 42 U.S.C. § 12101 et seq. Retrieved July 22, 2022 from https://www.ada.gov/pubs/adastatute08.htm

Andresen, E. M., Peterson-Besse, J. J., Krahn, G. L., Walsh, E. S., Horner-Johnson, W., & Iezzoni, L. I. (2013). Pap, mammography, and clinical breast examination screening among women with disabilities: A systematic review. *Women's Health Issues*, *23*(4), e205–e214. doi:10.1016/j.whi.2013.04.002 PMID:23816150

Association of American Medical Colleges. (2015). *Helping Medical Schools Assist Students with Disabilities*. AAMC. https://www.aamc.org/professional-development/affinity-groups/gsa/webinars/assist-students-with-disabilities

Battalova, A., Bulk, L., Nimmon, L., Hole, R., Krupa, T., Lee, M., Mayer, Y., & Jarus, T. (2020, November). "I Can Understand Where They're Coming From": How Clinicians' Disability Experiences Shape Their Interaction With Clients. *Qualitative Health Research*, *30*(13), 2064–2076. doi:10.1177/1049732320922193 PMID:32449447

Bulk, L. Y., Easterbrook, A., Roberts, E., Groening, M., Murphy, S., Lee, M., Ghanouni, P., Gagnon, J., & Jarus, T. (2017). 'We are not anything alike': Marginalization of health professionals with disabilities. *Disability & Society*, *32*(5), 615–634. doi:10.1080/09687599.2017.1308247

Bulk, L. Y., Tikhonova, J., Gagnon, J. M., Battalova, A., Mayer, Y., Krupa, T., Lee, M., Nimmon, L., & Jarus, T. (2020). Disabled healthcare professionals' diverse, embodied, and socially embedded experiences. *Advances in Health Sciences Education: Theory and Practice*, *25*(1), 111–129. doi:10.100710459-019-09912-6 PMID:31538268

Carmona, R. H., & McCabe, J. (2005). Improving the health and wellness of persons with disabilities: A call to action. *American Journal of Public Health*, *95*(11), 1883–1883. doi:10.2105/AJPH.95.11.1883 PMID:16254229

Centers for Disease Control and Prevention. (2020). *Autism Case Training: A Developmental-Behavioral Pediatrics Curriculum*. CDC. https://www.cdc.gov/ncbddd/actearly/autism/curriculum/class.html

Centers for Disease Control and Prevention. (January 14, 2022). *Autism and Developmental Disabilities Monitoring (ADDM) Network*. CDC. https://www.cdc.gov/ncbddd/autism/addm.html

Centers for Medicare and Medicaid Services Office of Minority Health. (2022). *Improving Communication Access For Individuals Who Are Blind Or Have Low Vision*. CMS. https://www.cms.gov/files/document/omh-visual-sensory-disabilities-brochure-508c.pdf

Commission on Dental Accreditation. (2021). *Accreditation Standards for Dental Education Programs*. CODA. https://coda.ada.org/~/media/CODA/Files/2022_predoc_standards.pdf?la=en

DeJong, G., Palsbo, S. E., & Beatty, P. W. (2002). The organization and financing of health services for persons with disabilities. *The Milbank Quarterly*, *80*(2), 261–301. doi:10.1111/1468-0009.t01-1-00004 PMID:12101873

Doebrich, A., Quirici, M., & Lunsford, C. (2020). COVID-19 and the need for disability conscious medical education, training, and practice. *Journal of Pediatric Rehabilitation Medicine*, *13*(3), 393–404. doi:10.3233/PRM-200763 PMID:33252100

Gofine, M., Mielenz, T. J., Vasan, S., & Lebwohl, B. (2018). Use of colorectal cancer screening among people with mobility disability. *Journal of Clinical Gastroenterology*, *52*(9), 789–795. doi:10.1097/MCG.0000000000000835 PMID:28723854

Iezzoni, L. I. (2022). Cancer detection, diagnosis, and treatment for adults with disabilities. *The Lancet. Oncology*, *23*(4), e164–e173. doi:10.1016/S1470-2045(22)00018-3 PMID:35358465

Iezzoni, L. I., & Agaronnik, N. D. (2020). Healthcare disparities for individuals with disability: informing the practice. In *Disability as Diversity* (pp. 15–31). Springer. doi:10.1007/978-3-030-46187-4_2

Iezzoni, L. I., Kurtz, S. G., & Rao, S. R. (2015). Trends in mammography over time for women with and without chronic disability. *Journal of Women's Health*, *24*(7), 593–601. doi:10.1089/jwh.2014.5181 PMID:26083235

Iezzoni, L. I., Kurtz, S. G., & Rao, S. R. (2016). Trends in pap testing over time for women with and without chronic disability. *American Journal of Preventive Medicine*, *50*(2), 210–219. doi:10.1016/j.amepre.2015.06.031 PMID:26372417

Iezzoni, L. I., Ngo, L. H., Li, D., Roetzheim, R. G., Drews, R. E., & McCarthy, E. P. (2008). Treatment disparities for disabled medicare beneficiaries with stage I non-small cell lung cancer. *Archives of Physical Medicine and Rehabilitation*, *89*(4), 595–601. doi:10.1016/j.apmr.2007.09.042 PMID:18373987

Iezzoni, L. I., Rao, S. R., Ressalam, J., Bolcic-Jankovic, D., Agaronnik, N. D., Donelan, K., Lagu, T., & Campbell, E. G. (2021). Physicians' Perceptions Of People With Disability And Their Health Care: Study reports the results of a survey of physicians' perceptions of people with disability. *Health Affairs*, *40*(2), 297–306. doi:10.1377/hlthaff.2020.01452 PMID:33523739

Iezzoni, L. I., Rao, S. R., Ressalam, J., Bolcic-Jankovic, D., Agaronnik, N. D., Lagu, T., Pendo, E., & Campbell, E. G. (2022). US Physicians' Knowledge About The Americans With Disabilities Act And Accommodation Of Patients With Disability: Study examines what physicians know about the Americans With Disabilities Act and what is done to accommodate patients with a disability. *Health Affairs*, *41*(1), 96–104. doi:10.1377/hlthaff.2021.01136 PMID:34982624

Iezzoni, L. I., Rao, S. R., Ressalam, J., Bolcic-Jankovic, D., & Campbell, E. G. (2022). Incidence of accommodations for patients with significant vision limitations in physicians' offices in the US. *JAMA Ophthalmology*, *140*(1), 79–84. doi:10.1001/jamaophthalmol.2021.5072 PMID:34854912

Jarus, T., Bezati, R., Trivett, S., Lee, M., Bulk, L. Y., Battalova, A., Mayer, Y., Murphy, S., Gerber, P., & Drynan, D. (2020). Professionalism and disabled clinicians: The client's perspective. *Disability & Society*, *35*(7), 1085–1102. doi:10.1080/09687599.2019.1669436

Juster, F., & Edwards, K. (2001). A rotation in chronic-care pediatrics with a focus on children and their families in the community. *Academic Medicine*, *76*(5), 568. doi:10.1097/00001888-200105000-00118 PMID:11346625

Krahn, G. L., Walker, D. K., & Correa-De-Araujo, R. (2015, April). Persons with disabilities as an unrecognized health disparity population. *American Journal of Public Health*, *105*(S2, Suppl 2), S198–S206. doi:10.2105/AJPH.2014.302182 PMID:25689212

Levy, A., & Perry, A. (2011). Outcomes in adolescents and adults with autism: A review of the literature. *Research in Autism Spectrum Disorders*, *5*(4), 1271–1282. doi:10.1016/j.rasd.2011.01.023

Magence, A., Gross, J., Wilson, J., Juster, F., Edwards, K., & Petersen, K. (2021). *Year one: Reflections on implementation of a disabilities curriculum for medical students*. AMA Research Challenge.

Mahoney, S. (2022). *Caring for adults with intellectual and developmental disabilities*. AAMC. https://www.aamc.org/news-insights/caring-adults-intellectual-and-developmental-disabilities

Meeks, L. M., Case, B., Herzer, K., Plegue, M., & Swenor, B. K. (2019). Change in prevalence of disabilities and accommodation practices among US medical schools, 2016 vs 2019. *Journal of the American Medical Association*, *322*(20), 2022–2024. doi:10.1001/jama.2019.15372 PMID:31769816

Meeks, L. M., Case, B., Plegue, M., Moreland, C. J., Jain, S., & Taylor, N. (2020). National prevalence of disability and clinical accommodations in medical education. *Journal of Medical Education and Curricular Development*, *7*, 2382120520965249. doi:10.1177/2382120520965249 PMID:33178890

Meeks, L. M., & Jain, N. (2018). *Accessibility, inclusion, and action in medical education: lived experiences of learners and physicians with disabilities*. Association of American Medical Colleges.

Meeks, L. M., Stergiopoulos, E., & Petersen, K. H. (2022). Institutional accountability for students with disabilities: A call for liaison committee on medical education action. *Academic Medicine*, *97*(3), 341–345. doi:10.1097/ACM.0000000000004471 PMID:34670236

Meeks, L. (2019). *The disabilities we don't see*. AAMC. https://www.aamc.org/news-insights/disabilities-we-dont-see

Miller, A. N., Todd, A., Toledo, R., & Duvuuri, V. N. S. (2022). The Relationship of Ethnic, Racial, and Cultural Concordance to Physician–Patient Communication: A Mixed-Methods Systematic Review Protocol. *Health Communication*, 1–7. doi:10.1080/10410236.2022.2070449 PMID:35502565

National Institutes of Health. (November 15, 2018). *Surgeon Chris McCulloh Stands Up to Disability*. National Institute of General Medical Sciences. https://biobeat.nigms.nih.gov/2018/11/surgeon-chris-mcculloh-stands-up-to-disability/

New York Medical College. (June 30, 2022). *Expanded Disabilities Curriculum at New York Medical College Receives Enthusiastic Student Response*. New York Medical College. https://www.nymc.edu/news-and-events/news-archives/expanded-disabilities-curriculum-at-new-york-medical-college-receives-enthusiastic-student-response.php

Nouri, Z., Dill, M. J., Conrad, S. S., Moreland, C. J., & Meeks, L. M. (2021). Estimated Prevalence of US Physicians With Disabilities. *JAMA Network Open*, *4*(3), e211254–e211254. doi:10.1001/jamanetworkopen.2021.1254 PMID:33710286

Office of the Surgeon General. (2005). *The Surgeon General's Call to Action to Improve the Health and Wellness of Persons with Disabilities*. U.S. Department of Health and Human Services, Office of the Surgeon General.

Okoro, C. A., Hollis, N. D., Cyrus, A. C., & Griffin-Blake, S. (2018). Prevalence of disabilities and health care access by disability status and type among adults—United States, 2016. *Morbidity and Mortality Weekly Report*, *67*(32), 882–887. doi:10.15585/mmwr.mm6732a3 PMID:30114005

Powell, P. S., Pazol, K., Wiggins, L. D., Daniels, J. L., Dichter, G. S., Bradley, C. B., Pretzel, R., Kloetzer, J., McKenzie, C., Scott, A., Robinson, B., Sims, A. S., Kasten, E. P., Fallin, M. D., Levy, S. E., Dietz, P. M., & Cogswell, M. E. (2021). Health Status and Health Care Use Among Adolescents Identified With and Without Autism in Early Childhood—Four US Sites, 2018–2020. *Morbidity and Mortality Weekly Report*, *70*(17), 605–611. doi:10.15585/mmwr.mm7017a1 PMID:33914722

Sarmiento, C., Miller, S. R., Chang, E., Zazove, P., & Kumagai, A. K. (2016). From impairment to empowerment: A longitudinal medical school curriculum on disabilities. *Academic Medicine*, *91*(7), 954–957. doi:10.1097/ACM.0000000000000935 PMID:26422593

Shapiro, J. (2008). Walking a mile in their patients' shoes: Empathy and othering in medical students' education. *Philosophy, Ethics, and Humanities in Medicine; PEHM*, *3*(1), 1–11. doi:10.1186/1747-5341-3-10 PMID:18336719

Smith, D. L. (2009). Disparities in patient-physician communication for persons with a disability from the 2006 Medical Expenditure Panel Survey (MEPS). *Disability and Health Journal*, *2*(4), 206–215. doi:10.1016/j.dhjo.2009.06.002 PMID:21122761

Sullivan, W. F., Diepstra, H., Heng, J., Ally, S., Bradley, E., Casson, I., Hennen, B., Kelly, M., Korossy, M., McNeil, K., Abells, D., Amaria, K., Boyd, K., Gemmill, M., Grier, E., Kennie-Kaulbach, N., Ketchell, M., Ladouceur, J., Lepp, A., Lunsky, Y., McMillan, S., Niel, U., Sacks, S., Shea, S., Stringer, K., Sue, K., & Witherbee, S. (2018). Primary care of adults with intellectual and developmental disabilities. *2018 Canadian consensus guidelines, 64*(4), 254-279.

Symons, A. B., McGuigan, D., & Akl, E. A. (2009). A curriculum to teach medical students to care for people with disabilities: Development and initial implementation. *BMC Medical Education*, *9*(1), 1–7. doi:10.1186/1472-6920-9-1 PMID:20042110

USDHHS. (2012). *Healthy People 2010 Final Review*. U.S. Department of Health and Human Services, National Center for Heatlh Statistics.

White, P. H., Cooley, W. C., Boudreau, A. D. A., Cyr, M., Davis, B. E., Dreyfus, D. E., Forlenza, E., Friedland, A., Greenlee, C., Mann, M., McManus, M., Meleis, A. I., & Pickler, L.Transitions Clinical Report Authoring Group. (2018). Supporting the Health Care Transition From Adolescence to Adulthood in the Medical Home. *Pediatrics*, *142*(5), e20182587. doi:10.1542/peds.2018-2587 PMID:30348754

World Health Organization. (November 24, 2021). *Disability and health*. WHO. https://www.who.int/news-room/fact-sheets/detail/disability-and-health

ENDNOTE

1 Disclaimer: This chapter took part in the double-blind peer review process and was not compromised due to the authors also being an editor. A non-author editor managed all of the editorial aspects of the chapter.

Chapter 3
Size Inclusivity in Medicine:
Barriers to Healthcare Access for Patients With Obesity

Amal Shibli-Rahhal
University of Iowa Carver College of Medicine, USA

Amie Ogunsakin
University of Iowa Carver College of Medicine, USA

Kathleen M. Robinson
https://orcid.org/0000-0002-5697-6323
University of Iowa Carver College of Medicine, USA

EXECUTIVE SUMMARY

The most recent estimates by the Center for Disease Control indicate that obesity is present in up to 41.9% of adults living in the United States, with a prevalence of severe obesity reaching 9.2%. Consequently, healthcare providers and healthcare systems in general will often interact with and provide care to individuals with obesity. However, weight stigma is common within the healthcare system, often presenting as a poorly equipped healthcare environment, and insufficient proficiency in communicating with and examining individuals with obesity. Most concerning, however, is how anti-obesity bias leads to stereotyping with premature closure and over-attribution of disease when treating patients with obesity. These factors can lead to discrimination and inequity in delivery of healthcare to individuals with obesity and result in healthcare avoidance by these patients. This chapter examines discriminatory practices affecting healthcare delivery to individuals with obesity and discusses approaches to address them.

DOI: 10.4018/978-1-6684-5493-0.ch003

INTRODUCTION

The World Health Organization defines obesity as an "abnormal or excessive fat accumulation that presents a risk to health." It is typically defined as a body mass index (BMI) of 30kg/m^2 or higher (World Health Organization). Obesity is multifactorial, with contributions from genetics, underlying disease, medication use, mental disorders, lifestyle and socioeconomic factors (Hill et al., 2013; van der Valk et al., 2019). The prevalence of obesity among adults in the United States (US) has increased from 13% in the 1960s to 41.9% in 2017 (Centers for Disease Control and Prevention). At a population level, obesity is associated with type 2 diabetes, cardiovascular disease, osteoarthritis, steatohepatitis, and certain cancers (Bluher, 2019). Globally in 2017, high BMI was associated with 4.7 million deaths and 165.6 million disability-adjusted life years lost (Dai et al., 2020).

The rise in obesity rates has been paralleled by an increase in weight stigma (Andreyeva et al., 2008). Weight stigma is the "social devaluation and denigration of individuals because of their excess body weight, [which] can lead to negative attitudes, stereotypes, prejudice, and discrimination" (Rubino et al., 2020). Approximately 40-60% of individuals with obesity experience weight teasing or discrimination (Prunty et al., 2020; Puhl, Lessard, Himmelstein, et al., 2021). Weight stigma manifests widely in multiple domains including the media, educational settings, interpersonal relationships, workplaces, and the structural environment (Alimoradi et al., 2020). The media often portrays individuals with obesity as disheveled, unorganized, undesirable, or as the appropriate subjects of humor (Eisenberg et al., 2015; Karsay, 2019). Social media outlets serve as forums for stigmatizing and misogynistic sentiments related to weight (Chou et al., 2014; Jeon et al., 2018; Wanniarachchi et al., 2022).

Similar to what is seen in society at large, weight stigma in healthcare is common. Physicians often hold negative or stereotypical attitudes toward patients with obesity. These biases may be explicit or more subtle or implicit (Foster et al., 2003; Harvey & Hill, 2001; Puhl & Brownell, 2001). Other healthcare professionals and trainees also manifest such attitudes, including nurses, medical and nursing students, dietitians, and psychologists, further contributing to an environment that is hostile to people with obesity (Budd et al., 2011). As we explore later, healthcare practitioners and trainees often do not understand the etiology or complexity of obesity, and how to treat it (Budd et al., 2011; Butsch et al., 2020; Foster et al., 2003; Katz et al., 2022; Metcalf et al., 2017). This may contribute to reluctance to care for people with obesity, and pessimism about their adherence to therapy and potential for weight loss success (Amy et al., 2006; Wigton & McGaghie, 2001). Furthermore, lack of knowledge and bias may lead to cognitive errors, such as over-attribution of disease to obesity, and premature diagnostic closure.

Another important potential source of weight stigma in healthcare is the misuse of BMI as a metric. Although BMI holds validity at a population level, it does not reflect levels of aerobic fitness, body composition, body fat distribution, the metabolic activity of adipose tissue, or overall health status (Bray et al., 2018; Humphreys, 2010; Muller et al., 2016). Indeed, significant debate remains regarding whether there may be a form of metabolically healthy obesity, essentially, individuals with obesity who do not have elevated risk of disease (Bluher, 2020). Current recommendations encourage the use BMI as a screening measure, coupled with further evaluation of individual patients for the presence of disease or risk for disease without over-reliance on this measure (Garvey et al., 2016).

Weight stigma in healthcare carries significant consequences. Women with overweight and obesity may feel dismissed and "not quite human," experiencing their healthcare as embarrassing or demeaning (Merrill & Grassley, 2008). Such negative experiences erode trust in the healthcare system and encourage "doctor shopping' in search of better care (Alberga et al., 2019). For women, pregnancy and the peripartum period can be times of vulnerability to weight stigma (Incollingo Rodriguez et al., 2020). As explored in Case 1, experiences of weight stigma are also associated with psychological distress, depression, anxiety, reduced weight loss, binge eating, exercise avoidance, worsening of metabolic health, and increased mortality (Alimoradi et al., 2020; Daly et al., 2019; Fruh et al., 2016; Hatzenbuehler et al., 2009; Jackson & Steptoe, 2017; O'Brien et al., 2016; Sutin et al., 2015; Udo et al., 2016; Vadiveloo & Mattei, 2017). Additionally, weight stigma has been associated with increased risk of cigarette smoking, driving while intoxicated, and risky sexual/drug use behaviors (Sutin & Terracciano, 2017). As explored in Case 2, at a system-wide level, effective therapies for obesity are available but are often under-utilized due to bias, lack of clinician knowledge and limited insurance coverage.

In addition to experiencing weight stigma from others, around 40% of individuals with obesity display weight bias internalization (WBI) (Puhl et al., 2018). This "occurs when individuals engage in self-blame and self-directed weight stigma because of their weight, [and] includes agreement with weight-based stereotypes and application of these stereotypes to oneself and self-devaluation" (Rubino et al., 2020). WBI is thought to mediate some of the negative consequences of weight stigma, including disordered eating, healthcare avoidance, and exercise avoidance (Mensinger et al., 2018; O'Brien et al., 2016; Pearl et al., 2015).

Although data regarding the pervasiveness of weight stigma and its detrimental effects are sobering, mitigation strategies are available and under development. Medical training must be improved to include education around weight stigma. As discussed in Case 1, current educational and communication strategies have shown promise for reducing weight stigma in a wide array of healthcare trainees and practitioners (Albury et al., 2020; Gayer et al., 2017; Vitolins et al., 2012). Additionally, programs are being developed to reduce WBI. A particularly promising intervention, utilizing a cognitive-behavioral intervention in combination with a weight loss program, was associated with significant reductions in WBI (Pearl et al., 2020).

At a societal level, further progress is needed to reduce weight stigma, and to protect people with obesity from discrimination. Improvements in media portrayals may be helpful in changing popular views (Pearl et al., 2012). Policy change is also needed. To date, within the US only Michigan and a few other localities have laws in place protecting people with obesity from discrimination (Puhl et al., 2015), but greater progress is required at a systemic level to effect change (Hill et al., 2021; Puhl, Lessard, Pearl, et al., 2021).

CASE 1: SHORTNESS OF BREATH

Goal

This case portrays examples of weight bias/stigma in the healthcare system and the effect that weight stigma has on the individual.

Learning Outcomes

1. Discuss weight stigma in healthcare and stereotypes applied to people with obesity.
2. Identify weight stigma in the clinical environment and ways to address it.
3. Review consequences of weight stigma in healthcare on health outcomes.

4. Recognize the key elements of appropriate communication and physical examination when caring for a person with obesity.

Case

Loretta is a 47-year-old-woman with type 2 diabetes mellitus, hypertension, and obesity (BMI 52kg/m^2) presenting to her primary care clinic for shortness of breath and palpitations. After check-in, she is directed to the waiting lobby where the chairs are narrow and have arms that further restrict their size. She struggles into a seat. Fifteen minutes later, a nursing assistant (NA) calls her name and when she notices her in the narrow chair she jokingly says, "we need to get larger chairs for people like you, don't we?" Loretta smiles nervously as other patients look at her. She follows the NA into the exam room. Outside the room, the NA asks Loretta what her weight is to record it in her chart. Loretta says she has not weighed herself in a while and asks the NA to just weigh her. The NA responds, "That is ok, we can skip the weight. I do not want you to break the scale." She then proceeds to measure Loretta's blood pressure, using a small cuff that pinches Loretta's skin. Loretta complains and asks for a larger blood pressure cuff. The NA sighs and walks to a locked cabinet, rummages in it then pulls out a larger cuff.

Next the medical resident, Dr. K., walks in and introduces himself then says, "I notice that you have not been to clinic in over 2 years and that you have cancelled several of your appointments." Loretta answers, "Sorry for that, it is just hard to come here." After asking a few more questions about Loretta's symptoms, Dr. K. motions to the exam table which again is too narrow. As Loretta struggles to sit on the table, he casually says, "You know this would be much easier if you lost weight." Dr. K. checks Loretta's pulse and listens to her heart and lungs without removing her clothing, then calls his attending physician, Dr. M. Dr. M. introduces herself to Loretta who is still sitting on the exam table and asks her if she prefers to sit back in her chair, which Loretta does. Dr. M. then asks Dr. K. to present the patient and Dr. K. says, "This is a 47-year-old morbidly obese woman presenting because of shortness of breath and palpitations …" When Dr. K. finishes his presentation, Dr. M. says: "So to summarize, this is a 47-year-old woman with type 2 diabetes, hypertension and obesity who is here for shortness of breath and palpitations." Dr. M. then asks if she can examine Loretta and asks her to change into an exam gown while she and Dr. K. wait outside the room. When Loretta invites the physicians back into the room, Dr. M. apologizes for the inadequate exam table and offers her hand to assist Loretta as she climbs onto the table again. She listens to Loretta's lungs and heart sounds, making sure she gently moves excess tissue as she positions the stethoscope against the skin. At the end of the consultation, Loretta asks to speak with Dr. M. privately and shares her concerns regarding the treatment that she has received from the NA and the resident. At the end of the clinic day, Dr. M. convenes the clinic team to "review some best clinical practice guidelines."

QUESTIONS AND ANSWERS

1. Discuss weight stigma in healthcare and describe how it manifests in this case.

Several studies have evaluated weight stigma among healthcare providers and demonstrated a significant prevalence of negative stereotypical views regarding individuals with obesity, including the beliefs that they lack self-control, are lazy and unmotivated to be healthier, and that they are responsible for their condition (Budd et al., 2011; Foster et al., 2003; Harvey & Hill, 2001; Persky & Eccleston, 2011; Price et al., 1987). In addition, a large proportion of healthcare providers view patients with obesity as unattractive, ugly and awkward (Foster et al., 2003; Harvey & Hill, 2001; Puhl & Brownell, 2001). Notably, in a study assessing physician-patient communication, physicians reported low respect toward 39% of the study patients; and these patients had a higher BMI than those who received high respect. Reported respect was inversely proportional to the patient's BMI, independent of sex, age and race (Huizinga et al., 2009). Furthermore, physicians participating in this study felt that 45% of the patients were non-adherent to medications, and higher BMI was directly correlated with this perception (Huizinga et al., 2010). In a survey of 4,732 medical students matriculating into 49 medical schools across the US in 2010, 74% and 67% of the students respectively manifested implicit and explicit weight bias (Phelan et al., 2014).

In this case, weight stigma manifests in the physical environment of the clinic and communication with the patient from nursing and medical staff.

Physical environment: The clinical environment in this case is not equipped to accommodate patients with obesity. The waiting lobby chairs are narrow and have arms that further constrict space, making them uncomfortable or even not useful for patients with obesity. The exam room table is narrow, another source of discomfort and possibly humiliation for the patient. The NA used a small cuff to measure the patient's blood pressure, causing pain and discomfort. While the clinic is equipped with a larger cuff, it is placed in a locked cabinet and not readily visible or accessible, discouraging people from using it. Furthermore, the NA mentioned that she did not want to weigh Loretta for fear of breaking the scale. It is unclear what the weight capacity of the scale is, but if it is indeed a scale that cannot accommodate heavier patients, this in of itself would be an additional manifestation of weight stigma and discrimination.

Provider-patient communication: This started with the embarrassing comment/joke that the NA made *("we need to get larger chairs for people like you")*. Later, the NA referred to Loretta's weight by saying *"I do not want you to break the scale,"* a statement that lays blame on the patient and further alienates her. The NA further manifests bias through ineffective non-verbal communication when she chose to use a too-small cuff to measure Loretta's blood pressure then manifested annoyance (sighed) at having to get the larger cuff.

Dr. K., manifests weight stigma both verbally and non-verbally. He does not offer to assist Loretta as she struggles to move to the exam table. He later leaves her sitting on the uncomfortable table while he finds his attending. He also casually approaches Loretta's weight without invitation or permission, using judgmental/blaming language *("you know this would be much easier if you lost weight")*. When presenting the patient to his attending, Dr. K. refers to Loretta as a "morbidly obese woman" a statement that associates obesity with the patient's identity in an undesirable way.

Several studies have in fact addressed the issue of language used by healthcare providers when referring to obesity. Patient surveys indicate a strong aversion to the words "fat" and "morbid obesity/morbidly obese" and most patients also rate the words "obese" and "obesity" as undesirable (Auckburally et al., 2021; Dutton et al., 2010; Gray et al., 2011; Lydecker et al., 2016; Puhl et al., 2013; Puhl, 2020; Volger et al., 2012).

In reference to the clinical environment, it is often designed with no attention to the comfort and dignity of patients with obesity. Waiting rooms often only offer chairs too narrow to be comfortable, with arms that restrict movement. Additionally, waiting room literature typically relies on magazines with negative body-size messages. Physical exam gowns may be too small, providing inadequate coverage. Exam tables and beds are frequently too narrow, and medical equipment does not always accommodate higher body weights, including blood pressure cuffs, scales, and imaging machines (Kaminsky &

Gadaleta, 2002; Merrill & Grassley, 2008; Pryor, 2002). For example, standard computed tomography (CT) and magnetic resonance imaging (MRI) machines often come with a weight limit of 450 pounds, effectively denying imaging to many patients with obesity. In one recent study, only 28% of academic hospitals had access to large weight capacity CT machines and 10% had access to large weight capacity MRI machines, with lower availability at non-academic and critical access hospitals (Ginde et al., 2008).

2. What are the effects of weight stigma on the health of individuals?

Weight stigma is associated with negative effects on physical and psychological health. A cross-sectional survey of 22,231 adults in the US showed strong correlations between perceived weight discrimination and mood disorders, anxiety disorders and substance use disorders after correction for BMI, sociodemographic variables, and perceived stress (Hatzenbuehler et al., 2009). Numerous studies have demonstrated positive correlations between weight stigma and maladaptive eating behaviors (such as emotional and binge eating) and physical inactivity/exercise avoidance that are independent of BMI (Puhl et al., 2020). Weight stigma is also associated with higher glycated hemoglobin (HbA1c) measurements, a higher risk of type 2 diabetes mellitus (Puhl et al., 2020), and systemic markers of stress and inflammation, including elevated cortisol and c-reactive protein (Himmelstein et al., 2015; Jackson et al., 2016; Jackson & Steptoe, 2017; McCleary-Gaddy et al., 2019; Sutin et al., 2014; Tomiyama et al., 2014). In combination, these disturbances are thought to lead to further weight gain (Tomiyama, 2014).

An increasing body of evidence has examined the effect of weight bias internalization (WBI) on health. A recent systematic review identified 30 studies that evaluated the relationship between depression and WBI, 28 of which demonstrated a positive correlation. Likewise, of 11 studies evaluating the relationship between anxiety and WBI, 10 found a positive correlation (Pearl & Puhl, 2018). In addition, high levels of WBI were found to be associated with higher odds of metabolic syndrome (Pearl et al., 2017).

While these studies do not separate the effects of weight stigma in general from weight stigma within healthcare, a survey of 600 adults with overweight and obesity showed that those who perceived weight discrimination from their healthcare providers were less likely to trust the provider, which can negatively affect quality of care and treatment adherence (Gudzune et al., 2014). A recent scoping review of studies on weight bias and healthcare utilization identified 7 studies on healthcare avoidance among patients with obesity. Unsolicited weight-related discussions, inadequate equipment, and embarrassment from being weighed or having to expose their body were the main reasons for healthcare avoidance (Alberga et al., 2019). This avoidance may extend into preventative care, particularly gynecologic and breast cancer screening (Aldrich & Hackley, 2010; Amy et al., 2006; Wee et al., 2000). In addition, healthcare professionals themselves may be less likely to recommend gynecological cancer screening to women with obesity (Ferrante et al., 2007). Although the consequences of such delays are difficult to determine, women with obesity are more likely to receive a diagnosis of cervical cancer rather than pre-cancer (Clarke et al., 2018).

3. Discuss best practices to eliminate weight stigma from the healthcare environment.

Several interventions and practice guidelines have explored ways to mitigate weight stigma in healthcare. The physical environment should be designed/re-designed to honor the comfort and dignity of patients with obesity. Examples include waiting rooms with couches, benches, and larger chairs with no movement-restricting arms, and diverse waiting room literature with less emphasis on publications that further stigmatize obesity. Examination tools and gowns of all sizes should be readily available. Exam tables and beds should be wider, and mattresses should provide adequate support. Medical equipment with high weight capacity, including imaging machines and scales, should be readily available and all scales should be placed in private areas, so weight measurements are not witnessed by others (Albury et al., 2020; Fruh et al., 2021; Fruh et al., 2016). Given the high prevalence of obesity, a recent international consensus statement called for the adoption of an appropriate infrastructure as a requirement for the accreditation of medical institutions (Rubino et al., 2020).

However, environmental changes are only one step in addressing healthcare-related weight stigma. Equally or possibly more important is the language used when providers communicate with patients. Earlier we described that the words "fat", "morbid" and "obese" are generally disliked by patients and generally considered hurtful and demeaning, so such words are to be avoided (Albury et al., 2020; Fruh et al., 2021; Rubino et al., 2020). People-first language should be used when referring to obesity, so as not to equate the person with their medical condition. Recommended terms include "person with obesity" or "person living with obesity" rather than "obese person" (Albury et al., 2020; American Medical Association, 2017; Fruh et al., 2021; Obesity Action Coalition). Uninvited references to obesity during conversation are often cited as a source of perceived discrimination and even as a factor that leads patients to avoid seeking healthcare. Healthcare providers should seek patient permission prior to starting a weight-related discussion, especially when obesity is not the main reason for the clinical visit. Open ended questions asking the patient what they think about their weight is one acceptable approach (Albury et al., 2020). Alternatively, direct permission-seeking questions such as "can we discuss your weight?" may be used (Fruh et al., 2021; Fruh et al., 2016; Ward et al., 2009). Finally, "fat humor" is not acceptable, even when not in the presence of the patient. In addition, non-verbal behaviors carry the same importance as words in the medical encounter and are linked to patient outcomes (Roter et al., 2006; Ward et al., 2009). Regardless of body size, healthcare providers should display attention to patient comfort and dignity, using words and actions that demonstrate respect, genuine care, and validation.

A discussion of clinical skills is incomplete without approaching the question of physical examination. Although obesity may decrease the accuracy of the clinical examination, providers can still modify the exam to maximize its yield (Beer et al., 2021; Gilat et al., 2022; Silk & McTigue, 2011). Unfortunately, most medical curricula do not prepare learners to perform an adequate physical examination on patients with obesity. As a matter of fact, medical education has not kept pace with most aspects of obesity education including foundational and clinical sciences and clinical skills (Butsch et al., 2020; Katz et al., 2022; Metcalf et al., 2017; Vitolins et al., 2012). As an example, 55% of body donation programs in the United States have a BMI or weight limit with an average of 240 pounds (Elzie & Cruz, 2020). However, a few recent interventions have explored educational approaches to weight-based stigma that promise to improve the attitude of healthcare providers toward obesity. For example, a recent study showed that the introduction of an obesity curriculum (including lectures and case study simulations) improved obesity-related knowledge and attitudes of osteopathic medical students (Gayer et al., 2017). Likewise, an educational intervention on communication skills with patients regarding obesity led to decreased stereotyping and increased empathy among medical students (Kushner et al., 2014).

Epilogue

This case examines the pervasiveness of weight stigma in healthcare and the different ways it presents, including non-accommodating physical environments and poor communication. It also discusses the ill-effects that weight stigma has on the mental and physical well-being of patients with obesity and how it affects their relationships and interactions with healthcare providers and healthcare in general. Research has identified ways to mitigate many of these shortcomings, and several approaches to improving the healthcare environment and providers' communication in relation to obesity are discussed. While the clinical approach to the patients' presenting symptoms was not addressed in this case study, it will be discussed in Case 2.

CASE 2: MISSED DIAGNOSIS

Goal

This case highlights the difficulties that individuals with obesity encounter in accessing quality medical care.

Learning Outcomes

1. Describe how implicit bias affects medical care of patients with obesity
2. Discuss consequences of premature closure and over-attribution of disease in the management of patients with obesity.
3. Discuss barriers to obesity care in clinical practice.

Case

Michael is a 50-year-old man with obesity (BMI $64kg/m^2$) who presents to his primary care clinic for a check-up. He has gained 10 pounds in the last 6 months and reports new onset of shortness of breath. No physical examination is performed, and some laboratory tests are obtained, showing new elevation in liver enzymes. Review of old records shows an abdominal ultrasound obtained within the past year for abdominal pain to be normal. Michael is informed that the elevated liver enzymes indicate fatty liver disease which is common in individuals with obesity. The physician recommends increased physical activity, diet modifications, and a liver elastography.

When Michael presents a few weeks later for the liver elastography, the ultrasound technician explains that an ultrasound probe will be used to deliver low frequency sound waves to the right upper abdomen to determine liver stiffness. He is informed that he will need to lay flat for about 10 minutes to complete the test and that the study may be suboptimal in quality, due to the extent of the abdominal fat present which may interfere with passage of the sound waves.

Michael replies that he will not be able to lay flat due to his shortness of breath and explains that he sleeps in a recliner. The technician and supervising radiologist discuss this concern and determine that the shortness of breath is likely due to obesity and that the patient should still attempt to lie down for the study. Michael declines the procedure, and the appointment is marked as "patient unable to perform test."

Michael returns to his primary care clinic four months later and is noted to have further weight gain and visible shortness of breath while walking a short distance to the exam room. His oxygen saturation and blood pressure are low. He is transferred to the emergency room where he is diagnosed with acute congestive heart failure. He is hospitalized and treated for congestive heart failure with subsequent improvement of the shortness of breath and liver function abnormalities. Upon discharge from the hospital, Michael is again advised to lose weight. He walks away not understanding his options for weight loss as those were not discussed and he has already made multiple unsuccessful attempts at weight loss.

QUESTIONS AND ANSWERS

1. How does implicit bias lead to inadequate clinical care or denial of care in individuals with obesity?

Implicit bias refers to preference, aversion to, or stereotypes about a certain group of people on an unconscious level. It can affect clinical communication, assessments, and healthcare delivery with often untoward consequences (Carels et al., 2010; Jungnickel et al., 2022; Lane, 2007). This case illustrates implicit bias within the context of obesity. Michael was automatically assumed to have shortness of breath because of obesity, a manifestation of a common stereotype. His clinical assessment, including the physical examination, was incomplete resulting in the non-consideration of alternative explanations by the physician. Even the patient's statement of his inability to lay supine - a pathognomonic feature of congestive heart failure - did not lead healthcare providers (in this case the radiology technician and supervising radiologist) to question the initial clinical impression.

Here, the implicit anti-obesity bias led to a delay in diagnosis, with prolongation of patient suffering and potential for serious harm had the delay been longer. This pattern has been documented in several studies that suggest that implicit bias leads to less time spent on the clinical assessment, counseling of the patient and rapport building leading to delays in diagnosis and treatments (Gudzune et al., 2014; Phelan et al., 2015; Puhl & Brownell, 2001; Tilburt et al., 2019).

Such bias may also manifest as reduced access to other forms of care, such as surgery where access may be restricted to patients below a certain BMI. Although elevated BMI is associated with surgical complications, in many cases the absolute risk increase remains minimal. Moreover, surgical risk does not dramatically increase at a certain BMI, making hard cutoffs arbitrary (Ricciardi et al., 2019). Perhaps most problematically, BMI is treated as a modifiable risk factor. In fact, few patients meet the required weight benchmarks, effectively denying these patients surgical care (Springer, 2019). The restriction of organ transplants to individuals with obesity is another area which raises ethical concerns. Transplant listing practices for solid organs are variable across the United States, with insufficient transparency, and obesity is often cited as a reason for refusal due to increased risk of complications and death (Kovesdy & Molnar, 2014; Wall et al., 2019).

General practitioners are expected to address obesity as part of the routine medical care of patients with high BMI. However, less than optimal obesity-related care often occurs in primary care settings due to a lack of capability, know-how, time and resources (Rhee et al., 2018; Story et al., 2002). In our patient scenario, care was inadvertently withheld as there was no discussion of other potential treatment options for obesity beyond diet and exercise.

Yet another common manifestation of bias presents when important diagnostic tests are withheld from patients who exceed a certain weight limit. This is commonly encountered with dual x-ray absorptiometry (DXA) scans in the setting of osteoporosis diagnosis. MRI and CT machines are another common example where serious diagnoses may be missed due to inability to accommodate the patient's weight. While machines that can accommodate higher weights are available, these are still missing in most clinical settings (Ginde et al., 2008), possibly representing an underlying bias leading to lack of interest in investing in these newer technologies.

Conscious efforts are required to mitigate implicit bias. Healthcare professionals must recognize that this bias is difficult to change and must be educated to understand its negative impacts. A multi-step framework has been proposed to integrate recognition of implicit bias into medical education. This framework aims to empower the learner to recognize their individual biases within a safe learning environment, understand the scientific underpinnings of implicit bias and mitigate its ill-effects on healthcare delivery (Sukhera & Watling, 2018). A similar framework was recently adopted by the Association of American Medical Colleges (AAMC) as part of its *Diversity, Equity and Inclusion Competencies Across the Learning Continuum* (Domain I, competency 1) (Association of American Medical Colleges, 2022). As it is still unclear whether such interventions will impact healthcare provider behaviors and patient outcomes, future research in this area is needed.

2. How does premature closure and over attribution of disease impact patients with obesity?

Premature closure is a common form of cognitive diagnostic bias wherein the clinician stops considering alternative diagnoses once a reasonable conclusion or explanation for the patient's symptoms is present (Norman & Eva, 2010; Phelan et al., 2015; Puhl & Brownell, 2001; Redelmeier, 2005). Over-attribution bias occurs when people attribute human behavior to whichever causal factor is most available to them (Darity, 2008). Over-attribution is often seen in the clinical care of patients with obesity, where healthcare providers are quick to assume that patients' symptoms are weight related. Because obesity offers a plausible explanation for many clinical symptoms and presentations (weakness, falls, joint pain, shortness of breath, palpitations, weight gain etc.), this leads to premature diagnostic closure, missed diagnoses (Phelan et al., 2015), and medical errors (Croskerry, 2003).

In our case, the clinician attributed the patient's abnormal liver function tests to nonalcoholic steatohepatitis without considering other possibilities and despite the normal recent abdominal ultrasound. This was likely driven by the rather high prevalence of nonalcoholic steatohepatitis in individuals with obesity. So, obesity in this case offered a readily available reasonable explanation for the patient's shortness of breath and abnormal liver tests (over-attribution), leading to non-consideration of other potential explanations, such as fluid overload that can lead to similar findings (premature closure).

It is critical for healthcare providers to recognize these caveats to clinical diagnosis in patients with obesity and to learn to question their impressions and assumptions. While obesity may cause a multitude of symptoms and physical findings, patients with obesity are not immune to other health conditions that too can explain their clinical presentations. A detailed clinical evaluation and examination of inconsistencies may present important clues to alternate diagnoses.

3. What are some of the barriers to obesity treatment?

Obesity treatment is multifaceted and includes nutritional therapy, exercise, pharmacotherapy and - in some instances - bariatric surgery. A detailed discussion of obesity therapy is beyond the scope of this chapter, but several recent reviews provide a comprehensive description of available treatment approaches (Angelidi et al., 2022; Ruban et al., 2019). However, a major barrier to effective treatment of obesity is that most healthcare providers do not fully understand the pathophysiology of obesity and consider it to be an issue of lifestyle and behavior choice, leading to reluctance to offer therapy (ECRI

Institute, 2013; Kelleher et al., 2013). Individuals with obesity perceive a lack of education, training and knowledge among health professionals on weight management treatment and best practices (Amy et al., 2006; Forhan et al., 2013; Russell & Carryer, 2013).

Additionally, medical education has not kept pace with the scientific advances made in this field; as a result many healthcare providers are not fully aware of available therapies and their application. In a 2018 cross-sectional survey of U.S. family medicine residency programs, 39% of programs surveyed reported little to no training on obesity management and very few programs covered pharmacological treatment of obesity (10%). Lack of curriculum and faculty expertise were reported as the greatest barriers to obesity education during residency (Orjuela-Grimm et al., 2021); these deficits result in healthcare providers who are ill-equipped and less than proficient in treating patients with obesity.

For example, and while pharmacotherapy and obesity surgery are increasingly being covered by healthcare insurance providers in the US, healthcare providers are often unaware of these options or do not fully understand their efficacy, risks and benefits (Woolford et al., 2010; Zevin et al., 2022). In a study of primary care providers in a community-based academic hospital system, concerns regarding surgical safety and effectiveness were the main reasons for provider reluctance to refer patients to bariatric surgery (Conaty et al., 2020). In this case study example, there was no discussion regarding anti-obesity management or metabolic surgery even when the patient's clinical presentation was assumed to be caused by obesity.

In addition to the above limitations in provider knowledge and attitudes, significant financial and logistical barriers may exist that limit patient access to effective therapy. In certain cases, medication costs may be prohibitive, or health insurance companies may mandate the use of cheaper, less effective agents with undesirable side effect profiles before approving more effective options. For example, Semaglutide is a new effective anti-obesity medication (Kim et al., 2022) but is largely not covered by health insurance (Andrews, 2015). Likewise, patients who are otherwise adequate candidates for bariatric surgery are often asked to meet challenging pre-surgical requirements, including attaining a specific weight loss goal within a determined timeframe for surgery to be approved. Due to the physiology of obesity, some patients may not be able achieve the required pre-surgical weight loss despite their best efforts at lifestyle modifications, thus not qualifying for an effective intervention that would have otherwise changed clinical outcomes. In this sense, obesity is one of the few chronic diseases where the onus is placed on the patient to help themselves, before being eligible for treatments (Kovesdy & Molnar, 2014; Wall et al., 2019).

The process for medication/procedure approval or authorization by health insurance is often time- and resource-consuming, presenting a disincentive for the healthcare professional to prescribe them. The complexity of these processes and the length of time they require may also act as a deterrent to weight loss efforts by the patient (Greenapple & Ngai, 2010; Verger et al., 2010).

Epilogue

Healthcare providers are important advocates for their patients and should be aware of biases that may impact the care of patients with obesity and appropriate mitigation strategies. This case highlights how over-attribution bias and premature diagnostic closure can affect the clinical care of patients with obesity and emphasizes the importance of diagnostic diligence. These cognitive errors may represent an underlying anti-obesity implicit bias. While implicit biases may not be eliminated, they can be mitigated. Systematic frameworks and competencies have been proposed in recent years to help healthcare providers understand and address such biases. The efficacy of these approaches has not been proven yet, and continued research and scholarship on this topic are needed. In addition, a fundamental provider understanding of the physiology of obesity and available treatment options will increase empathy, enhance the care of patients, and increase their access to effective therapies. Finally, numerous regulatory and financial barriers to the treatment of obesity still exist and ongoing advocacy for system change will be necessary.

REFERENCES

Alberga, A. S., Edache, I. Y., Forhan, M., & Russell-Mayhew, S. (2019). Weight bias and health care utilization: A scoping review. *Primary Health Care Research and Development*, *20*, e116. doi:10.1017/S1463423619000227 PMID:32800008

Albury, C., Strain, W. D., Brocq, S. L., Logue, J., Lloyd, C., & Tahrani, A. (2020). The importance of language in engagement between health-care professionals and people living with obesity: A joint consensus statement. *The Lancet. Diabetes & Endocrinology*, *8*(5), 447–455. doi:10.1016/S2213-8587(20)30102-9 PMID:32333880

Aldrich, T., & Hackley, B. (2010). The impact of obesity on gynecologic cancer screening: An integrative literature review. *Journal of Midwifery & Women's Health*, *55*(4), 344–356. doi:10.1016/j.jmwh.2009.10.001 PMID:20630361

Alimoradi, Z., Golboni, F., Griffiths, M. D., Brostrom, A., Lin, C.-Y., & Pakpour, A. H. (2020). Weight-related stigma and psychological distress: A systematic review and meta-analysis. *Clinical Nutrition (Edinburgh, Scotland)*, *39*(7), 2001–2013. doi:10.1016/j.clnu.2019.10.016 PMID:31732288

American Medical Association. (2017). *Person-First Language for Obesity H-440.821*. AMA. https://policysearch.ama-assn.org/policyfinder/detail/obesity?uri=%2FAMADoc%2FHOD.xml-H-440.821.xml

Amy, N. K., Aalborg, A., Lyons, P., & Keranen, L. (2006). Barriers to routine gynecological cancer screening for White and African-American obese women. *International Journal of Obesity*, *30*(1), 147–155. doi:10.1038j.ijo.0803105 PMID:16231037

Andrews, M. (2015). *Many Insurers Don't Cover Drugs For Weight Loss*. NPR. https://www.npr.org/sections/health-shots/2015/01/06/375198217/many-insurers-dont-cover-drugs-for-weight-loss

Andreyeva, T., Puhl, R. M., & Brownell, K. D. (2008). Changes in perceived weight discrimination among Americans, 1995-1996 through 2004-2006. *Obesity (Silver Spring, Md.)*, *16*(5), 1129–1134. doi:10.1038/oby.2008.35 PMID:18356847

Angelidi, A. M., Belanger, M. J., Kokkinos, A., Koliaki, C. C., & Montzoros, C. S. (2022). Novel noninvasive approaches to the treatment of obesity: From pharmacotherapy to gene therapy. *Endocrine Reviews*, *43*(3), 507–557. doi:10.1210/endrev/bnab034 PMID:35552683

Association of American Medical Colleges. (2022). *New and Emerging Areas in Medicine Series. Diversity, Equity, and Inclusion Competencies Across the Learning Continuum*. AAMC. https://store.aamc.org/downloadable/download/sample/sample_id/512/

Auckburally, S., Davies, E., & Logue, J. (2021). The Use of Effective Language and Communication in the Management of Obesity: The Challenge for Healthcare Professionals. *Current Obesity Reports*, *10*(3), 274–281. doi:10.100713679-021-00441-1 PMID:34003446

Beer, Y., Gilat, R., Ner, E. B., Shohat, N., Atoun, E., Lindner, D., & Agar, G. (2021). Impact of Body Mass Index on the Accuracy of Physical Examination and MRI of the Shoulder. *Orthopaedic Journal of Sports Medicine*, *9*(2), 2325967120985643. doi:10.1177/2325967120985643 PMID:33709009

Bluher, M. (2019). Obesity: Global epidemiology and pathogenesis. *Nature Reviews. Endocrinology*, *15*(5), 288–298. doi:10.103841574-019-0176-8 PMID:30814686

Bluher, M. (2020). Metabolically Healthy Obesity. *Endocrine Reviews*, *41*(3), bnaa004. doi:10.1210/endrev/bnaa004 PMID:32128581

Bray, G. A., Heisel, W. E., Afshin, A., Jensen, M. D., Dietz, W. H., Long, M., Kushner, R. F., Daniels, S. R., Wadden, T. A., Tsai, A. G., Hu, F. B., Jakicic, J. M., Ryan, D. H., Wolfe, B. M., & Inge, T. H. (2018). The Science of Obesity Management: An Endocrine Society Scientific Statement. *Endocrine Reviews*, *39*(2), 79–132. doi:10.1210/er.2017-00253 PMID:29518206

Budd, G. M., Mariotti, M., Graff, D., & Falkenstein, K. (2011). Health care professionals' attitudes about obesity: An integrative review. *Applied Nursing Research*, *24*(3), 127–137. doi:10.1016/j.apnr.2009.05.001 PMID:20974067

Butsch, W. S., Robison, K., Sharma, R., Knecht, J., & Smolarz, B. G. (2020). Medicine Residents are Unprepared to Effectively Treat Patients with Obesity: Results from a U.S. Internal Medicine Residency Survey. *Journal of Medical Education and Curricular Development*, *7*, 2382120520973206. doi:10.1177/2382120520973206 PMID:33283047

Carels, R. A., Wott, C. B., Young, K. M., Gumble, A., Koball, A., & Oehlhof, M. W. (2010). Implicit, explicit, and internalized weight bias and psychosocial maladjustment among treatment-seeking adults. *Eating Behaviors*, *11*(3), 180–185. doi:10.1016/j.eatbeh.2010.03.002 PMID:20434066

Centers for Disease Control and Prevention. (2022). *Adult Obesity Facts*. CDC. https://www.cdc.gov/obesity/data/adult.html

Chou, W. Y., Prestin, A., & Kunath, S. (2014). Obesity in social media: A mixed methods analysis. *Translational Behavioral Medicine*, *4*(3), 314–323. doi:10.100713142-014-0256-1 PMID:25264470

Clarke, M. A., Fetterman, B., Cheung, L. C., Wentzensen, N., Gage, J. C., Katki, H. A., Befano, B., Demarco, M., Schussler, J., Kinney, W. K., Raine-Bennett, T. R., Lorey, T. S., Poitras, N. E., Castle, P. E., & Schiffman, M. (2018). Epidemiologic Evidence That Excess Body Weight Increases Risk of Cervical Cancer by Decreased Detection of Precancer. *Journal of Clinical Oncology*, *36*(12), 1184–1191. doi:10.1200/JCO.2017.75.3442 PMID:29356609

Conaty, E. A., Denham, W., Haggerty, S. P., Linn, J. G., Joehl, R. J., & Ujiki, M. B. (2020). Primary Care Physicians' Perceptions of Bariatric Surgery and Major Barriers to Referral. *Obesity Surgery*, *30*(2), 521–526. doi:10.100711695-019-04204-9 PMID:31625056

Croskerry, P. (2003). The importance of cognitive errors in diagnosis and strategies to minimize them. *Academic Medicine*, *78*(8), 775–780. doi:10.1097/00001888-200308000-00003 PMID:12915363

Dai, H., Alsalhe, T. A., Chalghaf, N., Ricco, M., Bragazzi, N. L., & Wu, J. (2020). The global burden of disease attributable to high body mass index in 195 countries and territories, 1990-2017: An analysis of the Global Burden of Disease Study. *PLoS Medicine*, *17*(7), e1003198. doi:10.1371/journal.pmed.1003198 PMID:32722671

Daly, M., Sutin, A. R., & Robinson, E. (2019). Perceived Weight Discrimination Mediates the Prospective Association Between Obesity and Physiological Dysregulation: Evidence From a Population-Based Cohort. *Psychological Science*, *30*(7), 1030–1039. doi:10.1177/0956797619849440 PMID:31158067

Darity, W. A. J. (2008). Over-Attribution Bias. In W. A. J. Darity (Ed.), *International Encyclopedia of the Social Sciences* (2nd ed., pp. 88–89). https://link-gale-com.proxy.lib.uiowa.edu/apps/pub/1PAV/GVRL?u=uiowa_main&sid=bookmark-GVRL

Dutton, G. R., Tan, F., Perri, M. G., Stine, C. C., Dancer-Brown, M., Goble, M., & Van Vessem, N. (2010). What words should we use when discussing excess weight? *Journal of the American Board of Family Medicine*, *23*(5), 606–613. doi:10.3122/jabfm.2010.05.100024 PMID:20823355

ECRI Institute. (2013). Priority Area 10: Obesity. *AHRQ Healthcare Horizon Scanning System - Potential High-Impact Interventions Report.* https://effectivehealthcare.ahrq.gov/sites/default/files/obesity-horizon-scan-high-impact-1306.pdf

Eisenberg, M. E., Carlson-McGuire, A., Gollust, S. E., & Neumark-Sztainer, D. (2015). A content analysis of weight stigmatization in popular television programming for adolescents. *International Journal of Eating Disorders*, *48*(6), 759–766. doi:10.1002/eat.22348 PMID:25139262

Elzie, C., & Cruz, B. (2020). Comprehensive analysis of policies of whole body donor programs within the United States. *The FASEB Journal*, *34*(S1), 1–1. doi:10.1096/fasebj.2020.34.s1.05176

Ferrante, J. M., Chen, P. H., Crabtree, B. F., & Wartenberg, D. (2007). Cancer screening in women: Body mass index and adherence to physician recommendations. *American Journal of Preventive Medicine*, *32*(6), 525–531. doi:10.1016/j.amepre.2007.02.004 PMID:17533069

Forhan, M., Risdon, C., & Solomon, P. (2013). Contributors to patient engagement in primary health care: Perceptions of patients with obesity. *Primary Health Care Research and Development*, *14*(4), 367–372. doi:10.1017/S1463423612000643 PMID:23237022

Foster, G. D., Wadden, T. A., Makris, A. P., Davidson, D., Sanderson, R. S., Allison, D. B., & Kessler, A. (2003). Primary care physicians' attitudes about obesity and its treatment. *Obesity Research*, *11*(10), 1168–1177. doi:10.1038/oby.2003.161 PMID:14569041

Fruh, S. M., Graves, R. J., Hauff, C., Williams, S. G., & Hall, H. R. (2021). Weight Bias and Stigma: Impact on Health. *The Nursing Clinics of North America*, *56*(4), 479–493. doi:10.1016/j.cnur.2021.07.001 PMID:34749889

Fruh, S. M., Nadglowski, J., Hall, H. R., Davis, S. L., Crook, E. D., & Zlomke, K. (2016). Obesity Stigma and Bias. *The Journal for Nurse Practitioners*, *12*(7), 425–432. doi:10.1016/j.nurpra.2016.05.013 PMID:28408862

Garvey, W. T., Mechanick, J. I., Brett, E. M., Garber, A. J., Hurley, D. L., Jastreboff, A. M., Nadolsky, K., Pessah-Pollack, R., & Plodkowski, R. (2016). American Association of Clinical Endocrinologists and American College of Endocrinology Comprehensive Clinical Practice Guidelines for Medical Care of Patients with Obesity. *Endocrine Practice*, *22*(Suppl 3), 1–203. doi:10.4158/EP161365.GL PMID:27219496

Gayer, G. G., Weiss, J., & Clearfield, M. (2017). Fundamentals for an Osteopathic Obesity Designed Study: The Effects of Education on Osteopathic Medical Students' Attitudes Regarding Obesity. *The Journal of the American Osteopathic Association*, *117*(8), 495–502. PMID:28759091

Gilat, R., Mitchnik, I. Y., Moriah, A., Levi, A., Cohen, O., Lindner, D., Beer, Y., & Agar, G. (2022). The impact of body mass index on the accuracy of the physical examination of the knee. *International Orthopaedics*, *46*(4), 831–836. doi:10.100700264-021-05277-x PMID:34993555

Ginde, A. A., Foianini, A., Renner, D. M., Valley, M., & Camargo, C. A. Jr. (2008). The challenge of CT and MRI imaging of obese individuals who present to the emergency department: A national survey. *Obesity (Silver Spring, Md.)*, *16*(11), 2549–2551. doi:10.1038/oby.2008.410 PMID:18787528

Gray, C. M., Hunt, K., Lorimer, K., Anderson, A. S., Benzeval, M., & Wyke, S. (2011). Words matter: A qualitative investigation of which weight status terms are acceptable and motivate weight loss when used by health professionals. *BMC Public Health*, *11*(1), 513. doi:10.1186/1471-2458-11-513 PMID:21714892

Greenapple, R., & Ngai, J. (2010). Obesity: Effective treatment requires change in payers' perspective. *American Health & Drug Benefits*, *3*(2), 88–94. https://www.ncbi.nlm.nih.gov/pubmed/25126310 PMID:25126310

Gudzune, K. A., Bennett, W. L., Cooper, L. A., & Bleich, S. N. (2014). Patients who feel judged about their weight have lower trust in their primary care providers. *Patient Education and Counseling*, *97*(1), 128–131. doi:10.1016/j.pec.2014.06.019 PMID:25049164

Harvey, E. L., & Hill, A. J. (2001). Health professionals' views of overweight people and smokers. *International Journal of Obesity and Related Metabolic Disorders*, *25*(8), 1253–1261. doi:10.1038j.ijo.0801647 PMID:11477512

Hatzenbuehler, M. L., Keyes, K. M., & Hasin, D. S. (2009). Associations between perceived weight discrimination and the prevalence of psychiatric disorders in the general population. *Obesity (Silver Spring, Md.)*, *17*(11), 2033–2039. doi:10.1038/oby.2009.131 PMID:19390520

Hill, B., Bergmeier, H., Incollingo Rodriguez, A. C., Barlow, F. K., Chung, A., Ramachandran, D., Savaglio, M., & Skouteris, H. (2021). Weight stigma and obesity-related policies: A systematic review of the state of the literature. *Obesity Reviews*, *22*(11), e13333. doi:10.1111/obr.13333 PMID:34505334

Hill, J. O., Galloway, J. M., Goley, A., Marrero, D. G., Minners, R., Montgomery, B., Peterson, G. E., Ratner, R. E., Sanchez, E., & Aroda, V. R. (2013). Scientific statement: Socioecological determinants of prediabetes and type 2 diabetes. *Diabetes Care*, *36*(8), 2430–2439. doi:10.2337/dc13-1161 PMID:23788649

Himmelstein, M. S., Incollingo Belsky, A. C., & Tomiyama, A. J. (2015). The weight of stigma: Cortisol reactivity to manipulated weight stigma. *Obesity (Silver Spring, Md.)*, *23*(2), 368–374. doi:10.1002/oby.20959 PMID:25522347

Huizinga, M. M., Bleich, S. N., Beach, M. C., Clark, J. M., & Cooper, L. A. (2010). Disparity in physician perception of patients' adherence to medications by obesity status. *Obesity (Silver Spring, Md.)*, *18*(10), 1932–1937. doi:10.1038/oby.2010.35 PMID:20186132

Huizinga, M. M., Cooper, L. A., Bleich, S. N., Clark, J. M., & Beach, M. C. (2009). Physician respect for patients with obesity. *Journal of General Internal Medicine*, *24*(11), 1236–1239. doi:10.100711606-009-1104-8 PMID:19763700

Humphreys, S. (2010). The unethical use of BMI in contemporary general practice. *The British Journal of General Practice*, *60*(578), 696–697. doi:10.3399/bjgp10X515548 PMID:20849708

Incollingo Rodriguez, A. C., Dunkel Schetter, C., & Tomiyama, A. J. (2020). Weight stigma among pregnant and postpartum women: A new context of stigmatization. *Stigma and Health*, *5*(2), 209–216. doi:10.1037ah0000191

Jackson, S. E., Kirschbaum, C., & Steptoe, A. (2016). Perceived weight discrimination and chronic biochemical stress: A population-based study using cortisol in scalp hair. *Obesity (Silver Spring, Md.)*, *24*(12), 2515–2521. doi:10.1002/oby.21657 PMID:27740706

Jackson, S. E., & Steptoe, A. (2017). Association between perceived weight discrimination and physical activity: A population-based study among English middle-aged and older adults. *BMJ Open*, *7*(3), e014592. doi:10.1136/bmjopen-2016-014592 PMID:28270391

Jeon, Y. A., Hale, B., Knackmuhs, E., & Mackert, M. (2018). Weight Stigma Goes Viral on the Internet: Systematic Assessment of YouTube Comments Attacking Overweight Men and Women. *Interactive Journal of Medical Research*, *7*(1), e6. doi:10.2196/ijmr.9182 PMID:29559426

Jungnickel, T., von Jan, U., Engeli, S., & Albrecht, U. V. (2022). Exploring the weight bias of professionals working in the field of obesity with a mobile IAT: A pilot study. *Therapeutic Advances in Endocrinology and Metabolism*, *13*, 20420188221098881. doi:10.1177/20420188221098881 PMID:35592657

Kaminsky, J., & Gadaleta, D. (2002). A study of discrimination within the medical community as viewed by obese patients [Article]. *Obesity Surgery*, *12*(1), 14–18. doi:10.1381/096089202321144513 PMID:11868290

Karsay, K. S., & Schmuck, D. (2019). "Weak, Sad, and Lazy Fatties": Adolescents' Explicit and Implicit Weight Bias Following Exposure to Weight Loss Reality TV Shows. *Media Psychology*, *22*(1), 60–81. doi:10.1080/15213269.2017.1396903

Katz, N. J., Lovrics, O., & Zevin, B. (2022). A Canadian survey of medical students and undergraduate deans on the management of patients living with obesity. *BMC Medical Education*, *22*(1), 562. doi:10.118612909-022-03636-9 PMID:35864483

Kelleher, D. C., Merrill, C. T., Cottrell, L. T., Nadler, E. P., & Burd, R. S. (2013). Recent national trends in the use of adolescent inpatient bariatric surgery: 2000 through 2009. *JAMA Pediatrics*, *167*(2), 126–132. doi:10.1001/2013.jamapediatrics.286 PMID:23247297

Kim, N., Wang, J., Burudpakdee, C., Song, Y., Ramasamy, A., Xie, Y., Sun, R., Kumar, N., Wu, E. Q., & Sullivan, S. D. (2022). Cost-effectiveness analysis of semaglutide 2.4 mg for the treatment of adult patients with overweight and obesity in the United States. *Journal of Managed Care & Specialty Pharmacy*, *28*(7), 740–752. PMID:35737858

Kovesdy, C. P., & Molnar, M. Z. (2014). Restricting kidney transplant wait-listing for obese patients: Let's stop defending the indefensible. *Seminars in Dialysis*, *27*(1), 1–3. doi:10.1111di.12157 PMID:24400798

Kushner, R. F., Zeiss, D. M., Feinglass, J. M., & Yelen, M. (2014). An obesity educational intervention for medical students addressing weight bias and communication skills using standardized patients. *BMC Medical Education*, *14*(1), 53. doi:10.1186/1472-6920-14-53 PMID:24636594

Lane, K. A. B., Mahzarin, R., Nosek, B. A., Greenwald, A. G. (2007). Understanding and Using the Implicit Association Test: IV. In B. S. Wittenbrink, Norbert (Ed.), Implicit Measures of Attitudes (pp. 59-102). Guilford Publications.

Lydecker, J. A., Galbraith, K., Ivezaj, V., White, M. A., Barnes, R. D., Roberto, C. A., & Grilo, C. M. (2016). Words will never hurt me? Preferred terms for describing obesity and binge eating. *International Journal of Clinical Practice*, *70*(8), 682–690. doi:10.1111/ijcp.12835 PMID:27354290

McCleary-Gaddy, A. T., Miller, C. T., Grover, K. W., Hodge, J. J., & Major, B. (2019). Weight Stigma and Hypothalamic-Pituitary-Adrenocortical Axis Reactivity in Individuals Who Are Overweight. *Annals of Behavioral Medicine: a Publication of the Society of Behavioral Medicine*, *53*(4), 392–398. doi:10.1093/abm/kay042 PMID:29917036

Mensinger, J. L., Tylka, T. L., & Calamari, M. E. (2018). Mechanisms underlying weight status and healthcare avoidance in women: A study of weight stigma, body-related shame and guilt, and healthcare stress. *Body Image*, *25*, 139–147. doi:10.1016/j.bodyim.2018.03.001 PMID:29574257

Merrill, E., & Grassley, J. (2008). Women's stories of their experiences as overweight patients. *Journal of Advanced Nursing*, *64*(2), 139–146. doi:10.1111/j.1365-2648.2008.04794.x PMID:18764854

Metcalf, M., Rossie, K., Stokes, K., & Tanner, B. (2017). The Perceptions of Medical School Students and Faculty Toward Obesity Medicine Education: Survey and Needs Analysis. *JMIR Medical Education*, *3*(2), e22. doi:10.2196/mededu.7361 PMID:29122740

Muller, M. J., Braun, W., Enderle, J., & Bosy-Westphal, A. (2016). Beyond BMI: Conceptual Issues Related to Overweight and Obese Patients. *Obesity Facts*, *9*(3), 193–205. doi:10.1159/000445380 PMID:27286962

Norman, G. R., & Eva, K. W. (2010). Diagnostic error and clinical reasoning. *Medical Education*, *44*(1), 94–100. doi:10.1111/j.1365-2923.2009.03507.x PMID:20078760

O'Brien, K. S., Latner, J. D., Puhl, R. M., Vartanian, L. R., Giles, C., Griva, K., Carter, A., & O'Brien, K. S. (2016). The relationship between weight stigma and eating behavior is explained by weight bias internalization and psychological distress. *Appetite*, *102*, 70–76. doi:10.1016/j.appet.2016.02.032 PMID:26898319

Obesity Action Coalition. (2022). *People-First Language for Obesity*. OAC. https://www.obesityaction.org/wp-content/uploads/People-First.pdf

Orjuela-Grimm, M., Butsch, W. S., Bhatt-Carreno, S., Smolarz, B. G., & Rao, G. (2021). Benchmarking of provider competencies and current training for prevention and management of obesity among family medicine residency programs: A cross-sectional survey. *BMC Family Practice*, *22*(1), 132. doi:10.118612875-021-01484-y PMID:34167487

Pearl, R. L., & Puhl, R. M. (2018). Weight bias internalization and health: A systematic review [Review]. *Obesity Reviews*, *19*(8), 1141–1163. doi:10.1111/obr.12701 PMID:29788533

Pearl, R. L., Puhl, R. M., & Brownell, K. D. (2012). Positive media portrayals of obese persons: Impact on attitudes and image preferences. *Health Psychology*, *31*(6), 821–829. doi:10.1037/a0027189 PMID:22309884

Pearl, R. L., Puhl, R. M., & Dovidio, J. F. (2015). Differential effects of weight bias experiences and internalization on exercise among women with overweight and obesity. *Journal of Health Psychology*, *20*(12), 1626–1632. doi:10.1177/1359105313520338 PMID:24505060

Pearl, R. L., Wadden, T. A., Bach, C., Gruber, K., Leonard, S., Walsh, O. A., Tronieri, J. S., & Berkowitz, R. I. (2020). Effects of a cognitive-behavioral intervention targeting weight stigma: A randomized controlled trial. *Journal of Consulting and Clinical Psychology*, *88*(5), 470–480. doi:10.1037/ccp0000480 PMID:31971410

Pearl, R. L., Wadden, T. A., Hopkins, C. M., Shaw, J. A., Hayes, M. R., Bakizada, Z. M., Alfaris, N., Chao, A. M., Pinkasavage, E., Berkowitz, R. I., & Alamuddin, N. (2017). Association between weight bias internalization and metabolic syndrome among treatment-seeking individuals with obesity. *Obesity (Silver Spring, Md.)*, *25*(2), 317–322. doi:10.1002/oby.21716 PMID:28124502

Persky, S., & Eccleston, C. P. (2011). Medical student bias and care recommendations for an obese versus non-obese virtual patient. *International Journal of Obesity*, *35*(5), 728–735. doi:10.1038/ijo.2010.173 PMID:20820169

Phelan, S. M., Burgess, D. J., Yeazel, M. W., Hellerstedt, W. L., Griffin, J. M., & van Ryn, M. (2015). Impact of weight bias and stigma on quality of care and outcomes for patients with obesity. *Obesity Reviews*, *16*(4), 319–326. doi:10.1111/obr.12266 PMID:25752756

Phelan, S. M., Dovidio, J. F., Puhl, R. M., Burgess, D. J., Nelson, D. B., Yeazel, M. W., Hardeman, R., Perry, S., & van Ryn, M. (2014). Implicit and explicit weight bias in a national sample of 4,732 medical students: the medical student CHANGES study. *Obesity (19307381)*, *22*(4), 1201-1208.

Price, J. H., Desmond, S. M., Krol, R. A., Snyder, F. F., & O'Connell, J. K. (1987). Family practice physicians' beliefs, attitudes, and practices regarding obesity. *American Journal of Preventive Medicine*, *3*(6), 339–345. doi:10.1016/S0749-3797(18)31234-0 PMID:3452374

Prunty, A., Clark, M. K., Hahn, A., Edmonds, S., & O'Shea, A. (2020). Enacted weight stigma and weight self stigma prevalence among 3821 adults. *Obesity Research & Clinical Practice*, *14*(5), 421–427. doi:10.1016/j.orcp.2020.09.003 PMID:32952068

Pryor, W. (2002). The health care disadvantages of being obese. *New South Wales Public Health Bulletin*, *13*(7), 163–165. doi:10.1071/NB02066 PMID:12451413

Puhl, R., & Brownell, K. D. (2001). Bias, discrimination, and obesity. *Obesity Research*, *9*(12), 788–805. doi:10.1038/oby.2001.108 PMID:11743063

Puhl, R., Peterson, J. L., & Luedicke, J. (2013). Motivating or stigmatizing? Public perceptions of weight-related language used by health providers. *International Journal of Obesity (2005)*, *37*(4), 612-619.

Puhl, R. M. (2020). What words should we use to talk about weight? A systematic review of quantitative and qualitative studies examining preferences for weight-related terminology. *Obesity Reviews*, *21*(6), e13008. doi:10.1111/obr.13008 PMID:32048465

Puhl, R. M., Himmelstein, M. S., & Pearl, R. L. (2020). Weight stigma as a psychosocial contributor to obesity. *The American Psychologist*, *75*(2), 274–289. doi:10.1037/amp0000538 PMID:32053000

Puhl, R. M., Himmelstein, M. S., & Quinn, D. M. (2018). Internalizing Weight Stigma: Prevalence and Sociodemographic Considerations in US Adults. *Obesity (Silver Spring, Md.)*, *26*(1), 167–175. doi:10.1002/oby.22029 PMID:29082666

Puhl, R. M., Latner, J. D., O'Brien, K. S., Luedicke, J., Danielsdottir, S., & Salas, X. R. (2015). Potential Policies and Laws to Prohibit Weight Discrimination: Public Views from 4 Countries. *The Milbank Quarterly*, *93*(4), 691–731. doi:10.1111/1468-0009.12162 PMID:26626983

Puhl, R. M., Lessard, L. M., Himmelstein, M. S., & Foster, G. D. (2021). The roles of experienced and internalized weight stigma in healthcare experiences: Perspectives of adults engaged in weight management across six countries. *PLoS One*, *16*(6), e0251566. doi:10.1371/journal.pone.0251566 PMID:34061867

Puhl, R. M., Lessard, L. M., Pearl, R. L., Grupski, A., & Foster, G. D. (2021). Policies to address weight discrimination and bullying: Perspectives of adults engaged in weight management from six nations. *Obesity (Silver Spring, Md.)*, *29*(11), 1787–1798. doi:10.1002/oby.23275 PMID:34612007

Redelmeier, D. A. (2005). Improving patient care. The cognitive psychology of missed diagnoses. *Annals of Internal Medicine*, *142*(2), 115–120. doi:10.7326/0003-4819-142-2-200501180-00010 PMID:15657159

Rhee, K. E., Kessl, S., Lindback, S., Littman, M., & El-Kareh, R. E. (2018). Provider views on childhood obesity management in primary care settings: A mixed methods analysis. *BMC Health Services Research*, *18*(1), 55. doi:10.118612913-018-2870-y PMID:29378579

Ricciardi, B. F., Giori, N. J., & Fehring, T. K. (2019). Clinical Faceoff: Should Orthopaedic Surgeons Have Strict BMI Cutoffs for Performing Primary TKA and THA? *Clinical Orthopaedics and Related Research*, *477*(12), 2629–2634. doi:10.1097/CORR.0000000000001017 PMID:31764323

Roter, D. L., Frankel, R. M., Hall, J. A., & Sluyter, D. (2006). The expression of emotion through nonverbal behavior in medical visits. Mechanisms and outcomes. *Journal of General Internal Medicine*, *21*(S1, Suppl 1), S28–S34. doi:10.1111/j.1525-1497.2006.00306.x PMID:16405706

Ruban, A., Stoenchev, K., Ashrafian, H., & Teare, J. (2019). Current treatments for obesity. *Clinical Medicine (London, England)*, *19*(3), 205–212. doi:10.7861/clinmedicine.19-3-205 PMID:31092512

Rubino, F., Puhl, R. M., Cummings, D. E., Eckel, R. H., Ryan, D. H., Mechanick, J. I., Nadglowski, J., Ramos Salas, X., Schauer, P. R., Twenefour, D., Apovian, C. M., Aronne, L. J., Batterham, R. L., Berthoud, H. R., Boza, C., Busetto, L., Dicker, D., De Groot, M., Eisenberg, D., & Dixon, J. B. (2020). Joint international consensus statement for ending stigma of obesity. *Nature Medicine*, *26*(4), 485–497. doi:10.103841591-020-0803-x PMID:32127716

Russell, N., & Carryer, J. (2013). Living large: The experiences of large-bodied women when accessing general practice services. *Journal of Primary Health Care*, *5*(3), 199–205. doi:10.1071/HC13199 PMID:23998170

Silk, A. W., & McTigue, K. M. (2011). Reexamining the physical examination for obese patients. *Journal of the American Medical Association*, *305*(2), 193–194. doi:10.1001/jama.2010.1950 PMID:21191004

Springer, B. D. (2019). Management of the Bariatric Patient. What Are the Implications of Obesity and Total Joint Arthroplasty: The Orthopedic Surgeon's Perspective? *The Journal of Arthroplasty*, *34*(7, 7S), S30–S32. doi:10.1016/j.arth.2018.12.021 PMID:30638728

Story, M. T., Neumark-Stzainer, D. R., Sherwood, N. E., Holt, K., Sofka, D., Trowbridge, F. L., & Barlow, S. E. (2002). Management of child and adolescent obesity: Attitudes, barriers, skills, and training needs among health care professionals. *Pediatrics*, *110*(1 Pt 2, Supplement_1), 210–214. doi:10.1542/peds.110.S1.210 PMID:12093997

Sukhera, J., & Watling, C. (2018). A Framework for Integrating Implicit Bias Recognition Into Health Professions Education. *Academic Medicine*, *93*(1), 35–40. doi:10.1097/ACM.0000000000001819 PMID:28658015

Sutin, A. R., Stephan, Y., Luchetti, M., & Terracciano, A. (2014). Perceived weight discrimination and C-reactive protein. *Obesity (Silver Spring, Md.)*, *22*(9), 1959–1961. doi:10.1002/oby.20789 PMID:24828961

Sutin, A. R., Stephan, Y., & Terracciano, A. (2015). Weight Discrimination and Risk of Mortality. *Psychological Science*, *26*(11), 1803–1811. doi:10.1177/0956797615601103 PMID:26420442

Sutin, A. R., & Terracciano, A. (2017). Perceived weight discrimination and high-risk health-related behaviors. *Obesity (19307381)*, *25*(7), 1183-1186.

Tilburt, J. C., O Byrne, T., Branda, M. E., & Phelan, S. (2019). Higher BMI associated with shorter visits in male oncology patients: An exploratory analysis. *Patient Education and Counseling*, *102*(12), 2353–2357. doi:10.1016/j.pec.2019.07.009 PMID:31331706

Tomiyama, A. J. (2014). Weight stigma is stressful. A review of evidence for the Cyclic Obesity/Weight-Based Stigma model. *Appetite*, *82*, 8–15. doi:10.1016/j.appet.2014.06.108 PMID:24997407

Tomiyama, A. J., Epel, E. S., McClatchey, T. M., Poelke, G., Kemeny, M. E., McCoy, S. K., & Daubenmier, J. (2014). Associations of weight stigma with cortisol and oxidative stress independent of adiposity. *Health Psychology: Official Journal of the Division of Health Psychology, American Psychological Association*, *33*(8), 862–867. doi:10.1037/hea0000107 PMID:25068456

Udo, T., Purcell, K., & Grilo, C. M. (2016). Perceived weight discrimination and chronic medical conditions in adults with overweight and obesity. *International Journal of Clinical Practice*, *70*(12), 1003–1011. doi:10.1111/ijcp.12902 PMID:28032427

Vadiveloo, M., & Mattei, J. (2017). Perceived Weight Discrimination and 10-Year Risk of Allostatic Load Among US Adults. *Annals of Behavioral Medicine: a Publication of the Society of Behavioral Medicine*, *51*(1), 94–104. doi:10.100712160-016-9831-7 PMID:27553775

van der Valk, E. S., van den Akker, E. L. T., Savas, M., Kleinendorst, L., Visser, J. A., Van Haelst, M. M., Sharma, A. M., & van Rossum, E. F. C. (2019). A comprehensive diagnostic approach to detect underlying causes of obesity in adults. *Obesity Reviews*, *20*(6), 795–804. doi:10.1111/obr.12836 PMID:30821060

Verger, P., Rolland, S., Paraponaris, A., Bouvenot, J., & Ventelou, B. (2010). Drug reimbursement and GPs' prescribing decisions: a randomized case-vignette study about the pharmacotherapy of obesity associated with type 2 diabetes: how GPs react to drug reimbursement. *Fundamental & Clinical Pharmacology*, *24*(4), 509–516. doi:10.1111/j.1472-8206.2009.00779.x PMID:19840120

Vitolins, M. Z., Crandall, S., Miller, D., Ip, E., Marion, G., & Spangler, J. G. (2012). Obesity educational interventions in U.S. medical schools: A systematic review and identified gaps. *Teaching and Learning in Medicine*, *24*(3), 267–272. doi:10.1080/10401334.2012.692286 PMID:22775792

Volger, S., Vetter, M. L., Dougherty, M., Panigrahi, E., Egner, R., Webb, V., Thomas, J. G., Sarwer, D. B., & Wadden, T. A. (2012). Patients' preferred terms for describing their excess weight: Discussing obesity in clinical practice. *Obesity (Silver Spring, Md.)*, *20*(1), 147–150. doi:10.1038/oby.2011.217 PMID:21760637

Wall, A., Lee, G. H., Maldonado, J., & Magnus, D. (2019). Medical Contraindications to Transplant Listing in the USA: A Survey of Adult and Pediatric Heart, Kidney, Liver, and Lung Programs. *World Journal of Surgery*, *43*(9), 2300–2308. doi:10.100700268-019-05030-x PMID:31111229

Wanniarachchi, V. U., Scogings, C., Susnjak, T., & Mathrani, A. (2022). Fat stigma and body objectification: A text analysis approach using social media content. *Digital Health*, *8*, 20552076221117404. doi:10.1177/20552076221117404 PMID:35990109

Ward, S. H., Gray, A. M., & Paranjape, A. (2009). African Americans' perceptions of physician attempts to address obesity in the primary care setting. *Journal of General Internal Medicine*, *24*(5), 579–584. doi:10.100711606-009-0922-z PMID:19277791

Wee, C. C., McCarthy, E. P., Davis, R. B., & Phillips, R. S. (2000). Screening for cervical and breast cancer: Is obesity an unrecognized barrier to preventive care? *Annals of Internal Medicine*, *132*(9), 697–704. doi:10.7326/0003-4819-132-9-200005020-00003 PMID:10787362

Wigton, R. S., & McGaghie, W. C. (2001). The effect of obesity on medical students' approach to patients with abdominal pain. *Journal of General Internal Medicine*, *16*(4), 262–265. doi:10.1046/j.1525-1497.2001.016004262.x PMID:11318928

Woolford, S. J., Clark, S. J., Gebremariam, A., Davis, M. M., & Freed, G. L. (2010). To cut or not to cut: Physicians' perspectives on referring adolescents for bariatric surgery. *Obesity Surgery*, *20*(7), 937–942. doi:10.100711695-010-0152-9 PMID:20401742

World Health Organization. (2022). *Obesity and Overweight.* https://www.who.int/news-room/fact-sheets/detail/obesity-and-overweight

Zevin, B., Sivapalan, N., Chan, L., Cofie, N., Dalgarno, N., & Barber, D. (2022). Factors influencing primary care provider referral for bariatric surgery: Systematic review. *Canadian Family Physician Medecin de Famille Canadien*, *68*(3), e107–e117. doi:10.46747/cfp.6803e107 PMID:35292475

Chapter 4
Ageism:
Care at the Extremes of Life

Samiksha Prasad
Nova Southeastern University Dr. Kiran C. Patel College of Allopathic Medicine, USA

Chasity O'Malley
Wright State University Boonshoft School of Medicine, USA

Arkene Levy
Nova Southeastern University Dr. Kiran C. Patel College of Allopathic Medicine, USA

EXECUTIVE SUMMARY

Individuals may experience ageism and age discrimination in numerous aspects of their lives. This typically refers to negative or indifferent attitudes towards people because of their age (old or young). The cases exemplified in this chapter portray both sides of the spectrum where age discrimination can occur. Case one discusses the challenges faced by an elderly patient in a healthcare setting due to their age. This form of age discrimination has been documented more commonly in the literature. These cases explore how the elderly population can experience dismissive attitudes and differential treatment. Another case involves a health professional student who is significantly younger than her peers and how this age gap impact her learning environment and the opportunities that she has missed due to it. While the scenarios of the cases demonstrate overt displays of age discrimination, it is also common for ageism to occur in more subtle instances.

INTRODUCTION

"Ageism," coined by R. Butler in the 1960s (Butler, 1969), refers to discrimination exhibited towards individuals based on being considered "of an advanced in age" or "old". However, more recently, the term "age discrimination" has a different focus, representing the arbitrary decisions made about an individual because of their age, (whether "young" or "advanced in age") (Davies, 2011; Marco *et. al.*, 2001). Ageism and age discrimination are terms used in best practice statements and in literature to

DOI: 10.4018/978-1-6684-5493-0.ch004

define negative or indifferent attitudes towards people because of their age - whether advanced in age or young. (Kydd and Fleming, 2015). Results from the national survey of US adults over age 45 by the American Association of Retired Persons (AARP), in 2017, reported that about 2 out of every 3 workers have experienced or witnessed age discrimination. About 55% of the participants reported that typically, the discrimination started at approximately 50 years of age (Perron, 2018). Despite the ubiquitous nature of age discrimination and strong evidence for its adverse social consequences, many institutions confine responses for tackling ageism typically to discrimination in the workplace (Stypinska and Turek, 2017). Ageism may present in different variations: (i) positive and negative ageism (Iversen *et. al.,* 2009, Palmore 1999), refers to the homogenization of populations based on favorable or unfavorable age-related stereotypes and connotations. (ii) implicit and explicit ageism (Blackburn 2006; Couto and Wentura, 2017; Malinen and Johnston, 2013), where implicit ageism refers to thoughts, feelings, and behaviors toward individuals of a particular age group that exist and operate without conscious awareness or control, implicit ageism also tends to be mostly negative (Levy, 2001; Perdue and Gurtman 1990). On the other hand, explicit ageism relates to conscious actions or thoughts towards a particular age group. (iii) personal and institutional ageism (Bytheway 1995; Palmore 1999; Palmore *et. al.*, 2005). Apart from an individual's viewpoint and actions related to ageism (personal ageism), institutional ageism may be defined as the laws, rules, social norms, policies, and practices of institutions that unfairly restrict opportunities and systematically disadvantage individuals because of their age. These different variations of ageism may have further subtypes, that can be are distinguished into: (a) interactive ageism (Minichiello et. al., 2000) which involves experiences at the interpersonal level, self-perceptions through interactions with others involves being seen and treated as "old" or "young" in ways which are more obviously defined as age-related; (b) compassionate ageism (Furunes and Mykletun 2010) a subtype of positive ageism, for example being overly compassionate for a particular age group that may can result in perpetuating a stigma/stereotype associated with that age group; (c) gendered ageism (Handy and Davy 2007) associated with ageism related to individuals of a particular gender. It is more prevalent in women and may display intersectionality between ageism and sexism.

It is important for health care clinician trainees to note that with older adults, universal healthcare insurance, such as Medicare (Medicare report, 2016), can be seen as a benefit, but these individuals often experience ageism when they attempt to use the insurance for specific services. Services can be limited or not covered as a systemic effort to reduce costs (Kane and Kane, 2005).

There have been limited studies conducted in the nursing and medical professions that focus attention on ageism and age discrimination. However, there is a paucity of literature concerning ageism among direct care workers (Eymard, and Douglas, 2012). This often neglected, yet critical population of health care providers is essential to the care of adults of advanced age. Recommendations regarding their training and mentoring need to be emphasized and incorporated into professional program curricula (Eymard, and Douglas, 2012). The Age Discrimination in Employment Act (ADEA) prohibits ageism towards people who are 40 years of age or older (US Equal Employment Opportunity Commission, 2022). However, there is no national law protecting individuals under 40 years of age, though some states do provide protection under state laws for younger workers (US Equal Employment Opportunity Commission, 2022).

Two notable theories have been put forth to explain the existence of ageism in healthcare: the social identity theory and terror management theory. Social identity theory suggests that to uphold one's own self-esteem, younger individuals identify more strongly with other younger individuals and push away those who are different (i.e., adults of advanced age) (North and Fiske, 2012). This phenomenon may be perpetuated by the value placed on belonging to the preferred social group in society and social settings (Chonody and Teater, 2016). According to social identity theory, those who belong to the younger group will promote negative attitudes and stereotypes about the advanced age groups, which promotes a more favorable perception of the younger group (Van Wicklin, 2020; Chonody and Teater, 2016). It is important to note that the negative viewpoint is primarily focused on the physical process of aging, and not the advanced-age itself (Van Wicklin, 2020; Bodner, 2009). On the other hand, the terror management theory states that when confronted with the realization of one's own mortality, it is easier to push away from reminders of their own death (i.e., adults of advanced age) (North and Fiske, 2012). Avoidance reduces the terror by allowing the individual to believe that "death is far into the future, distracting oneself from the threat, denying ones' vulnerability to death, or physically removing oneself from salient reminders of death" (Van Wicklin, 2020; Chonody and Teater, 2016).

It is important to note that ageism and age discrimination are intersectional in nature. Intersectional discrimination takes place when two or multiple grounds operate simultaneously and interact in an inseparable manner, producing distinct and specific forms of discrimination (Fredman, 2016; Cho *et. al.*, 2013; Beijing Declaration, United Nations, 1995). This means that individuals experiencing ageism or age discrimination may also experience discrimination in other areas of their lives. For instance, a young Hispanic female healthcare professional may experience marginalization based on age as well as race, ethnicity and gender. Another aspect to take note of is the population of marginalized young individuals who experience additional barriers when compared to same-aged peers. Future research is necessary to better understand the impact of intersecting multiple marginalized identities. Studies should also focus on potential solutions to better support marginalized young people's access to and engagement with healthcare (Robards, *et. al.*, 2018). A key policy priority should, therefore, should be to plan for age diversity teams where health-related professionals of various age groups may work together (Fairygodboss, 2019). Additionally, institutions and individuals need to prioritize the implementation of adequate training and access to resources to mitigate age discrimination. (Stypinska and Turek, 2017)

The cases included in this chapter aim to catalyze discussion of the issues surrounding ageism and age discrimination by providing healthcare professional learners and practitioners with the tools to identify ageism and age discrimination and its implications in the healthcare setting. The cases discuss ageism that may occur on both sides of the spectrum, i.e., age discrimination towards adults of advanced age as well as younger individuals. Furthermore, the chapter discusses actions that may be taken to spread awareness and strategies to mitigate ageism and age discrimination in the healthcare setting. It is important to note that workplace-associated age discrimination has received much less research attention than other forms of discrimination (Prazeres and Passos, 2021). Thus, there is a particular need for discussions pertaining to the significant implications of age discrimination.

CASE 1: DISORIENTED BEHAVIOR

Goal

This case exemplifies ageism related to a health care teams' communication with and treatment of an elderly person receiving patient care.

Learning Outcomes

1. Define ageism and recognize instances of it and discrimination in the clinical setting.
2. Discuss the nature of ageism and its impact on recipients and bystanders.
3. Explore how the recipient and the source may be viewing the situation differently.
4. Discuss responses to ageism that can build a climate of inclusivity, repair and re-establish relationships, and restore or protect reputations.

Case

Howard Fleur, a 70-year-old male, is brought into the emergency department by his 29-year-old granddaughter, Bethany. Howard recently started displaying some disoriented behavior, including forgetfulness, and "zoning-out" during conversations. Howard had spent the day at the amusement park with his family, when he started feeling unwell and having incoherent speech about an hour ago, which concerned Bethany, who is a nursing student.

Nurse Stout enters the room and introduces herself to Bethany, and asks why they are visiting the emergency department. Bethany explains that her grandfather was not feeling well, so she brought him in to be checked out. Nurse Stout then begins to fill out the intake forms and to examine Howard. During the initial patient intake and examination, Nurse Stout directs all of the questions to Bethany, asking her how long he has felt this way, what he has consumed recently, and if he is on any medications. Bethany answers the questions to the best of her ability, but consistently refers to her grandfather for confirmation of her answers.

When Nurse Stout begins to ask questions about Howard's medical history, Bethany is visibly uncomfortable and suggests that the questions be directed to her grandfather, stating "Grandpa is very private about his health matters, and this isn't something we talk about when I visit outside of me asking how he's doing. He hasn't had any major health issues that I know of, but you should definitely ask him rather than me to get accurate answers."

Nurse Stout rolls her eyes and turns to Howard to begin the questions again. In a very loud voice, she yells to him "DO YOU HAVE A HISTORY OF HEART DISEASE?". Howard flinches and grimaces, responding with "no". She continues "HAVE YOU EVER HAD A STROKE?"

This time, Howard politely asks "Would you please lower your voice a little? I have not had a stroke, but the whole floor doesn't need to hear this personal information."

Nurse Stout continues "I HAVE TO SPEAK LOUDLY SO THAT YOU CAN HEAR ME CORRECTLY."

Howard replies "I am not hearing impaired, so the speaking voice you used earlier with my granddaughter will be loud enough. I could understand you during that conversation. Please, stop yelling. You are hurting my ears and unnecessarily shouting information about my health where others can hear."

Nurse Stout is agitated, rolls her eyes, and leaves the room saying "I'll be right back."

Outside, Bethany overhears Nurse Stout saying "There's a grumpy old man in that room and I can't deal with him. You need to take over. I just can't deal with him anymore; he insists on answering the questions and I can't be too loud or too low. It's a mess, maybe better to talk to the granddaughter."

Unfortunately, the other nurses are unavailable to assist Nurse Stout so she goes back in the room. Bethany pretends not to have heard Nurse Stout's comments and is focused on making her grandfather feel better. Nurse Stout proceeds with the questioning of Howard.

Nurse Stout asks how long Howard has experienced dementia.

He replies "I have not been diagnosed with dementia, I'm just been a little disoriented this afternoon and Bethany insisted that we come here."

Nurse Stout continues to insist that this is an episode of dementia and documents it in his intake forms. She faces the granddaughter and says, "these are tell-tale signs and his age...., anyways he needs testing for confirmation".

Bethany feels extremely offended for herself and her grandfather. She states sternly "Thank you for your concern, we can follow-up on that later, but right now he needs assistance for the symptoms he is currently experiencing".

Nurse Stout replies, "Well time is ticking so don't wait too long," as she walks out of the room.

Bethany steps out into the hallway to find the Charge Nurse. Bethany explains how her grandfather has been treated and that she is concerned he isn't being taken seriously and is being mistreated by Nurse Stout. The Charge Nurse apologizes for the situation, explaining that "Nurse Stout sometimes has issues when interacting with elderly patients, and this is not the first time this concern has been brought up to her".

She continues "Nurse Stout clearly needs to get some further training."

Nurse Stout is then replaced by Nurse York. Nurse York introduces herself, reviews the intake form and proceeds to verify and fill in the information from Howard. The remainder of the visit goes smoothly, and Howard is examined by Doctor Oli.

Dr. Oli determines that Howard is dehydrated, likely from the time in the heat without enough fluids at the amusement park, and he is given intravenous fluids to help with dehydration. Dr. Oli also states that he does not need to follow-up for dementia testing, as his symptoms are likely caused by dehydration. However, if he experiences increased and more severe disorienting behavior, he should make an appointment for testing.

After Dr. Oli's is finished, he asks to talk to Nurse Stout when he sees her in the hallway. He asks her why was dementia mentioned on Mr. Fleur's notes. When Nurse Stout does not have a concrete response, Dr. Oli firmly reminds her that it is important to maintain accurate notes for each patient and refrain from doing a diagnosis without confirmation.

A couple hours later, Howard is feeling much better and is released from the emergency department with directions to rest and continue to rehydrate at home with electrolyte containing fluids and food as tolerated.

QUESTIONS AND ANSWERS

1. Discuss the assumptions made by Nurse Stout and how they affected Howard's care.

Nurse Stout assumed that Howard would have age related health conditions. She assumed he would be hard of hearing due to his age. Additionally, she assumed he had dementia due to his disorientation. With Nurse Stout preferring to speak to Howard's granddaughter Bethany, she made the assumption that Howard was unable to reply for himself. By assuming he was hard of hearing, she may have tended not to ask Howard questions which she thought Bethany could answer. By asking Bethany for information rather than Howard, there could be errors made to his medical history or to the status of how he is feeling with his current presentation. With the biases that Nurse Stout displayed towards Howard, his care could be affected by neglecting to attend to his symptoms and there could be potential delays in his care. These interactions also caused unnecessary distress to both Howard and Bethany.

2. Discuss if these assumptions could occur innocently or subconsciously and explain why they have negative connotations.

Ageism is a form of bias that is pervasive in society and is learned at an early age, often as early as childhood in many cases (Nuances of Ageism, 2022). Although ageism can occur across the lifespan of a person, this bias more often occurs in regards to advanced age. The biases of Nurse Stout could have occurred innocently through childhood ideologies that she learned at an early age. However, with the mannerisms displayed in the case, it is more likely that they are either from implicit bias towards patients of advanced age or from her past experiences with patients who were of similar age to Howard. This can perpetuate stereotypes and biases unknowingly if left unchecked. The negative connotations associated with these kinds of assumptions lie in the belief that elderly patients are not coherent or have conditions such as hearing loss irrespective of the true condition of the individual. This also diminishes the value and autonomy of the individual seeking care.

3. Discuss a potential appropriate immediate response from the Charge Nurse for the mishap.

The Charge Nurse acted appropriately by listening to the concerns of the patient's family and then finding an alternative person to assume the care of the patient. Additionally, the Charge Nurse stated that she would talk to Nurse Stout about her behavior and take appropriate steps to ensure it does not continue. However, from the discussion, it is implied that this is not the first incident where Nurse Stout has mistreated a patient due to their age. That information should not have been shared with the patient. Moreover, there should be standardized protocols put in place to address and avoid such issues in the future.

4. Discuss a potential appropriate immediate response from Bethany to the overheard hallway conversation.

Initially, Bethany reacted by ignoring a comment as her priority was to obtain a quick response and care for her grandfather. However, due to escalation in the behavior, she later reported and sought assistance from the Charge Nurse to ensure her grandfather received appropriate care and Nurse Stout's concerning behavior was mentioned. This method ensured minimal conflict and proper reporting of the issue. Another approach could have been to have a non-confrontational conversation with Nurse Stout to let her know that her comments were heard and how her behavior was disrespectful, emphasizing that her grandfather needs unbiased care.

5. How can Nurse Stout's actions towards Mr. Fleur have the potential to lead to medical errors?

Any instances in which misinformation or incorrect information is added to a patient's file, it has the potential to lead to medical errors if appropriate checks are not in place. These instances can occur by human error as well as implicit biases or microaggressions. Such medical errors have been reported to lead to unnecessary tests, misdirection of treatment, accidental dissipation of resources, time and money. Taken to the extreme, these situations may lead to serious and sometimes life-threatening consequences to the patient and legal repercussions for the healthcare institutions. In this scenario, Nurse Stout's biases may have led to Mr. Fleur being subjected to unnecessary testing for a condition (Dementia) he does not have, and attention being focused away from the condition he presented with (dehydration) for treatment to the Emergency Department.

6. What actions can be taken to prevent this type of scenario from occurring in the future?

One of the best ways to prevent this from occurring in the future is to provide the healthcare professionals with appropriate unconscious bias training. In this particular situation, it seems that Nurse Stout has a history of inappropriate behavior with elderly patients. Thus, she would likely benefit from empathy and bias training, as well as a plan for remediating her behavior to stop it from occurring in the future. Annual and refresher trainings are important to maintain an inclusive work environment.

Epilogue

This case presents an extreme case of age discrimination which unfortunately can occur in healthcare settings for elderly patients. Bethany's choice to be an advocate for better healthcare treatment for her grandfather ensured this issue was addressed and mitigated.

At the end of Nurse Stout's shift, the Charge Nurse calls for a meeting with her. She discusses how her behavior with Mr. Fleur was inappropriate and offensive to him and his granddaughter. She explains how, as a nurse at the emergency department, Nurse Stout should display compassion and patience, and treat all of her patients equally. While she does acknowledge that the emergency department is a fast-paced work environment which treats a wide variety of patients, spanning all ages, genders, nationalities, religions, and political beliefs, she reminds Nurse Stout that everyone should receive the same level of patience and compassionate care. Furthermore, the Charge Nurse emphasizes on how such attitudes may lead to medical errors due to the inability to communicate with patients effectively as well as biased assumptions. She also adds how this behavior may lead to limiting or diminish the patient autonomy. By providing examples the Charge Nurse explains how some healthcare professionals have lost licenses due to such medical errors.

She directs Nurse Stout to some professional development trainings and books on this subject. She mentions that Nurse Stout has 30 days to finish these trainings and schedules another meeting with her to follow up and allow her to provide her thoughts and reflections.

CASE 2: PLEASE MIND THE GAP

Goal

This case provides an example of ageism related to a student who is younger than her peers.

Learning Outcomes

1. Define ageism and age discrimination and recognize instances of them in the academic setting.
2. Assess methods that may be used to identify unintentional ageism.

3. Explore how the recipient and the source may be viewing the situation differently.
4. Formulate the components of an inclusive learning environment that prevents instances of age discrimination.

Case

Emma is a 20-year-old Physician's Assistant (PA) student. She finished high school at the age of 15 due to enrollment in advanced classes and is the youngest enrolled PA student at the university. During a Team-Based Learning (TBL) session, Emma is in a team with 4 other students (Melissa- age 26; Varun- age 25; Jackson- age 28; and Maria- age 26).

During the TBL session, there is a question related to diabetes and the team is debating between answers.

Emma remarks to the group "I think the answer is Type I diabetes mellitus."

However, the other students think it is Type II diabetes mellitus and don't give Emma an opportunity to explain how she came to that conclusion. When Emma tries to interject and explain her reasoning, Varun says "Of course you would say Type I, that's the juvenile form, which is all you'd be familiar with."

The rest of the group laughed and ignored Emma, talking over her as she continued to try to explain her thoughts.

When the time came for group reporting of the answer, the team went with the majority answer of Type II diabetes mellitus, which was incorrect. As the other teams' answer came in, it was clear that Emma had correctly identified the answer, but the team did not give her the courtesy of listening to her explanation.

As the faculty facilitator continues to discuss the question and ask for the reasoning, Emma is called on to walk the class through the answer choices. She eloquently explains the reasons why the other choices are incorrect and why Type I diabetes is correct answer. The facilitator then questions why their group didn't get the question correct, especially with that well thought out answer. Emma replies, "I don't know" and sinks into her seat.

Later that day, the students receive their anonymous peer feedback reviews. Emma is upset as she sees statements related to her young age and her peers citing her as immature. From her perspective, she behaves in a more mature manner than her peers and she is hurt by their statements.

In the reviews written by Emma for her peers, she tactfully brought up the way that the group doesn't provide her with opportunities to share her thoughts and knowledge. She also explained how active listening is a skill that her peers could work toward improving, especially when listening to each other in group discussions during small group sessions.

Two days later, in the next TBL session on the topic of birth control, there is another question where the other students in the group choose one answer while Emma defends a different answer.

Maria says "We should let Emma speak. We all know she was the one who said that their contributions aren't valued in our reviews."

Emma begins to explain the answer choice, sharing specific facts and data she remembered from the reading. Melissa interrupts Emma, asking her "How would you know about this topic at all? You're young and clearly don't have the life experience for this conversation."

Maria responds with "I think she may be right about the side effects of estrogen in the birth control pills. There was a whole page on the side effects and potential consequences of taking them while nursing.

I can't remember the specific details, but Emma is right about it being really detailed in the book. Does anyone remember why nursing moms shouldn't take estrogen containing birth control if they can help it?"

Emma hesitates, but then replies "The estrogen reduces milk supply by inhibiting milk production. It blocks the release of prolactin which is what leads to milk production."

Maria says, "That sounds right."

The group submits the answer choice chosen by Emma, then thanks Maria for coming through and helping them arrive at the correct answer, not acknowledging Emma's contribution to the discussion.

QUESTIONS AND ANSWERS

1. Discuss the assumptions made by the members of the TBL group. Do these assumptions occur innocently or are they associated or directed with a purposeful negative connotation?

The members of the TBL group assumed that Emma was immature and would not understand adult themed topics due to her young age. These assumptions may have been innocent, though they are often due to microaggressions (a verbal or nonverbal contumelious behavior towards individuals who might identify as being from a marginalized or nonmainstream community). Emma assumed that she would be treated as an equal by the members of her group. It is not unreasonable to expect to be treated in a fair and equitable manner by peers.

2. Discuss an appropriate and immediate response from Emma to the TBL group members in the first session (on diabetes).

In the case, Emma chose to remain quiet when the group would not listen to her. She could have chosen to discuss the situation with the group or to make a point of calling out. However, with the behavior of the group being to talk over her and ignore her, her choice to stay quiet can also be supported. She chose not to make an issue into a larger situation during class time. Although she did write the peers feedback stating that they talk over her, she could have chosen to ask for a discussion with the group after the session.

3. Discuss an appropriate and immediate response from Emma to the facilitator in the first session (on diabetes). How could the faculty facilitator mediate the situation occurring for Emma?

During the session, Emma again chose to remain quiet when the facilitator questioned the group's choice. She could have used this moment to state that there was some debate between the answers. After the session, Emma could have chosen to discuss her learning environment with her facilitator. She could have reached out to ask for intervention or for advice on how to handle the situation. The faculty facilitator could then make an effort to facilitate that group's interactions during the next session, ensuring that each member is able to speak.

4. What actions can be taken to prevent this type of scenario from taking place in the future?

One important step would be to ensure that bias training occurs at the onset of the school year for every student entering the program. By recognizing biases that exist, the students would then be able to recognize when their behaviors are influenced by bias and make corrective actions. Another aspect that could be helpful is using anonymous reporting systems through which students can submit encounters of biases they witnessed or experienced themselves. Another important strategy to mitigate such instances of biased behavior would be to encourage facilitated discussions with the student body, faculty, staff, and administration. Training on mediation and bias mitigation would also be very helpful to faculty and staff to help students navigate through the tough situations and conversations that may arise along the way.

5. How do the interactions of classmates affect the overall learning environment? Discuss an action plan for use during situations similar to those depicted in the case.

The interactions of classmates play a huge role in the overall learning environment, especially in an active learning style classroom. When biases affect the way that individuals are treated, individuals can feel excluded and not get the full benefit from participating in discussions. As was demonstrated in this case, Emma was ignored during the group discussions and as a result, she shut down. Everyone could have benefited from her speaking up and participating in discussions. In the second TBL, she did speak up, but some members of the group didn't trust her information because of her age and lack of life experience. However, her rationale for answering the TBL question was correct, her participation could have contributed to a deeper enriched discussion if the group had allowed it. The group did go with her answer, but gave the credit for that answer to Maria who supported Emma's rationale, once again confirming Emma's feelings of isolation.

6. How can the university play a role in reducing bias among students?

To reduce bias, the University can cultivate an awareness of bias by providing training to help identify biases, and by fostering an inclusive environment which allows for supportive discussions as individuals try to mitigate their biases. The institution should prioritize fostering an environment where empathy is encouraged and displayed by leadership. They may also consider providing mindfulness training to help promote mindfulness among students and faculty. In addition, it is critical that the institution maintains professionalism competencies for all health professions programs to ensure that a professional environment is maintained consistently within the administration, faculty, staff, and students.

Epilogue

This case presents a scenario of ageism in a younger person, which is not highlighted as often when discussing ageism. Emma's choice to use a peer feedback form as a means to call attention to it is one useful approach to help call attention to her concerns regarding ageism.

After the first year, during her summer break, Emma is visiting her hometown and catching up with her high school friends. She mentions to them the challenges she has faced during her first year due to being the youngest in her class. She explains how she was talked over and dismissed, mainly because she was the youngest in the group. She definitely feels she missed out on some leadership opportunities such as chairing the dermatology interest group, due to how marginalized she felt for a big portion of the year. However, she mentions that she spoke up to the group and that she did feel that there had been a shift in attitudes towards her since she voiced her opinions. She plans to start the second year fresh and hopes her peers will do the same.

CASE 3: THE ADMISSIONS COMMITTEE

Goal

This case provides an example of ageism related to the admissions process for a medical school.

Learning Outcomes

1. Recognize how ageism can manifest in selection processes for academic programs.
2. Assess the impact of ageism on the careers of individuals.
3. Explore how individuals may be viewing the situation differently.
4. Characterize the importance of being an advocate to mitigate ageism.

Case

The medical school admissions committee is meeting for their bimonthly candidate review session. On the agenda are 4 candidates, including Andrew Paige who is a 52-year-old, former paramedic, applying to the doctor of medicine program. The committee has reviewed all four candidates' application packets individually and they are meeting to discuss them as a group. Andrew's application packet was received well and the letters of recommendation from practicing physicians were quite impressive.

Dr. Gupta, the faculty member assigned to lead the discussion for Andrew's packet begins by summarizing his file:

"Mr. Andrew Paige had a 3.9 GPA from his undergraduate institution and a 4.0 from the thesis-track Masters in Biological Sciences program. His MCAT is a 515 and he has a lot of experience working with underserved populations through his years of service with the Peace Corps after college. He is currently working as a paramedic and desires to attend medical school."

The committee spends a couple of minutes looking over his file and reviewing the feedback notes from the in-person interview that took place 2 weeks ago.

Dr. Walters, the Professor and Chair of Pre-clerkship Curriculum, asks "In reviewing his file, there were some concerning reviewer feedback statements received from the in-person interview that we should discuss. Point one is the comment that states "His life experience will help him in Geriatrics". From the file, I do not see this experience reflected in the application materials. Can anyone elaborate on this comment?"

Dr. Sloan, a Professor in Pharmacology and member of the admissions committee responds "Actually, it was me who interviewed the candidate." Dr. Sloan proceeds to say "If I remember correctly, I think I made the comment after a discussion with respect to his age."

Dr. Walters replies "Thank you for clarifying that there wasn't an omission in the applicant's packet. I'd like to remind everyone on the committee to refrain from making vague statements based on external factors that are not interview prompts on the feedback forms."

To this, Dr. Sloan replies "Honestly, it was my impression that this candidate would only be appropriate for a career in Geriatrics, that is if we are even considering admitting a student of his age. There's so little time left for him to practice if he makes it through medical school. I doubt he'd even match for a residency program."

Dr. Stafford, a committee member who is the chair of Internal Medicine, asks "Well that seems a bit harsh. I'm sure the situation isn't that dire. How old do you think he was?"

Dr. Sloan replies "He looked at least mid-sixties. With school and residency, he'll be 70 by the time he makes it to practice."

Dr. Stafford replies "Wow, that does seem like quite an age difference from our standard applicants. I wonder what his end goal is?"

During this conversation, the demeanor of several committee members changes. These members are of a more advanced age and are visibly uncomfortable with the conversation.

Dr. Gupta notices this and attempts to refocus the group. "As a reminder to everyone, a person's age is not a factor we consider when reviewing applicants. We specifically remove that piece of information from their files before the applicant packets are distributed to the committee members to maintain a level playing field for those types of factors that may be used to discriminate. How about we continue to review the candidate, striking the age-related comments from the record. He deserves a fair evaluation, regardless of age. From my understanding, this particular candidate received excellent initial scores for their application packet and was being considered as one of the top choices for the program."

Dr. Gupta continues "I do however see the single low score for the in-person interview portion of the process. Dr. Sloan, were there any particular responses to the interview prompts provided that resulted in a low score during the in-person interview?"

Dr. Sloan simply replies "It was based on my overall impression of the candidate and his ability to become a physician as his new career path. Our program has limited seats which I think would be more useful to candidates with more longevity in their careers."

Dr. Gupta lets out a long sigh and addresses the entire committee. "It appears that our committee members need to have a refresher on the do's and don'ts of interviews and the admissions process. I would like to clearly state that this note on Mr. Andrew Paige's file was inappropriate, as were the comments discussed today regarding this candidate's age and we will not be considering age as a factor to admission to our program."

The meeting continued, with all four candidates being reviewed and assessed for admission.

QUESTIONS AND ANSWERS

1. Discuss the assumptions made by the members of the admissions committee.

Dr. Gupta assumed that everyone would approach candidates in a nonbiased and professional manner. Dr. Gupta and Dr. Walters assumed that each member of the committee would take the time to review each candidate's application packet prior to the meeting.

Dr. Sloan assumed that others might agree with the interpretation and assessment of the candidate that he wouldn't have a long career in medicine and that it would only be in Geriatrics. Dr. Sloan also assumed that residency programs would not accept a candidate of advanced age. These assumptions were likely based on implicit bias related to candidates with advanced age for medical school. Dr. Stafford assumed that all of the candidates would be reviewed using an unbiased approach; however, unfortunately the committee members were easily influenced by Dr. Sloan.

2. Discuss how the language used by Dr. Sloan could have affected those in the room.

The language individuals use can be taken by others in various ways, depending on their own personal life histories, experiences, and biases. Sloan's comments regarding the candidate's age may have inadvertently offended others. Alternatively, Dr. Sloan's choice of words may have also given confirmation to others holding some of the same unconscious biases. Dr. Stafford's viewpoint towards the candidate's profile and appropriateness for the program seemed to have been impacted by Dr. Sloan's comments. It is clear from the scenario that some committee members appeared uncomfortable after Dr. Sloan's comments related to the age of the candidate.

3. Discuss the response of Dr. Gupta to the committee and Dr. Sloan.

When Dr. Gupta reminded the committee of the protocol for evaluating candidates during the admissions process, this was a clear and appropriate response to Dr. Sloan's comments. The response would have reset the tone of the continued discussions as well as ensuring that the proper protocol is used. Dr. Gupta's response to Dr. Sloan's language and comments was professional and responsible in the committee meeting.

4. Discuss additional measures that could have been taken related to the situation if you were in Dr. Gupta's position.

Although Dr. Gupta's response was appropriate, there are some additional steps that could have been taken. One approach could be to remind the committee of the candidate review guidelines briefly at the start of each session. Secondly, Dr. Sloan could be referred to additional training for implicit biases. It is also helpful to ensure that an annual implicit bias training is given to all committee members to help identify and mitigate these biases to prevent them from impacting a candidate's review. Moreover, having institutional support and resources available to protect vulnerable groups is vital for maintaining equity and inclusivity in the applicant selection process.

5. Deliberate the impact of being in an environment of implicit bias if nothing was done to correct the situation.

Although each member of the committee is entitled to their individual opinions, it is important that those opinions be free of bias when impacting the potential future career prospects of applicants to health professions programs. If the committee had been influenced or persuaded by Dr. Sloan's comments regarding Andrew, and there was no opposition to them, Andrew may not have been given a fair chance to expand his knowledge in the field of medicine. This equitable chance should be provided to any candidate, prior to review of scores and grades.

6. Elucidate the intersectionality of ageism with other forms of marginalization/discrimination.

Ageism is one of the few forms of discrimination that, if all other things were equal, any individual could experience as they are younger in age and as they advance in age. When other factors are added to age, such as gender, race, sexuality, or disability status, the impact is magnified (Nash *et. al.,* 2020).

The American Geriatrics Society (AGS) has been actively addressing the intersection of racism and ageism since 2020. As part of their review, an AGS working group has identified five target areas to reduce the intersectionality of ageism with other forms of discrimination (Hollman, 2021). These areas included:

- working at the intersection of structural racism and ageism
- advancing diversity in research
- incorporating diversity into professionalism, education, and training
- developing our own skills as advocates
- increasing professional and public awareness

These targeted areas will assist in reducing intersectional? discrimination so that it no longer may influence healthcare access, quality, and health outcomes for populations of advanced age and their caregivers (Hollman, 2021).

Epilogue

This case demonstrates an explicit bias towards adults with advanced age in the setting of an applicant for medical school. However, the scenario could also be extrapolated towards individuals entering the workplace.

After the meeting, Dr. Gupta requested a meeting with Dr. Sloan to discuss the situation that occurred. During the meeting, Dr. Gupta refers Dr. Sloan to the Age Discrimination Act of 1975 which prohibits discrimination on the basis of age in programs and activities receiving federal financial assistance (US Department of Labor, 2022).

"Moreover," Dr. Gupta continues, "there is also the Age Discrimination in Employment Act of 1967 (ADEA) which protects applicants and employees 40 years of age and older from discrimination on the basis of age (US Department of Labor, 2022). These laws protect not just the applicants for our program, but also them as physicians in their future careers. Furthermore, your comments were not representative of the mission and values of our college or the University. I understand that you were coming from a place of 'practicality', but nonetheless, it was inappropriate and cannot bear an impact on the candidate's strengths or weaknesses."

Mr. Andrew Paige was admitted to the program, ranked second in his class overall, matched in his preferred residency program of Internal Medicine, and received a standing ovation at the commencement ceremony. He was a mentor to many peers in the program and inspired them to never stop learning and reaching for their goals.

Dr. Sloan, after much self-reflection, realized a blind spot towards age needed some attention. Dr. Sloan drew inspiration for this watching Andrew succeed in the program, be admired by both peers and faculty, and carry on with his career goals.

REFERENCES

Blackburn, R. (2006). The Global Pension Crisis: From Gray Capitalism to Responsible Accumulation. *Politics & Society*, *34*(2), 135–186. doi:10.1177/0032329206288150

Bodner, E. (2009). On the origins of ageism among older and younger adults. *International Psychogeriatrics*, *21*(6), 1003–1014. doi:10.1017/S104161020999055X PMID:19619389

Butler, R. N. (1969). Age-ism: Another form of bigotry. *The Gerontologist*, *9*(4), 243–246. doi:10.1093/geront/9.4_Part_1.243 PMID:5366225

Cho, S., Crenshaw, K. W., & McCall, L. (2013). Toward a Field of Intersectionality Studies: Theory, Applications, and Praxis. *Signs (Chicago, Ill.)*, *38*(4), 785–810. doi:10.1086/669608

Chonody, J. M., & Teater, B. (2016). Why do I dread looking old?: A test of social identity theory, terror management theory, and the double standard of aging. *Journal of Women & Aging*, *28*(2), 112–126. doi:10.1080/08952841.2014.950533 PMID:26716474

Couto, M. C. P. de P., & Wentura, D. (2017). Implicit Ageism. In *Ageism*. The MIT Press., doi:10.7551/mitpress/10679.003.0006

Davies, N. (2011). Reducing inequalities in healthcare provision for older adults. Nursing standard (Royal College of Nursing (Great Britain): 1987), 25(41), 49–58. doi:10.7748/ns2011.06.25.41.49.c8573

De Marco, M., Thorburn, S., & Zhao, W. (2008). Perceived discrimination during prenatal care, labor, and delivery: An examination of data from the Oregon Pregnancy Risk Assessment Monitoring System, 1998-1999, 2000, and 2001. *American Journal of Public Health*, *98*(10), 1818–1822. doi:10.2105/AJPH.2007.123687 PMID:18703444

Eymard, A. S., & Douglas, D. H. (2012). Ageism among health care providers and interventions to improve their attitudes toward older adults: An integrative review. *Journal of Gerontological Nursing*, *38*(5), 26–35. doi:10.3928/00989134-20120307-09 PMID:22420518

Fairygodboss. (2019). Ageism in the workplace. *Fairygodboss*. https://d207ibygpg2z1x.cloudfront.net/image/upload/v1564675149/files/Ageism_in_the_Workplace.pdf

Fredman, S. (2016). Directorate-General for Justice and Consumers, Intersectional discrimination in EU gender equality and non-discrimination law. *Publications Office*. https://data.europa.eu/doi/10.2838/241520

Furunes, T., & Mykletun, R. J. (2010). Age discrimination in the workplace: Validation of the Nordic Age Discrimination Scale (NADS). *Scandinavian Journal of Psychology*, *51*(1), 23–30. doi:10.1111/j.1467-9450.2009.00738.x PMID:19694986

Handy, J., & Davy, D. (2007). Gendered ageism: Older women's experiences of employment agency practices. *Asia Pacific Journal of Human Resources*, *45*(1), 85–99. doi:10.1177/1038411107073606

Hollmann, P. (2021). Charting our first steps: An update on the AGS initiative to address the intersection of structural racism and ageism. *Geriatric Nursing (New York, N.Y.)*, *42*(4), 961–962. doi:10.1016/j.gerinurse.2021.06.025 PMID:34229872

Iversen, T. J., Larsen, L., & Solem, P. E. (2009). A conceptual analysis of Ageism. *Nordic Psychology, 61*(3), 3, 4–22. doi:10.1027/1901-2276.61.3.4

Kane, R. L., & Kane, R. A. (2005). Ageism in Healthcare and Long-Term Care. *Generations: Journal of the American Society on Aging, 29*(3), 49–54. https://www.jstor.org/stable/26555410

Kydd, A., & Fleming, A. (2015). Ageism and age discrimination in health care: Fact or fiction? A narrative review of the literature. *Maturitas, 81*(4), 432–438. doi:10.1016/j.maturitas.2015.05.002 PMID:26044073

Levy, B. R. (2001). Eradication of ageism requires addressing the enemy within. *The Gerontologist, 41*(5), 578–580. doi:10.1093/geront/41.5.578 PMID:11574700

Malinen, S., & Johnston, L. (2013). Workplace ageism: Discovering hidden bias. *Experimental Aging Research, 39*(4), 445–465. doi:10.1080/0361073X.2013.808111 PMID:23875840

Minichiello, V., Browne, J., & Kendig, H. (2000). Perceptions and consequences of ageism: Views of older people. *Ageing and Society, 20*(3), 253–278. doi:10.1017/S0144686X99007710

Nash, P., Taylor, T., & Levy, B. (2020). The Intersectionality of Ageism. *Innovation in Aging, 4*(Suppl 1), 846–847. doi:10.1093/geroni/igaa057.3105

North, M. S., & Fiske, S. T. (2012). An inconvenienced youth? Ageism and its potential intergenerational roots. *Psychological Bulletin, 138*(5), 982–997. doi:10.1037/a0027843 PMID:22448913

Palmore, E. B. (1990). Ageism: Negative and positive. *Springer Publishing Company*. https://www.scirp.org/(S(oyulxb452alnt1aej1nfow45))/reference/ReferencesPapers.aspx?ReferenceID=1987593

Palmore, E. B., Branch, L., & Harris, D. K. (Eds.). (2005). *Encyclopedia of ageism*. Haworth Pastoral Press. doi:10.4324/9781315043975

Perdue, C. W., & Gurtman, M. B. (1990). Evidence for the automaticity of ageism. *Journal of Experimental Social Psychology, 26*(3), 199–216. doi:10.1016/0022-1031(90)90035-K

Perron, R. (2018). *The Value of Experience: AARP Multicultural Work and Jobs Study*. AARP Research. https://www.aarp.org/research/topics/economics/info-2018/multicultural-work-jobs.html

Prazeres, F., & Passos, L. (2021). Age discrimination at work against health-related professionals in Portugal. *Work (Reading, Mass.), 70*(3), 929–935. doi:10.3233/WOR-213612 PMID:34744039

Robards, F., Kang, M., Usherwood, T., & Sanci, L. (2018). How Marginalized Young People Access, Engage With, and Navigate Health-Care Systems in the Digital Age: Systematic Review. *The Journal of adolescent health: official publication of the Society for Adolescent Medicine, 62*(4), 365–381. doi:10.1016/j.jadohealth.2017.10.018

RTOERO. (2022). *Nuances of Ageism*. RTOERO. https://rtoero.ca/wp-content/uploads/2022/01/Nuances-of-ageism-whitepaper-RTOERO-2021.pdf

Sandra, F. (2016) *Intersectional discrimination in EU gender equality and non-discrimination law.* European Commission. https://data.europa.eu/doi/10.2838/241520

Stypinska, J., & Turek, K. (2017). Hard and soft age discrimination: The dual nature of workplace discrimination. *European Journal of Ageing*, *14*(1), 49–61. doi:10.100710433-016-0407-y PMID:28804394

UN Women. (2015). *Beijing Declaration and Platform for Action.* United Nations Entity for Gender Equality and the Empowerment of Women (UN Women). https://www.unwomen.org/en/digital-library/publications/2015/01/beijing-declaration

U.S Centers for Medicare & Medicaid Services. (2016) *Medicare.gov: the official U.S. government site for Medicare*. Medicare. http://medicare.gov

U.S. Department of Labor. (2022) Age *Discrimination.* USDL. https://www.dol.gov/general/topic/discrimination/agedisc#:~:text=The%20Age%20Discrimination%20in%20Employment,conditions%20or%20privileges%20of%20employment

U.S. Equal Employment Opportunity Commission. (2022) *Age Discrimination | U.S. Equal Employment Opportunity Commission*. EEOC. https://www.eeoc.gov/age-discrimination#:~:text=Age%20discrimination%20involves%20treating%20an,are%20age%2040%20or%20older

Van Wicklin, S. A. (2020). Ageism in Nursing. *Plastic surgical nursing: official journal of the American Society of Plastic and Reconstructive Surgical Nurses*, *40*(1), 20–24. doi:10.1097/PSN.0000000000000290

ENDNOTE

1 Disclaimer: This chapter took part in the double-blind peer review process and was not compromised due to the authors also being an editor. A non-author editor managed all of the editorial aspects of the chapter.

Chapter 5
Race and Racism and the Healthcare Professional Perspectives

Gabriella Dauer
Nova Southeastern University Dr. Kiran C. Patel College of Allopathic Medicine, USA

William James Dawson
Nova Southeastern University Dr. Kiran C. Patel College of Allopathic Medicine, USA

Heejung Kim
Nova Southeastern University Dr. Kiran C. Patel College of Allopathic Medicine, USA

Arkene Levy
Nova Southeastern University Dr. Kiran C. Patel College of Allopathic Medicine, USA

Kevin Kuang
Nova Southeastern University Dr. Kiran C. Patel College of Allopathic Medicine, USA

Samiksha Prasad
Nova Southeastern University Dr. Kiran C. Patel College of Allopathic Medicine, USA

EXECUTIVE SUMMARY

The American Psychological Association defines racism as a construct that is 'structural, institutional, interpersonal, and internalized.' The marginalization of persons of color due to blatant racism is a pervasive social issue that has historically held negative consequences for the health of these individuals, and evidence links racism to the higher levels of morbidity and mortality, seen especially among Blacks/African Americans (Paradies, 2015). The effort and movement to reduce marginalization of minorities through healthcare professional education is upon us. Providing health professional learners and practitioners with tools to understand manifestations and implications of racial acts and microaggressions in the healthcare setting is imperative, as is training medical professionals to recognize and mitigate their biases. This chapter highlights cases of varying levels of racism from the healthcare professionals' view and experience in the clinical setting.

DOI: 10.4018/978-1-6684-5493-0.ch005

INTRODUCTION

Racial biases are not always overt and can manifest in subtle ways through microaggressions. Racial microaggressions can be chronic or episodic daily race-related hassles that occur in the form of subtle degradations against people of color (Slaughter, 2015; Sue 2007). An example of racial microaggressions include when Asian Americans and Latino Americans are assumed to be foreign-born and a statement such as "You speak good English." is made which implies that the individual is not American (Wing, 2007). Another example is the pathologizing of cultural values or communication styles of persons of color with the underlying perception that the values and communication styles of the dominant White culture are ideal (Wing, 2007). A classical representation of this is asking an individual who identifies as Black "Why do you have to be so animated?" or asking an individual who identifies as Asian "Why are you so quiet?" (Wing, 2007). These statements indirectly imply that these individuals should assimilate to the dominant culture. Although microaggressions might be subtle occurrences, their effects can create barriers to appropriate healthcare as they may negatively impact patient-centered care by preventing the formation of a positive patient-provider relationship (Cuffee, 2013). This is important as patient satisfaction with their provider and healthcare interactions correlates with health outcomes (Cuffee, 2013).

Furthermore, microaggressions and racist acts are commonly overlooked when directed to communities who may phenotypically present as 'White' such as experienced by the Asian population. It is imperative to note that many minority groups in the United States have continuously faced prejudice and discrimination in healthcare (Huang, 2020). While each group has had its own traditional stereotypes, one association for Asians is that they are carriers of disease (Hussain, 2020). Repeatedly, this association was revitalized, most prominently during disease outbreaks. The recent COVID-19 outbreak has again, brought back previous racist stereotypes and thrown Asian-Americans into the national spotlight. Even while many Asian-Americans actively worked in the healthcare field to combat COVID-19, this did not mitigate prejudice and discrimination. In fact, many Asian-American healthcare workers have reported an increased amount of racism from their patients. Our second case scenario in this chapter aims to highlight the obvious and subliminal methods people may convey prejudice and discrimination against Asian healthcare workers, the causes or motivations behind their actions and words, the effects these situations may have on all parties involved, and any actions bystanders may take.

Finally, the third case of this chapter will explore how typifying a diagnosis to a specific race can be a form of racial bias. Studies have exemplified and supported medical educators in moving away from using specific racial or ethnic identifiers in patient summaries or case frames, proving that these diagnostic stereotypes can delay proper diagnosis and incite misdiagnosis of minorities, especially patients who identify as Black (Darshali, 2020). A stark example of typifying diagnosis to race in identifying Lyme Disease to be an infectious tick-borne illness that affects primarily White Americans, leading to delay in diagnosis of the typical target-like rash that appears early in the disease process, and leaving many Black patients undiagnosed until they exemplify symptoms of later disease such as arthritis. Many textbooks have also traditionally exampled cases on specific race or skin types, especially Dermatological diseases portrayed commonly as rashes imaged upon White skin (Yousuf, 2022). It is imperative to change the narrative with education of the healthcare professional to affect their clinical experience and exposure, which can indirectly benefit the experience of our underrepresented and underserved minorities.

CASE 1: DR. A'S BLUNDER

Goal

This case exemplifies a medical resident team member witnessing a microaggression of racist etiology, as a bystander while on rounds with their attending, a hierarchical superior.

Learning Outcomes

1. Define microaggressions and recognize instances of microaggressions and discrimination in the clinical setting.
2. Explain the nature of microaggressions and its impact on recipients and bystanders.
3. Identify how the recipient and the source may be viewing the microaggression situation differently.
4. Recommend responses to microaggression that can build a climate of inclusive excellence, repair and re-establish relationships, and restore or protect reputations.

Case

You are part of a large medical team that has begun rounding on a patient admitted to the inpatient floor for an acute illness. As the team gathers at the patient's door, you see the attending and residents preparing for the presentation of the patient. This resident team has been working with Dr. A for two weeks on a four-week rotation. The resident team is comprised of two Black female physicians, Dr. D (Danielle) and Dr. C (Chantal), and one White male resident physician, Dr. O (Oliver). The attending physician, Dr. A (Allison), is an older White female and is directing rounds:

Dr. A: "Good morning. Let's start our adolescent rounds with patient in room 28A. The nurse has noted he is in discomfort and has had worsening diarrhea as of this morning."

Dr. A is looking to resident Danielle and states: "Chantal, why don't you go ahead and start presenting overnight events for this patient."

Danielle looks surprised at being referred to as her colleague's name and replies, "I am not Chantal, I'm Danielle." Chantal is equally visibly uncomfortable by Dr. A's mistaking her colleague for her.

Dr. A quickly and subtly murmurs, "Well you two really shouldn't be standing next to one another, it's confusing." Dr. A chuckles embarrassingly and proceeds to direct the conversation at the correct resident: "Ok, Chantal, go ahead with the overnight events."

After rounds, Danielle and Chantal return to their resident work room. Both seem to hold a heaviness and sadness to their demeanor and decide to discuss the statements of Dr. A. Both feel the statements were hurtful and unnecessary. They immediately converse with their chief residents who set up an urgent meeting for Chantal and Danielle to report the incident to the program director.

QUESTIONS AND ANSWERS

1. Discuss the error made by Dr. A in mistaking one resident for her colleague. Discuss if this initial mishap could occur innocently, or innately has negative connotation.

Mistaking one resident for another on medical rounds by calling them by a colleague's name is a common occurrence. Attending physicians and residents interact for a short period of time during the day and the residents rotate through subspecialty fields with great frequency, affording attendings minimal time to personally interact with residents outside of rounds. However, the fact that the two students who were mixed up by Dr. A were both Black females brings into question whether there was an innate racist microaggression on behalf of Dr. A's error. If there was another female on the team who perhaps was White with which this error occurred, the concern for racial microaggression may not be in question.

2. Discuss how the error is more likely to be a racial microaggression after Dr. A comment on how the two residents should stand separately on rounds.

Dr. A's statement that they should not stand next to each other helped give more credence to it being a racial microaggression that led to her confusion of the names. Though this comment could have also been related to the gender of the residents, the fact that both residents are persons of color further implicates Dr. A in holding an unconscious bias that persons of color look similar and therefore can be easily confused for one another. The behavior and aspect of her language, with the murmuring of comments, indicates that Dr. A recognizes that what she was thinking and saying was not appropriate, but that she was saying it, nonetheless.

3. Discuss a potential appropriate immediate response from Dr. A for the mishap.

Dr. A is unlikely to recognize her own statement in real-time as offensive or racially micro-aggressive. In the case that an immediate re-do is available, one can immediately stop rounds, turn around, and face the group and openly recognize that the statement was not appropriate and apologize. A statement of example could be, "Team, I am realizing that my statement was not appropriate for several reasons." And looking at the residents to whom it was directed noting, "I sincerely apologize. Please let me know if you would like to speak about this more after rounds."

4. Discuss a potential appropriate immediate response from Danielle and Chantal respectively.

Either Dr. D or Dr. C can stop rounds and approach Dr. A about the comment. Whether the resident would like to respond within the context of rounds with other participants present or want to step aside with Dr. A is their personal choice for the comfort level of the resident. After such a statement, the resident could state, "Dr. A, can we please take a minute to chat?". The duo can move aside and Dr. D or C can note the following: "Dr. A, that comment was very hurtful. When you say that the two of us should not stand next to one another, I am not sure what you mean. To me, it means that because of the color of my skin, you are confusing myself for my co-resident who shares the same shade of skin tone. Is that what was meant by your statement? If so, that is very hurtful." Opening the conversation with the resident's emotion to the statement is appropriate to elicit Dr. A's response in etiology for the statement.

5. Discuss how a bystander may respond to the situation. For example, a potential response from the third White male resident.

A bystander can also comment on the scenario if there is discomfort. They can do so immediately or report the scenario to their program director. The White male resident upon recognition of hurt from Dr. D and Dr. C could console them and assure that he heard and felt the comment to be hurtful for his two co-residents. Dr. O or a bystander could also address the situation with Dr. A directly as follows in this alternate scenario: After rounds, Dr. O catches Dr. A on her way back to her office. He asks her if she has a minute to talk about the rounds they just performed. She has a few minutes before her next patient and agrees to talk for a few minutes. They step into her office and Dr. O begins with, "Dr. A, I'm not sure how to approach this, but I think your confusion of Dr. C and Dr. D may have caused some unintended discomfort for them."

6. Discuss potential escalation of this incident to your supervisor.

This type of scenario is often difficult to immediately reflect on and respond to. If early recognition and attention is given to the scenario, the immediate feedback is most effective for the receiver of feedback. After the event, it is also appropriate to escalate these types of events when witnesses or partaking members feel necessary. Escalating supervisor attention can offer a more experienced view and also document such instances and infractions to assure repeat offenders are remediated with respect to their actions. In this scenario, it is appropriate for the medical student, resident, nurse or any other person on rounds witnessing the event, to bring this to their respective hierarchy for advice and guidance. Upon bringing this scenario to the program director, a meeting between program leadership and Dr. A was scheduled where the scenario was discussed from her perspective. Dr. A becomes tearful in her recognition that her comments were hurtful and could be taken as a racially charged microaggression. The program director discussed the event with Dr. A from the perspective of the resident and Dr. A feels remorseful and acknowledges that she will be more mindful with her words. The program director then meets with the resident to close the loop of communication and assure the resident physician knows her concerns are sound and taken seriously.

Epilogue

Racial microaggressions can present subtly and in many ways in the field of health professions. In this scenario, Dr. A has worked with her resident team for two weeks and arrives at medical rounds having mistaken one of her residents for the other. This could have been an innocent error, however Dr. A then comments on how the two residents should stand physically separated on rounds. This follow up comment denotes that Dr. A mistakenly referred to Danielle as Chantal likely because the color of her skin being similar to that of her colleague. Many times, these comments are delivered without conscious effort and are expressions of subtle or unconscious biases. These statements, though swift and seemingly mild on the surface, are harmful and perpetuate structural racism. Upon recognition by any member of the team, including the person delivering the comments, the scenario should be directed to immediate remediation. Recognition of the harmful statement and subsequent apology with intent to modify behavior by the person who delivered the statement. This can be done immediately during or after the event with self-direction or with advocacy and support of a supervisor. Reconciliation with the person(s) to whom the statement was directed is imperative.

CASE 2: A PANDEMIC BEYOND THE VIRUS

Goal

This case explores a situation in which an Asian healthcare professional experiences prejudice and discrimination due to generalized hysteria and misinformation surrounding the COVID-19 pandemic (Coronavirus disease 2019, due to SARS-CoV-2).

Learning Outcomes

1. Recognize the prevalence of racism and discrimination against Asian Americans in clinical settings.
2. Explain the nature of the proceeding discrimination and its impact on the patient, the healthcare providers, and the recipients and bystanders.
3. Summarize strategies to navigate scenarios that involve differences in patients' values and beliefs expressed as racist remarks or actions.
4. Explain the importance of allyship in promoting safe work environments.

Case

You are a health professional student rotating through an inpatient Internal Medicine unit during the height of the COVID-19 pandemic. One of your new patients was admitted from her assisted living facility with concern for septic shock after a diagnosis of a urinary tract infection. The patient was stabilized with intravenous fluids and antibiotics in the emergency room and is now on the inpatient unit for continued management. Your team decides to round on her first. Your team consists of an Asian-American nurse, a White attending, and a Black resident. Following introductions, the attending physician steps out to round on other patients while the resident and Asian-American nurse are left to draw blood for culture and labs. The nurse steps to the front of the room to discard materials in the sharp objects container. You then witness the following interaction between the patient and the resident:

Patient, looking visibly nervous and pointing at the nurse: "Who is she? Am I going to be seeing a lot of her?"

Resident: "That is Taylor, she is a very experienced nurse who is going to be taking care of you today."

Patient: "Well, has she been vaccinated? Are all your nurses regularly tested for coronavirus and other diseases? I do not want to get that virus."

The resident is now also visibly uncomfortable with the nature and tone of this conversation. The nurse stays at the front of the room but can hear the dialogue between her patient and the resident. The resident responds in reassurance that the hospital staff and faculty fully understand the gravity of the pandemic and have implemented all personnel to don appropriate personal protective equipment such as N95 masks and gowns. The resident relays that the hospital has adopted a strict 'no sick' policy where staff and faculty who have been exposed to a sick contact or who themselves have any symptoms should remain at home until they test negative for COVID-10.

The patient almost does not let the resident finish her explanation of hospital safety policies and escalates the conversation by raising her voice.

Patient: "Well, you never know who she is talking to outside the hospital! Is there anyone else you can switch me to!? Please, it is my choice who cares for me, and I am sick, so I do not want to worry about added risks."

Resident: "I am sorry you feel this way. I completely understand these are frightening times. I assure you that you are in more than capable hands. I am happy to relay your concerns to our nurse manager so that we can work to make you as comfortable as possible during your stay. I do want you to know that it may not be possible to switch your nurse for the day as the unit is at full capacity"

Your patient scoffs and continues to say that 'a lot of [her] friends and family have become ill due to COVID in the past year, so [she is] very uncomfortable with her nurse caring for her." "Are you sure she has been regularly tested and vaccinated? Where is she from anyways?" she asks.

Resident: "I appreciate your concerns. I cannot answer that question but again will escalate your concerns to our nurse manager and to our patient care team. We are doing our best to assure patients in the hospital do not contract illnesses from staff, faculty, or other patients..."

The patient continues to become more upset, and she requests that you and the nurse leave the room immediately to let her rest. Nursing leadership and the patient care team are contacted to assist in conflict resolution. The nurse remains visibly upset throughout her shift after this interaction, and the patient has been told that no change will be made to staffing assignments. The patient is requesting that her children are contacted so that she can be moved to a different hospital.

QUESTIONS AND ANSWERS

1. Consider why racist acts against the Asian population may be less overtly publicized and spoken about? What cultural components, genetics, and phenotypic characteristics may have made us believe that our Asian colleagues are less affected by racism and how has COVID exposed this too be untrue?

Racial discrimination against Asian Americans during the Coronavirus Disease-2019 (COVID-19) pandemic cannot be fully understood without the context of the different forms of racial stereotyping and subsequent discrimination against Asian Americans throughout history. One stereotype is the Model Minority Myth (Sakamoto, 2012), which identifies Asian Americans as the minority group that has successfully achieved the "American Dream." Although this may seem harmless, it undoubtedly has harmful effects on Asian Americans. First, this stereotype denies and overlooks the diversity within the Asian American community. Different subtypes within the Asian American community have vastly different immigrant experiences that may not fit under the Model Minority stereotype, such as refugee families seeking asylum from their country of origin . In addition, the myth diminishes the racism and discrimination that Asian Americans experience in the United States. It is easy to extrapolate that this has, and continues to occur during the COVID-19 pandemic with minimization of discrimination of Asian Americans.

Another concept that shapes the Asian American experience is Yellow Peril, which is the idea that Asian Americans are considered foreigners and their practices largely deviate from common norms and practices of White culture (Kawai, 2005). As early as the 1800s, negative Asian racial biases were formed as large numbers of immigrant Chinese workers entered the country (Huang 2020). The association that Chinese people are "disease carriers" is old (Hussain, 2020). Unfortunately, the COVID-19 virus, which originated in Wuhan, China, likely only strengthened this association. At the beginning of the pandemic, news outlets contributed to this association by using stock photos of Asians in masks when reporting on emerging COVID-19 information (Burton, 2020; Walker, 2020).

Xenophobic thoughts turned into actions through discrimination and aggression. The AAPI released a report in April of 2020 documenting a total of 1497 reports of coronavirus discrimination on the CAA/A3PCON STOP AAPI HATE website from March 9th to April 15, 2020 (Jeung & Nham, 2020). Reports of anti-Asian discrimination included verbal harassment, shunning, physical assault, vandalism, and being barred from establishment or transportation (Jeung & Nham, 2020). Additionally, the FBI reported a 77% increase in anti-Asian hate crimes when comparing the year 2019 to 2020 ("2020 FBI," 2022). This has also been exemplified in Chinese American families reporting being directly targeted in COVID-19 racial discrimination; for example, experiencing Covid-19 related fears and racism while their children were admitted for an unrelated diagnosis. This higher level of racism against Asian Americans was also associated with declines in mental health of those affected (Cheah et al., 2020).

Being a healthcare worker did not eradicate xenophobia and discrimination. One Asian American ER physician, Dr. Alex Tran, reported that the increase in xenophobia amidst the COVID-19 pandemic made them feel like they no longer belonged in their hospital (Tran, 2020). An increase in the prevalence of mental health issues among healthcare workers can be attributed to COVID-19 (Spoorthy et al., 2020). Such issues include insomnia, stress, anxiety, and depression (Spoorthy et al., 2020). One study found that Asian American and Asian Canadian healthcare workers have reported an increase in racial microaggressions, threats of violence, and actual violence since the beginning of COVID-19 pandemic (Shang et al., 2021). Even as healthcare workers, especially at the beginning of the pandemic, were heralded as heroes, the effects of xenophobia could still be felt among Asian American healthcare workers.

2. In the spectrum of microaggression to macroaggression, define the above scenario.

Macroaggressions and microaggressions differ in that macroaggressions occur at a more systematic level whereas microaggressions occur at a more interpersonal level (Torres 2019). Different subtypes of microaggression exist in the healthcare field. The main types include microassaults, microinsults, and microinvalidations (Torres 2019). Microassaults involve remarks that are more overt and targeted toward individuals. Such remarks include, "You people are all the same, claiming your minority status to take the spots that belong to someone else." (Torres 2019). Microinsults include more subtle remarks that could be disparaging to the target regardless of the perpetrator's intention. Microinvalidations are characterized by diminishing the target's experiences by invalidating their experiences. Such examples could include remarks like "I don't see color" (Torres 2019).

Considering the above scenario, we can attempt to identify the type of microaggression that is occurring in this circumstance. Though there is a suspicion that the patient is refusing care from the Asian American nurse due to her ethnicity and a perceived link to the Coronavirus, it can only remain a suspicion because the patient did not outright say it. Another consideration is that the patient had targeted her remarks toward the individual rather than at a larger group. When the patient asks if "all" nurses have been vaccinated and tested, while not outright racist, can be seen as targeted toward the only nurse in the room. Additionally, asking where the nurse is from is not outwardly discriminatory and racist but still a pointed and targeted remark, as it highlights the concept of "othering" of Asian Americans. Given these considerations, the patient most likely was a perpetrator of a microinsult. The statement "Well, you never know who she is talking to outside the hospital!" may also be intended to cast a shadow on the nurse's personal choices and/or assume nefarious or unsafe associations, based only on the nurse's observed physical feature. Though it may have not been the patient's intention to disparage the nurse, her remarks reflect her assumptions and biases about the nurse's health and potentially her moral character, based on her ethnicity.

3. In the above scenario, consider where the patient's remarks could have been rooted in the context of the social climate during the pandemic.

The Coronavirus Disease-2019 (COVID-19) pandemic has been a time of uncertainty and fear for many individuals. As mentioned by the patient, many of her loved ones had been impacted by this disease. Given that at the beginning of the pandemic, inaccurate information had been widely spread, individuals still have varying understandings of this disease. One interpretation of this patient's response to the Asian American nurse includes the response of fear to misinformation. Given that certain media could often heighten fear of the unknown through misinformation and 'sensationalization', it is possible that the patient believes the disease is spread only by individuals of Asian descent. Similar phenomena have occurred in the past about other novel diseases. For example, the spread of HIV/AIDS in the 80's resulted in mass prejudice and discrimination against the LGBTQ+ community, or Ebola virus outbreaks in recent history inciting discrimination of Black Africans.

4. What are strategies that could help gain a deeper understanding of the patient's perspective?

At the time of this writing in 2022, the spread of misinformation due to technology is an impactful societal issue. Healthcare providers can be affected by the easy access to inaccurate medical and health information from news and social platforms. Compounding this issue is the fact that misinformation may come from people the patient trusts and respects such as friends, family, politicians, professional athletes or other celebrities. Therefore, in treating patients such as the one from the case study, it becomes critical to first understand what the patient knows about COVID-19, where the information is coming from, and why the patient is thinking the way they are. The key point during this conversation is to avoid confrontation and combative cues as the patient may become defensive, and instead, rely on a more understanding and compassionate attitude. Finally, the last component is to educate the patient on for example, how viruses spread, the uncertainty on the COVID-19 origins, and other available scientifically sound information. However, at times, the patient may remain set in their thinking and unwilling to change. What strategies can we employ as health professionals in educating our patients in hopes of mitigating prejudice and discriminatory behaviors due to novel diseases?

5. What are some strategies that health care professionals can utilize to advocate for the nurse in this scenario? How can a health professional, whether involved directly or as a bystander to these interactions, serve in allyship to the cause of removing prejudice from the healthcare system?

A senior hospital or health care team member in this position might find it most effective to draw more attention and focus on the nurse's competency and skills in patient care and away from her ethnicity. Therefore, one important advocacy strategy is to professionally explain why the nurse is qualified to be there, such as through previous patient reports and the healthcare team's opinion of her. Additionally, patient care excellence can be expressed by defining the hiring practices of the hospital in prioritizing performance and experience when selecting candidates, and how members of the healthcare team are assigned to each patient. Finally, the patient could be given a detailed outline of the hospital protocols for COVID-19, such as prevention and screening practices, and how they mitigate transmission from the healthcare team to the patients.

Most importantly, hierarchical professionals should reiterate to patients that the culture of the workplace is to perpetuate equal care to all patients and that racist prejudice and discrimination are not tolerated at the hospital. If the patient is refusing to comply, the hospital may need to further involve their patient care team and ethics team. The key behind this conversation is to establish trust in the hospital and the team working with the patient, and hope that through this trust, the patient will feel much more comfortable with the different healthcare professionals. The conversation is also meant to protect the healthcare team itself, from any prejudice and discriminatory actions.

Bystanders who may be within the vicinity of this type of interaction could also be of help under different circumstances. Bystanders can support the target by reporting the incident to their supervisor. This is more commonly practice if the perpetrator is a staff member as well. This is called allyship, which involves advocating for the target even though they may not share the same ethnic or social background. The work of an ally is impactful as they support the target as well as normalize the standard of standing up against racism and racist microaggressions.

Finally, the hospital system can be of support by implementing larger systemic changes to the institution. For example, employee education could raise awareness about multicultural competencies and minority experiences of racism with strategies for responding to microaggressions.

6. How could the nurse in this scenario be affected by the circumstances?

Microaggressions have negative effects on the target (Nadal, 2014). Apart from the obvious uncomfortableness that the nurse may experience because of those comments, there is an isolation of the individual in targeting a person for their skin color or ethnicity which can feel alienating. Beyond these immediate emotional responses, targets of microaggression have more lasting effects as well. Microaggressions have been shown to have detrimental effects on one's mental health, such as effects on self-esteem, alcohol use, depression, and anxiety (Blume, 2012; O'Keefe, 2015). Within their places of work, where Asian Americans sacrifice their safety for the sake of caring for patients during the pandemic, such encounters could negatively affect individuals' morale and happiness overall.

Epilogue

Asian Americans face a unique history of racism and discrimination in the United States. Given the background of that history delineated in this chapter as well as the above example of how microaggressions could manifest during the COVID-19 pandemic, we encourage readers to consider their current places of work. Microaggressions have an impact on the target but also could lead to implications for the larger social group. Lack of support and allyship to an individual could lead to others in the same ethnic group assuming they are lacking support as well. This type of practice normalizes perpetrating microaggressions and lack of accountability and growth. We hope that this chapter encouraged readers to become educated about the various influences that cause members of the Asian American communities to suffer and find practical strategies to fight against them.

CASE 3: RACIAL STEREOTYPING

Goal

Structural racism has plagued the healthcare received by persons of color for centuries. In this case, we will discuss the care of a Black woman with a specific diagnosis that may typically be associated with the white race. Exemplified will be the approach to treatment, process of hospitalization and care, and medical team commentary and biases.

Learning Outcomes

1. Define structural racism and identify components of the healthcare system that continue to be so.
2. Analyze examples of how persons of color have historically been cared for, or lack thereof, within the healthcare system.
3. Describe how depicting race in problem presentations can guide health professions educators and students to particular and/or incorrect diagnoses.
4. Evaluate how specific diagnoses have historically and socially been 'associated' with specific races.
5. Evaluate other components of the healthcare system and patient care process in which treatment of persons of color may differ from that of persons who identify as non-persons of color.

Case

The doors of the Emergency Room swing open and a young woman is pulled up to the front desk by her parents. She sulks in annoyance of being back to the place she likes least, the place which exemplifies the reality of her diagnosis.

Gaby is a 22-year-old female who has struggled with severe bulimia for years. She began her journey as a young teenager with body dysmorphia, anxiety, and occasional purging of meals. Her history is now marked by multiple hospitalizations for hypokalemia in the setting of chronic self-induced vomiting and metabolic acidosis from copious diarrhea secondary to laxative abuse. She returns now against her will, brought in by her parents. Her father is a renowned physician in the area, and her mother holds a law degree and works within the home. Her father sits her down to register her as her mother brings in a suitcase, knowing this hospitalization will be longer than the last with how thin Gaby has gotten. She is ushered into a bed in the Emergency Room bay and vitals and labs again confirm that she is sicker than ever: hypotensive, bradycardic, acidotic -- but her potassium is strangely normal despite her reporting persistent vomiting. She soon reports that her father had prescribed her potassium pills in an attempt to keep Gaby out of the hospital, citing disbelief that their daughter could 'actually be diagnosed with something like an eating disorder'.

STOP. REFLECT. At this point of the case, you have already developed an image of Gaby and a narrative of her story regarding where she 'comes from' and how this scenario 'plays out'. *What race is she?* Is she of an affluent background? What are her social determinants of health?

Gaby is a young Black woman. Her parents are also both Black.

She is admitted to the inpatient team for medical optimization with intravenous fluids and a nasogastric tube for adequate refeeding and calorie counting. She is booked for at least a week-long stay with lab monitoring and weight checks before she can be moved to the inpatient psychiatric ward.

She holds steady and compliant on Day 1 and 2 of hospitalization. The residents and medical students who take over her care seem surprised when her history is told as "A 22-year-old BLACK female with severe bulimia nervosa and electrolyte derangements admitted for monitoring of refeeding syndrome." Their shock comes with the narrative that Gaby is not a young white female to whom these scenarios occur in the movies.

Day 3 and 4 prove challenging for Gaby. She becomes irritable, and quickly deteriorates. By day 5 of her hospitalization, her food is given to her solely by a nasogastric tube as she is refusing any oral intake. All medications are given to her first-hand by the nurses and she is requiring as needed medications to calm her agitated state. Psychiatry is suspecting acute stress disorder and panic disorder. Then she breaks. Gaby, despite having a 1:1 care-person in the room 24/7, makes a run for the door. She grabs nothing but herself as her belongings have already been confiscated per Psychiatry and social work to facilitate her compliance. She makes it to the elevator before a medical resident physically blocks her as security drags her back to her room. She is moved to a locked unit, all clothing removed from her and she degenerates into acute psychosis and placed on multiple injectable antipsychotic medications per Psychiatry to facilitate a calm mood.

During her deterioration on Day 1 and 2, nurses strolling past her room comment on how rare it is for a young Black woman to have an eating disorder. On day 3 and 4, security guards from her code grey alert comment aloud on how this is "White level crazy." When she is moved to a locked room and placed on 24/7 constant observation by Psychiatry, her grandmother begins to question the medical teams diagnoses of mental illness as 'this doesn't happen in our community; Black children do not do this for no reason."

QUESTIONS AND ANSWERS

1. Discuss your initial reflection to the case prior to being given the fact that Gaby is a Black patient. Did you initially assume her diagnosis to be that which is more common in another race? Why?

All health professionals arrive in their education, training, and practice with preconceived notions regarding diagnoses based on their own life experiences. They then further develop a diagnosis profile within their education and practice. For example, if someone was introduced to the case of a patient with anorexia in education as always related to a case frame of a white female, they may move into practice with the notion that this disease is mostly prevalent in this patient population (Sonneville, 2018). The goal of decoupling race from diagnosis in education is to remove these associations and allow the health professional to explore the diagnosis within the individual patient before assigning the diagnosis a preconceived notion with respect to race.

2. What are some diagnoses within your field of training that have been systemically typified to a specific race? How can this be harmful for the patient?

Many diagnoses can be traced back to affiliates with a specific race or ethnicity based on one's life experiences and background. These relationships we develop are further typified by what we are exposed to in the healthcare setting, media, and in our education and training. For example, a diagnosis of histrionic personality disorder can be typified to a white or white-Hispanic female as this is the often portrayed as a common role in media. An example of perpetuated association in the medical field is that of the Black race with sickle cell disease. In preparing a case frame for a patient, the healthcare professions have noted race in their statements and presentations, often noting an opening one-liner to a case as "A 50 year old Black man with chest pain" which can lead a student or trainee down a line of diagnoses that may have nothing to do with the patient's race. Typifying a diagnosis to a race and vice versa can disrupt the relationship between the physician and the patient with implicit bias and lead to inappropriate differentials.

3. Can you think of a scenario where knowing the race of a patient with a specific diagnosis can be helpful to the patient? Why?

Medical education has harbored the notion that identifying the patient race may assist in navigating to a diagnosis in a more succinct manner. For example, in the case frame of a '50 year old Black man with severe chest pain,' one might move into the thought process of a potential aortic dissection as this diagnosis is more common in patient who identify as Black, and particularly those who have had tobacco exposure. Early recognition of this specific diagnosis is key to initiating life saving measures to correct a dissection before patient harm is caused. On the contrary, moving swiftly into this diagnosis and obtaining emergent imaging such as a CT angiogram of the chest can incur unnecessary cost and stress to the patient in the scenario that a patient may have severe chest pain from a more benign diagnosis such as a gastrointestinal ulceration.

4. Consider the scenario where a white and Black family both present to the same Emergency Room within one week for accidental ingestion of THC gummies by their toddler. The white family is given a consult with social services, a slap on the wrist, and told to better secure the gummies. The Black family has child protective services called.
    a. Describe the difference in care between these families and how race may have played a role on that difference.

The care received by the white family in this case was vastly different than that received by the Black family. Many instances in medicine lend themselves to healthcare providers assuming the worst of our Black families and giving harsher treatment as a result of bias and racism. The white family was given guidance, support, and education, while the Black family was given shame. This offers no opportunity to our Black families to learn from these instances where a child may be put in danger. More so, calling child protective services can further create tension between our Black families and their healthcare providers as doing so implies that this family potentially intended harm or neglect to their child, which may not be the case. Offering, education, support, and guidance to ALL families presenting for care in this situation is the only path we can pursue in medicine to provide equal care opportunities for children and families of all races and minorities.

    b. Describe other scenarios within the medical system where a patient of color or minority race may receive treatment that may differ from their white counterparts.

An anecdotal example of treatment differences with respect to race includes when and how a 'code grey' is called. A code grey in the hospital setting is typically a rapid and public overhead call for security personnel to arrive to a specific location. This 'code' is called for a variety of scenarios but most commonly ones where a patient may be escalating their aggression towards a healthcare provider, or a patient has begun to elope. Few studies have examined the actual numbers, but various news stories have gathered anecdotal evidence over the years and a recent controversial scenario in 2021 accused a Seattle hospital of calling security twice as often on Black families in comparison to their white counterparts. Instances that exemplify the racial differences in care from the diagnoses we treat to the care we provide can strengthen or harm the fiduciary relationship between the healthcare professional and the patient. Active awareness in asking ourselves if our actions or our management would be different if the patient was of a different minority, ethnicity, or race is crucial to the self-pursuit of recognition of implicit biases.

Epilogue

This case highlights the importance of understanding how a disease can present, how to diagnose it, and how to treat it, regardless of race. Typifying race to a diagnosis can harm everyone involved from the patient to the caregivers who may inflict their implicit biases unto their patients. In this case, despite the commentary from her healthcare team and family members, Gaby prevails. Her labs normalize as she sits behind a locked door. She smiles at her medical team from her window and her constant observation is removed as she adjusts to her new antipsychotic and antidepressant medications. She knows her road is long, but she sits hopeful that this is her last time being known as Gaby, the 22-year-old BLACK female with an eating disorder.

REFERENCES

Blume, A. W., Lovato, L. V., Thyken, B. N., & Denny, N. (2012). The relationship of microaggressions with alcohol use and anxiety among ethnic minority college students in a historically White institution. *Cultural Diversity & Ethnic Minority Psychology*, *18*(1), 45–54. https://doi.org/10.1037/a0025457

Burton, N. (2020, March 6). Why Asians in masks should not be the "face" of the coronavirus. *Vox*. https://www.vox.com/identities/2020/3/6/21166625/coronavirus-photos-racism

Cheah, C. S. L., Wang, C., Ren, H., Zong, X., Cho, H. S., & Xue, X. (2020). Covid-19 racism and Mental Health in Chinese American families. *Pediatrics*, *146*(5). https://doi.org/10.1542/peds.2020-021816

Cuffee, Y. L., Hargraves, J. L., Rosal, M., Briesacher, B. A., Schoenthaler, A., Person, S., Hullett, S., & Allison, J. (2013). Reported racial discrimination, trust in physicians, and medication adherence among inner-city African Americans with hypertension. *American Journal of Public Health*, *103*(11), e55–e62. https://doi.org/10.2105/AJPH.2013.301554

Huang, J., & Liu, R. (2020). Xenophobia in America in the age of coronavirus and beyond. *Journal of Vascular and Interventional Radiology*, *31*(7), 1187–1188. https://doi.org/10.1016/j.jvir.2020.04.020

Hussain, S. (2020, February 3). Fear of coronavirus fuels racist sentiment targeting Asians. *Los Angeles Times*. https://www.latimes.com/california/story/2020-02-03/fear-panic-around-the-coronavirus-fuels-racist-sentiment

Jeung, R., & Nham, K. (2020). *Incidents of coronavirus-related discrimination*. A3PCON. https://www.asianpacificpolicyandplanningcouncil.org/wp-content/uploads/STOP_AAPI_HATE_MONTHLY_REPORT_4_23_20.pdf

Kawai, Y. (2005). Stereotyping Asian Americans: The Dialectic of the Model Minority and the Yellow Peril. *The Howard Journal of Communications*, *16*(2), 109–130. https://doi.org/10.1080/10646170590948974

Nadal, K. L., Wong, Y., Griffin, K. E., Davidoff, K., & Sriken, J. (2014). The adverse impact of racial microaggressions on college students' self-esteem. *Journal of College Student Development*, *55*(5), 461–474.

O'Keefe, V. M., Wingate, L. R., Cole, A. B., Hollingsworth, D. W., & Tucker, R. P. (2015). Seemingly Harmless Racial Communications Are Not So Harmless: Racial Microaggressions Lead to Suicidal Ideation by Way of Depression Symptoms. *Suicide & Life-Threatening Behavior*, *45*(5), 567–576. https://doi.org/10.1111/sltb.12150

Paradies, Y., Ben, J., Denson, N., Elias, A., Priest, N., Pieterse, A., Gupta, A., Kelaher, M., & Gee, G. (2015). Racism as a Determinant of Health: A Systematic Review and Meta-Analysis. *PLoS One*, *10*(9), e0138511. https://doi.org/10.1371/journal.pone.0138511

Sakamoto, A., Takei, I., & Woo, H. (2012). The Myth of the Model Minority Myth. *Sociological Spectrum*, *32*(4), 309–321. https://doi.org/10.1080/02732173.2012.664042

Shang, Z., Kim, J. Y., & Cheng, S. O. (2021). Discrimination experienced by Asian Canadian and Asian American health care workers during the COVID-19 pandemic: A qualitative study. *CMAJ Open*, *9*(4). https://doi.org/10.9778/cmajo.20210090

Slaughter-Acey, J. C., Sealy-Jefferson, S., Helmkamp, L., Caldwell, C. H., Osypuk, T. L., Platt, R. W., Straughen, J. K., Dailey-Okezie, R. K., Abeysekara, P., & Misra, D. P. (2016). Racism in the form of micro aggressions and the risk of preterm birth among black women. *Annals of Epidemiology*, *26*(1), 7–13.e1. https://doi.org/10.1016/j.annepidem.2015.10.005

Sonneville, K. R., & Lipson, S. K. (2018). Disparities in eating disorder diagnosis and treatment according to weight status, race/ethnicity, socioeconomic background, and sex among college students. *International Journal of Eating Disorders*, *51*(6), 518–526. https://doi.org/10.1002/eat.22846

Spoorthy, M. S., Pratapa, S. K., & Mahant, S. (2020). Mental health problems faced by healthcare workers due to the COVID-19 pandemic–A Review. *Asian Journal of Psychiatry*, *51*, 102119. https://doi.org/10.1016/j.ajp.2020.102119

Sue, D. W., Capodilupo, C. M., Torino, G. C., Bucceri, J. M., Holder, A. M., Nadal, K. L., & Esquilin, M. (2007). Racial microaggressions in everyday life: Implications for clinical practice. *The American Psychologist*, *62*(4), 271–286. https://doi.org/10.1037/0003-066X.62.4.271

Torres, M. B., Salles, A., & Cochran, A. (2019). Recognizing and Reacting to Microaggressions in Medicine and Surgery. *JAMA Surgery*, *154*(9), 868–872. https://doi.org/10.1001/jamasurg.2019.1648

Tran, A. (2020, May 22). Hero and villain: An Asian American doctor's perspective on being viewed as the solution and the problem. *The Hill.* https://thehill.com/changing-america/opinion/499156-hero-and-villain-an-asian-american-doctors-perspective-on-being

USDJ. (2022). *2020 FBI Hate Crimes Statistics*. The United States Department of Justice. https://www.justice.gov/crs/highlights/2020-hate-crimes-statistics

Vyas, D. A., Eisenstein, L. G., & Jones, D. S. (2020). Hidden in Plain Sight - Reconsidering the Use of Race Correction in Clinical Algorithms. *The New England Journal of Medicine*, *383*(9), 874–882. https://doi.org/10.1056/NEJMms2004740

Walker, A. (2020, May 3). News outlets contribute to anti-Asian racism with careless stock photos on coronavirus coverage. *Media Matters for America*. https://www.mediamatters.org/coronavirus-covid-19/news-outlets-contribute-anti-asian-racism-careless-stock-photos-coronavirus

Yousuf, Y., & Yu, J. C. (2021). Improving Representation of Skin of Color in a Medical School Pre-clerkship Dermatology Curriculum. *Medical Science Educator*, *32*(1), 27–30. https://doi.org/10.1007/s40670-021-01473-x

ENDNOTE

1 Disclaimer: This chapter took part in the double-blind peer review process and was not compromised due to the authors also being an editor. A non-author editor managed all of the editorial aspects of the chapter.

Chapter 6
Cultural Competency by and for the Healthcare Professional

Gabriella Dauer
Nova Southeastern University Dr. Kiran C. Patel College of Allopathic Medicine, USA

Thura Al-Khayat
Nova Southeastern University Dr. Kiran C. Patel College of Allopathic Medicine, USA

EXECUTIVE SUMMARY

Healthcare and cultural competency are intimately intertwined concepts. Understanding how to provide the latter when caring for patients translates to better care. Transitioning between cultures and overcoming linguistic barriers can be challenging for healthcare workers. Differences in cultural norms can often be the cause of irritation and discontent for both patients and healthcare professionals, impeding the ease with which we are able to communicate and connect with our patients. Insufficient education and training on culturally competent care for patients renders our healthcare team unprepared for the challenges faced when practicing in culturally diverse clinical environments. In this chapter, the authors will explore how medical interpretation is vital to the care of patients with limited English-speaking proficiency (LEP), how healthcare professional's beliefs can affect their practice, and how to navigate working with healthcare professionals of various cultural backgrounds.

INTRODUCTION

Cultural competency encompasses working with and taking care of persons from various cultural backgrounds with respect to personal characteristics from race and ethnicity to education and financial status. Caring for persons of different backgrounds can be challenging for healthcare professionals without appropriate education, training, and exposure. Specific vulnerable populations we will address include patients with limited English proficiency (LEP), patients or providers with religious or spiritual beliefs other than our own, and providers or colleagues with foreign medical training.

DOI: 10.4018/978-1-6684-5493-0.ch006

The US Department of Health and Human Services predicts that as much as 10% of our patient population identifies as having LEP, prompting executive orders and other legal modalities to improve medical provider accountability in providing equal access and services to people with LEP. LEP as a definition accounts for persons with a non-English primary language who has any level of difficulty with communication, verbal and/or non-verbal, in the English language. However, medical interpretation is underutilized within the American healthcare system with limited clinician time and limited access to interpreter services identified as barriers to providing equal access and care. Furthermore, providers note preferentially utilizing video and telephone interpretation services-modalities that hold their own set of barriers in lacking non-verbal cues and communication (Hsieh, 2015). Prioritization of appropriate care of this vulnerable population with additional socio-economical stressors and burdening social determinants of health should further encourage medical providers to appropriately provide and utilize interpretation services to improve healthcare outcomes (Fischer, 2021).

Another contentious case of cultural acceptance and understanding lies within the realm of religious and spiritual belief differences. These differences can affect provider care practices depending on their state of practice. A stark example of provider religious beliefs affecting practice dates back to the 1973 case of Roe vs Wade where the Supreme Court established ruling against a women's right to abortion. In the case, a medical provider refused a Texan woman's request for aborting an unwanted pregnancy as it was deemed to not 'endanger' her life. In light of this case, the 'conscious clauses' were enacted giving healthcare providers the right to refuse to perform or assist in non-therapeutic abortions based on religious and moral objections. This eventually expanded to include various types of services in addition to abortion and broadened to include pharmacists as "indirect" providers of care (Martha, 2006). Legal support and mandating of medical provider practice variance with respect to their own cultural belief systems has and continues to affect our most vulnerable patient populations.

Finally, working with our diverse pool of healthcare professional colleagues can pose cross-cultural challenges. The National Resident Matching Program (NRMP) notes a continuous rise in the number of international and foreign graduates applying for work in the United States (US). In 2022, the rate of non-US International Medical Graduates (IMG) that matched into residency programs was 58.1%, up 3.3% from 2021, with studies from New York University estimating that 5.6 to 16 percent of our country's more than 3 million nurses were educated in another country. Despite many studies identifying internationally trained healthcare professionals as more resilient with an eagerness to learn, a lack of understanding and acceptance of provider communication skill and cultural differences persists (Gozu, 2009). Understanding provider and colleague differences is essential to achieving a team approach when working with persons from various backgrounds. Studies on cultural education and training for both foreign and native trained graduates have shown positive results with respect to reduction in transitional stress of a foreign medical graduate working in a new system, and acceptance and tolerance by native trainees (Porter, 2008). Such educational initiatives show just how cultural training and exposure can influence acceptance.

CASE 1: "HOLA DOCTORA, HABLA ESPAÑOL?"

Goal

To identify and describe vulnerability of non-English speaking patients in the primarily English-speaking American healthcare system.

Learning Outcomes

1. Identify the reasons why patients and families with limited English proficiency are a vulnerable patient population in Westernized medical systems and explain the importance of appropriate interpretation services for all encounters in this patient population.
2. Recognize that medical providers have a professional, ethical, and legal obligation to provide and utilize appropriate interpretation services with patients and families with LEP.
3. Identify that culturally competent care of the LEP patient population can improve healthcare outcomes.
4. Discuss how immigration and legal status can contribute to fear and distrust of the healthcare system in vulnerable populations such as patients with LEP.

Case

Marco is a 7-year-old boy admitted to the Pediatric Hospitalist service on an inpatient floor with Kawasaki disease. He has received appropriate treatment with aspirin and intravenous immunoglobulin (IVIG), but continues to have fever two days after therapy. With that in mind, secondary evidence-based therapies such as a repeat dose of IVIG are initiated. Marco continued to have fever and is classified as having refractory Kawasaki. On hospital day 4, he is on intravenous fluids for poor oral intake and daily aspirin and is being consulted upon by Pediatric Cardiology.

Marco and his father recently emigrated from Mexico. Marco's mother passed away in Mexico when Marco was a young child; no additional details were provided. Marco speaks some conversational English, but Marco's father is proficient in Spanish with limited understanding of the English spoken or written language. Upon rounding on Marco, the medical team consistently uses interpreter services for all interactions.

On the afternoon of hospital day 4, the pediatric nurse caring for Marco sees an attending from the Pediatric Hematology team entering his room and speaking extensively with the family. The Hematologist leaves the room and lets the nurse know that the patient has consented to take part in a study and will shortly be receiving a medication as part of a novel drug use trial. The nurse looks up the medication and sees that it is a medication commonly used in patients with liver disease but has not been approved for use in Kawasaki. The nurse also notes that there was no interpreter used for the conversation held between the physician and Marco and his father, and so calls the Pediatric Hospitalist for confirmation and further discussion.

After several conversations, the nurse and Pediatric Hospitalist address this with the Hematologist. It is elicited that in fact no interpreter was used, and the Hematologist has minimal working proficiency in Spanish and attempted to have this discourse with the child who himself does speak some English. The family was approached by the team and an interpreter was called to discuss consent as the patient's initial consent was inappropriately obtained. The father expressed minimal understanding of the drug and its' use for his son, does not understand that this is part of a novel trial, and is appropriately concerned about consenting for his son to participate in the trial. The father and son report that they were under the impression that the medication would help Marco feel better. The father is now refusing the novel medication to be trialed on his son and revokes consent for participation in the study. He angrily asks the Hematologist to leave the room and wants to speak to someone about the incident.

The team leaves the room, and the Hematologist mutters some words to the Hospitalist and nurse regarding 'how hard it is to enroll patients into this study as is' and how they had 'cost one less candidate to a study that could help other kids.' The team contacts the international review board (IRB) to report this incident, and appropriate educational action is arranged for the Hematologist, with patient relations support for the family.

QUESTIONS AND ANSWERS

1. Describe the benefits of appropriately utilizing medical interpretation services. In contrast, discuss the potential pitfalls, which could result from the misuse or nonuse of interpretation services in various clinical settings.

Benefits to appropriate use of interpretation services include decreasing adverse outcomes, improving adherence, and increasing patient satisfaction. Problems arising from lack of appropriate interpretation service use include but are not limited to lack of informed consent, avoidance of healthcare providers and the healthcare system, and aggression and anger, amongst other negative outcomes (Unger, 2014).

You can imagine the scenario of presenting to an emergency room or urgent care in a foreign country where the spoken language is not a language you are proficient in or one that is not your first language. The normal feelings of fear and despair often felt by patients experiencing an acute illness are now amplified by the additional hurdle of having to attempt communication regarding your condition in an unfamiliar language. This scenario can ensue with broken communication and a game of charades to come to a sense of a possible diagnosis; or could be mitigated by interpretation services and give you a sense of calm and comfort.

2. Use this case example to describe how immigrant populations and patients with LEP are innately vulnerable.

Immigrant populations and those with LEP have borne centuries of second-class care and negligence from the medical community. Historically practiced culturally incompetent care has sparked fear and distrust in our most vulnerable populations. Patients with LEP have multiple socioeconomic stressors when compared to their non-LEP counterparts and their concerns with payment and navigating the healthcare setting vary in etiology.

Consider social determinants of health, economic and psychosocial, that are more likely linked to the health disparities presenting in immigrant populations. Health professionals hold internal biases and one assumption that can be amplified in persons with LEP is in how we communicate patient education and shared decision making on healthcare plans (Green, 2017). In comparison to a patient with English as their first language who may be more likely to be viewed by providers as a partner in the patient's healthcare in making informed decisions and may be given appropriate patient education on their diagnoses, a person with LEP may be biased against and seen as 'less capable of understanding' these 'complex' conversations and not given the opportunity to partake in them. However, facilitation of these conversations via the use of interpreter services would render these biases insufficient as practitioners would recognize that the underlying misunderstanding is from a language barrier and not an intellectual barrier.

3. Identify and describe when to use interpretation services in the healthcare settings, identifying scenarios of medical and procedural consent to be prioritized.

Any medical encounter involving a healthcare provider who cannot fluently communicate in the same language as their patient should utilize interpretation services for every such encounter. This means that health care professionals who have working proficiency in a specific language should demonstrate medical working proficiency, not colloquial proficiency, in that language if they decide to not utilize interpretation services. Interpretation must be utilized for any medication or procedure when caring for patients with LEP. Healthcare areas of especially high contention include consent for any voluntary research study participation. In addition, interpretation should always be utilized in vulnerable scenarios such as when a minor is offered to interpret for a family member and for consent and explanation of physical examination of genitalia and/or rectal or pelvic exam in patients with LEP. Incorporation of minors into the interpretation process for their family members has led to medical legal complications and implications as a two-fold concern where the person interpreting is usually not an adult, and usually not able to understand the true etiology of consent.

Consider scenarios in your respective fields that would be deemed sensitive and especially require clear documentation of interpretation service use; for example, the placing of physical restraints on a patient with LEP by nursing without interpretation services to explain the process.

4. Discuss potential motives from the hematologists' perspective for NOT eliciting interpretation services.

Demands on the 21st century healthcare provider have limited the time available to spend with patients at the bedside and widened providers' attention to include finance, business, and production in medicine. Physicians and healthcare providers are working long hours and are often spending more time with technological 'advancements' such as the electronic health record than with their patients (Hsieh, 2015). External and internal stressors placed on the medical team express themselves through shortcomings such as in this case where a faster course of action was attempted to save time or to enroll yet another patient in institution-financed study. The physician may not have thought that she was directly harming the patient, but her 'cutting of corners' distracted the entire team from focusing on the child's care and on an irrelevant research study.

Discuss the emotions elicited in this case. Imagine the father's perspective-was his anger and dismay at the hematologist appropriate? Discuss also how witnessing and partaking in this situation could potentially affect the child's view of the healthcare system.

A parent or caregiver accompanying a hospitalized child or family member will have heightened awareness and responses to any scenario regarding their significant other's care. Patient and family mistrust and frustration with medical professionals have become familiar stressors to providers to a point of desensitization. In this case, the father's frustration should be viewed as a responsible and reflexive response to the egregious action of a physician-led decision to consent a LEP family without interpretation. In this scenario where a family member or patient displays emotions of anger or dismay with the medical team, patient representative services should be called immediately to rectify the situation.

5. Discuss the responsibilities of the bystanders to redirect the course of the event and report the event. How should team members respond in such an event?

In medicine, it is often best to address situations firsthand with your colleague in a non-confrontational manner. For anyone uncomfortable doing so, every hospital and healthcare workplace has a process of escalation for concerns of this nature. Any of the members of the healthcare team, or the patient and family/caregiver, can escalate concerns to their superiors or to patient support services. The nurse who witnessed such consent taken without interpretation appropriately reached out to the attending of service but could have also contacted her nursing supervisor or charge nurse to address potential next steps. If she wanted to remain anonymous, she could have contacted the IRB herself to report a claim as institutional and university review boards accept anonymous reports of research misconduct. The resident team and hospitalist could have escalated the concern to the residency program director or chief resident, and hospitalist medical directors respectively. This reflects that any healthcare professional who is part of the patient care process should feel comfortable interjecting into the scenario if they feel the patient may be in direct harm or escalating the case to their supervisors if time is allotted.

Epilogue

Cultural competency in appropriate care for patients with limited English proficiency is essential to assure better healthcare outcomes for this vulnerable population. Providing and utilizing interpreter services for such patients in all scenarios is an extremely important concept for all healthcare professionals, especially in highly contentious scenarios such as consent for research participation of a child. However, instances like our case prove these interactions as commonplace in our healthcare system. An analogous situation as recanted by Dr. Tonkin, a resident psychiatrist consulted on a non-English speaking patient for assumption of noncompliance to cancer therapies, highlighted this mislabeling of a patient as 'combative and refusing care,' when in fact the patient was coping with misunderstandings of her healthcare team because of a language barrier (Tonkin, 2017). Dr. Tonkin speaks on how resolution of a critical patient care scenario was mediated with appropriate communication in the patient's language.

This case further depicts how potential stressors and pressures of a clinician can result in errors such as consenting an ill, LEP child into a study without using interpreter services and without appropriate engagement with his father as legal guardian. This misstep then leads to a complex situation where other healthcare providers attempt to rectify patient trust, and anger and distrust from the family with regards to appropriate care by the medical team. This case scenario highlights the need for medical interpretation and culturally competent care provided from all parties of the medical team. In this case, discrimination towards and vulnerabilities of patients and families with limited English proficiency was exemplified through a scenario in which consent is obtained without appropriate interpretation and understanding. As a result of this interaction taking place without proper interpretation services, several parties of the medical team became emotionally and intimately involved in correcting the process, while the patient and his father eventually and unfortunately lost trust in their medical providers.

CASE 2: A DISPENSING DILEMMA

Goal

Increase awareness of health professions educators on laws and regulations of Pharmacist right to refuse dispensing of prescribed medications in lieu of personal beliefs, morals, and experiences.

Learning Outcomes

1. Recognize the circumstances during which health professionals may refuse provision of patient care.
2. Define Pharmacist Conscience Clauses that give pharmacists the right to refuse to perform certain services if it violates their religious or personal beliefs or values.
3. Discuss state clauses for healthcare providers to refuse to provide care related to family planning for religious or medical reasons.
4. Discuss women's reproductive health rights with respect to the healthcare provider's 'Right to Not Dispense'.
5. Explore factors that may shape a health professional's decision to dispense a medication, such as religious beliefs.

Case

You are a primary care provider in a busy clinic, and you receive a call from your front desk administrator noting that your patient has arrived without an appointment and is requesting to see you urgently; the patient is visibly upset with tears. You review your schedule and agree to see the patient as your review of her most recent visit elicits that her last visit with you was regarding an early unwanted pregnancy. You note that she was 7 weeks pregnant and for personal reasons had decided not to continue with the pregnancy. She had visited you for advice on next steps at which time she was provided detailed and careful counselling and referred to an OBGYN (Obstetrics and Gynecology) specialist who counselled her and provided her with options to terminate the pregnancy. The patient decided to take the abortion pill. She was given Mifepristone in the specialist's office and was provided a prescription for Misoprostol with instructions on how to administer the medicine, and when to return for a follow-up visit.

Today, your patient has returned and seems upset upon entering your exam room. She reports that the following interactions had taken place upon presenting to the pharmacy to pick up her prescription: The patient presented to the pharmacy and approached the desk with her prescription requesting to pick up her prescribed medication. She handed her prescription to the pharmacist who scrolled his eyes carefully over the Misoprostol script. The pharmacist then sighed and noted that he would be back in a few minutes and for the patient to have a seat.

After 15 minutes of patiently waiting, the patient stood up and requested that the pharmacy technician provide the medication so she could get to work on time. The technician leaves the counter to request the pharmacist return to speak with the patient.

The pharmacist begrudgingly returns to the front desk and reports that they will not be able to dispense this medication. Upon the patient prompting the pharmacist as to why they cannot do so, the pharmacist blurts out that this was not what they 'signed up for' and asks the patient how far along in the pregnancy she is. The patient notes that she is 7 weeks pregnant. The pharmacist further pries into the patient's personal medical history and now asks her to clarify if she would like to 'end the life of the baby growing inside of her?'

The patient shockingly steps back from the counter and is embarrassed by the tone and nature of the questioning, especially as the patrons beside her begin to look over at this awkward interaction. The patient again approaches the pharmacist and quietly asks them to dispense the medication as she and her provider already discussed the risks and benefits of this medication and the effects; understanding fully her entitled rights to end an unwanted pregnancy.

The pharmacist looks at the patient who is now saddened by this interaction and apologizes. The pharmacist further notes that they cannot dispense this medication as it would end the life of the unborn child, which already carries a heartbeat, and that within the pharmacist's cultural and religious beliefs, that is equivalent to ending the life of a child. Therefore, the pharmacist again declines to dispense the medication. The patient pleads for another provider to dispense the medication instead, but the second pharmacist in the practice is on leave. The pharmacist offers for her to return the next week when the other provider would return as they may have a different 'ethical code' and feel more comfortable in providing the medication. The patient is not provided with an alternative and would like this 'to be over as soon as possible,' yet leaves the store without the medication in hand.

Upon review of this scenario with your patient, you apologize for the stressful scenario she just endured at the pharmacy. You call another pharmacy in the area that takes her insurance and speak with the pharmacist directly to assure that the medication is readily available and that there will be no issues in dispensing the medication to the patient later this afternoon. You document the interaction in your note and your patient leaves your office relieved to be able to move forward with her decision to end her unwanted pregnancy.

QUESTIONS AND ANSWERS

1. Discuss the pharmacist's point of view. Was he right to refuse to dispense? Is there legal support for his actions?

The Pharmacist Conscience Clauses, a general set of statements pertinent to a Pharmacists' oath, grant pharmacists the right to refuse any service that violates their religious and/or personal beliefs or values. In the state of Florida however, the refusal laws have been generalized to all healthcare providers, therefore permitting a pharmacists' dispensing decisions to be made based on their personal religious beliefs and morals. In this case, the pharmacist could refrain from expressing their personal beliefs and imposing them on the patient. Asking her if she would like to 'end the life of the baby growing inside of her' was not professional behavior.

Actual national pharmacist practices may differ from our case as noted by a public code of ethics published by the association of pharmacists (ASHP) which further supports patient autonomy as follows:

"A pharmacist respects the autonomy and dignity of each patient...A pharmacist promotes the right of self-determination and recognizes individual self-worth by encouraging patients to participate in decisions about their health...In all cases, a pharmacist respects personal and cultural differences among patients."

2. Discuss the pharmacist's actions and behaviors with respect to facilitating care for the patient. Were they legally and medically appropriate?

The Pharmacist in this case chose to exercise his right to refuse to dispense Misoprostol on ethical bases even after the patient presented him a prescription from an OBGYN. The patient was presented with the option to "come back next week" when another pharmacist would be available who may have different ethics and beliefs. The patient had received Mifepristone and needed to take Misoprostol within the next 48 hours for the medicine to have its' full effect. Time was of essence. Therefore, the option she was provided with was not appropriate. A more appropriate solution would have been to delegate care to a nearby pharmacy, ensuring that another pharmacist(s) was available to dispense Misoprostol to the patient in need. Many states legally mandate providers to either perform essential healthcare acts themselves or to delegate them to another equal healthcare provider if the initial provider feels they are unable to carry out the request. It is important to understand such laws for your respective fields for the states which within you plan to practice.

3. Discuss the patient's position in this case. What might she have done in a situation like this to self-advocate?

According to the Planned Parenthood Federation of America, 1 in 4 women younger than 45 decide to have an abortion. This decision can be simple or can be complex and extremely difficult as many women might feel guilt or shame and are in fear of being criticized and judged for their decisions. Therefore, it is imperative that patients are extensively counseled regarding the decision to abort. This would include discussing in depth the reasons behind their decisions, providing and alternative options, and weighing the pros and cons of their choice. Nevertheless, and despite this vigorous process, women still shy away if they feel judged. In this case there is no wrong or right way for the patient to handle the situation. One option would be to persist and ask for the medicine to be dispensed despite the pharmacist's refusal. Another one would be to try a different pharmacy. This patient felt she had no choice but to visit her primary care physician without an appointment in hopes that they would assist in solving the issue.

4. How might the case plot differ if the patient was an adolescent?

Adolescents generally have limited decision-making rights when it comes to healthcare. However, in certain instances such as for a mature adolescent or emancipated minor, adolescents are allowed to give consent without their parents. The case of *Bellotti v. Baird* ruled that minors are able to have abortions without parental consent; however, the state can ask the court to authorize the capacity of the minor to do so. Therefore, an emancipated minor has the right to choose to have an abortion and does not need parental or court consent. In states that allow this legal plan of action, pharmacists may dispense the abortion pill if the emancipated minor provides a physician's prescription. If they chose not to do so, as in the case above, they are to follow their state's law when it comes to delegating care.

5. Think about the primary care physician's position. What could their course of action be with respect to the returning patient?

Depending on various state laws, a primary care physician has the right to refuse care if it contradicts with their personal ethical, religious, or moral beliefs. In this case the physician did not object to help solve the issue for the patient. The patient was aware of this, as this physician was the one who referred her to the OBGYN specialist and had seemed understanding and accepting of her decision. A major factor in timely response to such patient requests and issues are of physician availability and schedules. The physician in this case realized the urgency and timing of the situation at hand and was able to take the time to call another pharmacy in the area that takes her insurance and speak with the pharmacist directly to assure that the medication would be dispensed.

6. Discuss how various cultures and/or religions approach abortion as a choice?

Various cultures and religions have different views when it comes to legalization of abortion. Buddhism, Evangelical Lutheran Church in America, Unitarian Universalist Association, Episcopal Church, the United Church of Christ, and the Presbyterian Church of USA are examples of religions with official positions supporting the right of a woman to decide to terminate a pregnancy.

Some religious groups who consider abortion as unacceptable include the Assemblies of God, Greek Orthodox, Hinduism, Islam, Jehovah's Witnesses, Southern Baptist Convention, and the Catholic Church. Many religious groups often have no clear or external broad views on the topic and these include the Church of Jesus Christ of Latter-Day Saints, Judaism, National Baptist Convention, Seventh-Day Adventist Church, and the United Methodist Church.

7. Let's say that a bystander such as a pharmacy technician witnesses this discourse. How might they approach the pharmacist in addressing this scenario?

The pharmacy technician's primary role as a bystander would be to ensure that pharmacy protocols, procedures, and laws are not bypassed. One approach to intervene might be to approach the pharmacist immediately and privately to remind them that regardless of personal beliefs, this specific medication needs to be dispensed in a timely manner and that an alternative option should be provided to the patient. If they are unable to do so or if they are faced with resistance, the pharmacy technician may report the incident up their hierarchical ladder to ensure policy is accurately followed and that the patient is either provided with the medication or referred to another pharmacy for continued care.

8. Identify points of difficulty in the clinical scenario that could be refined and improved upon to create a more seamless process for the patient requesting an abortive medication to end her unwanted pregnancy?

Patients often seek initial abortive methods without prescription before asking for physician assistance. These methods can include using the 'morning after pill' from their local pharmacies, or attempting less supported and more natural methods such as using pineapple, papaya, cohosh, etc. Some women may opt to eventually seek abortions via unsafe practices when abortion is illegal in their states. Studies report that as high as 4-13% of maternal deaths occur each year from complications of unsafe abortions (Say, 2014). After a specific point of conception, the morning after pill and natural methods of abortion are non-functional, requiring a physician to prescribe either an oral or vaginal medication for abortive purposes. These prescriptions vary by state as to who can prescribe and dispense these medications; government funded clinics such as planned parenthood versus a subspecialist such as an OBGYN. In the case above, the patient may live in a state that requires a specialist to provide abortive services, rendering her primary care physician incapable of prescribing such medications. The need for her primary care physician to refer her to an OBGYN adds a level of complexity and another provider to the situation. Legislative change and improved general physician education on abortive methods, risks and benefits would have prevented an additional physician visit for this patient. Also, a pharmacy with dispensing ability of an available medication often has the right to refuse dispensing a medication based on a pharmacist's personal beliefs. However, that pharmacist may need to legally provide an immediate option for patient retrieval of the medication to not delay the process of ending an unwanted pregnancy which could result in requiring a surgical dilation and curettage for some pregnancies further alone than the first trimester. In providing an immediate alternative, the patient would have received her medication and would not have visited her primary care physician to amend the situation. Educating health professionals on their rights but also on ways to mitigate their personal and religious beliefs to deliver highest level of credible care is necessary.

9. Discuss other potential scenarios within your respective fields of study (nursing, physical therapy, optometry, among others) where a similar discussion could ensue regarding personal beliefs and morals directly affecting patient care.

Healthcare workers from all fields have ethical responsibilities towards their patients. They should do no harm (non-maleficence), always act within the best interest of the patient (beneficence), respect patient rights to make their own decisions (autonomy), and practice (justice) when deciding who receives what treatment. With that in mind, religious beliefs and morals can often cause disagreements between healthcare workers and their patients and can in some states legally direct healthcare professionals' practice. For example, in some states, a nurse who identifies as "prolife" may refuse to administer Mifepristone to a patient. State laws vary between granting or denying healthcare workers the right to refuse care and the conversation is ongoing. Ideally, in keeping the concepts of medical ethics in mind, healthcare workers have a professional obligation to avoid abandoning patients and should delegate care to another professional when their personal beliefs prevent them from caring for patients themselves.

Epilogue

This case discusses women's reproductive health rights with respect to the pharmacists' rights in refusing to dispense a specific prescribed medication to facilitate an abortion. The case reviews the rights pharmacists have when it comes to dispensing medications and exemplifies difficulties in doing so when personal beliefs may affect moral obligations to patients. Scenarios related to family planning offer the most difficult conversations as pharmacists are to dispense oral contraceptive pills or the abortion pill. Mifepristone is a medication commonly utilized to achieve early abortive effects by reducing the level of progesterone hormone needed to maintain healthy pregnancy growth. In combination with Misoprostol, which has a similar effect by causing the uterus to contract and eventually empty its contents, together they form the abortion pill that has been approved by the FDA to be used within 49 days of the last menstrual period. Mifepristone is given first, and Misoprostol is administered anytime within the next 48 hours. In this process, many providers play key roles from the primary care physician who can prescribe the medication or refer out to another provider or specialist, to the pharmacist who ultimately dispenses the medication. This last interaction is the key to the successful attainment of the medication, but each can be complicated when personal beliefs are involved.

Healthcare workers personal morals and religious beliefs often impede optimum patient care. In this case, a patient who has decided to have an abortion was seen and counselled on abortive options by her OBGYN. She proceeds with taking Mifepristone but then has to obtain the second component of the abortion pill from the pharmacy within 48 hours. However, when she went to pick up her medication the pharmacist refused dispense it to her based on personal beliefs and morals. The pharmacist chose to exercise their right based on the Pharmacist Conscience Clauses that grants pharmacists the right to refuse any service that violates their religious and/or personal beliefs or values. However, the pharmacist did not maintain patient protection by delegating care to someone else. A more appropriate solution would have been to delegate care to another pharmacy or provider. Ideally, healthcare workers should refrain from imposing their personal beliefs on patient care courses and keep the four components of medical ethics in mind when caring for patients.

CASE 3: MEDICINE BEYOND BORDERS

Goal

To increase awareness of the commonplace cultural educational biases in medicine as demonstrated by interprofessional colleagues.

Learning Outcomes

1. Recognize that more training on culturally competent interprofessional interactions is needed within medical education, specifically with respect to education and degrees received by our foreign medical graduate colleagues.
2. Identify how to address biases with relation to interprofessional colleagues with training and education from a culture or educational path different than what is experienced and taught in westernized medicine.
3. Understand that cultural competency with respect to the workplace translates to better care for patients, especially those who self-identify culturally and racially to their medical team.

Case

Upon entering a busy dental clinic in South Florida, Alana is greeted with familiar faces as she is a long-time patient of Dr. C.

Front desk administrator: "Here to get your annual check-up Alana?"

Alana responds in her practiced Spanish: "Si! Tu sabe, me gusta visitar con mi dentisto favorito," (Yes! You know, I love coming to see my favorite dentist), Alana exclaims in her practiced Spanish which she learned in grade school.

Alana is seated in the waiting room and is called upon by a new dental hygienist whom she has not met, Casey.

Casey: "Patient Alana Morris?"

Alana briskly stands, smiles, and moves to follow Casey into the patient room. Upon entering the room, Alana and Casey begin to chat about Alana's busy work schedule as a new ICU nurse. Casey also reveals the difficulties of working in a busy clinic as she also just graduated. After some small talk to establish rapport, Casey preps Alana for her cleaning and begins to express some concerns that sit uneasily with Alana.

Casey: "You know, it's been so hard working here. I'm from the area, so I get it- everyone speaks Spanish and a lot of the patients do too. But it is SO hard to understand Dr. C with his thick accent. He means well, but I truly don't know half of what he asks of me, so I feel like I am always prepping the wrong patient tools for him!"

Alana smiles and nods to these seemingly harmless comments as her teeth cleaning is underway.

Casey: "I have to tell you, there was even a time last week when he asked me to prep some solution for a cavity filling and I could swear this was something he concocted while practicing in Cuba because it is NOT standard of care here. I hope I don't have to learn Cuban dental medicine practices because then this would really be impossible!"

Alana gives no response to perpetuate the conversation. She is now sensing the trend of dismay in Casey's tone and comments and is disappointed and uncomfortable by them. The continuation of a one-sided dialogue persists as Alana cannot respond during the cleaning.

Casey: "Anyways, so I prep the solution and go on with my day thinking maybe I didn't hear him right with that accent. But it's really not going to work for me if that continues. I may have to tag along with the other practice partner Dr. P. People love Dr. P! No accent, easy to understand, communicates well. We even had a patient yesterday who asked me if he could see the 'American' dentist in the practice after meeting Dr. C and not being able to decipher his thick Cuban accent, and I don't blame him!"

Alana holds her palm up to prompt Casey to stop the cleaning. She sits up and is saddened by the negative comments made. Alana asks to be excused and steps out of the hygienist's room. She is uncomfortable with the situation and unsure of what her next steps should be.

QUESTIONS AND ANSWERS

1. Elaborate on how cultural competency between providers can enhance healthcare practices and patient care delivery.

Education and training in cultural competency and acceptance of the experiences and education of health professions colleagues can enhance the workplace in many ways. Any tension that arises within a workplace, regardless of etiology, can be palpable to the patient population and negatively affect the potential of the practice to thrive financially and reputably. Furthermore, if racist or culturally incompetent remarks are made to patients with respect to either colleagues or other patients' cultures, ethnicities, language ability, or backgrounds, these can lend themselves to litigation for the provider if a patient decides to sue based on receiving care differences secondary to racial or ethnic bias. Respecting and welcoming all educational and cultural practices creates a community within a healthcare practice and system of a growth mindset where all providers are willing to learn from their colleagues; this environment of positivity then transcends to the patient experience. Positive outcomes with respect to patient satisfaction and patient healthcare have been well studied and documented as a result.

2. Discuss how the comments made by Casey can be harmful to the dental practice and to patient care, and how they perpetuate xenophobia.

Comments with relation to a colleague's cultural or educational background can be offensive to many and can especially land on a patient's ears who identifies in a similar line with the foreign colleague. Casey would cause serious harm to the trust this patient has in Casey and in the practice. Moreso, personal feelings and comments with respect to how one is coping with their new workplace, especially in terms of cultural or ethnic differences, should not be placed upon the patient and should be discussed with colleagues so as to focus on the patient's illness entirely. This type of commentary can be overheard by other patients and can damage the reputation of the practice if people were to infer that other like-minded individuals may be working at this healthcare facility. These remarks can even be quoted in reviews of the practice and seen by other patrons seeking care, which could diminish monetary gain and respect for the practice. Also, many healthcare professionals are highly regarded and respected by patients as educated and esteemed members of society. Holding ourselves to the highest standards and modeling inclusive language is imperative as spewing racist or culturally competent remarks can perpetuate xenophobia.

3. How would you respond to another provider making such statements about a colleague with cultural practices and linguistic abilities different than their own? Think about foreign medical graduates who often obtain degrees from their home countries and institutions and then become board certified in other countries for practice.

There are many ways to respond as a patient or as a provider who witnesses indirectly or directly such actions or words. An example of an appropriate direct response to the person initiating the conversation would be to note that this is a professional workplace and this type of jargon with the patient is unprofessional and may be considered unethical and such issues should be taken back to a person of charge or hierarchy within the practice if they are cause for concern. A sample statement from the patient could look as follows: 'I'm sorry, but I am feel uncomfortable with some of your statements and I believe they are not part of the care process for my visit. Can we please proceed without the discussion of your personal feelings and beliefs regarding your colleagues? Thank you.' A similar statement could come from a colleague. An actionable statement from a colleague who hears these statements could look as follows: 'Casey, some of your statements are unprofessional, judgmental, and seem to be arising from cultural differences between yourself and Dr. C. I suggest you bring this up to your boss or Dr. C if they are causing barriers to your general patient care delivery.'

4. If you encountered a patient requesting an 'American doctor' similar to the example in the case, how could you mitigate this request?

Many times, physicians or other healthcare professionals are caught in the crossfire between a patient and their healthcare provider with respect to cultural or ethnical differences. An appropriate way to respond to a patient who is unhappy with their current care and requesting a different care provider within your system is with kindness, confidence, and education-but with a clear stance for support of the healthcare professional. A statement as such may be appropriate; 'I understand you may not be satisfied with the current care situation. I assure you, all staff and faculty within the practice are capable and appropriately educated within their field. We ask that all employees be respected by patients regardless of gender, race, or ethnicity as per our hospital culture and policy." If the patient continues to escalate the conversation, one can recommend the patient speak with the patient care center for patient experience. Maintaining professionalism and not engaging with such statements from patients is the best course of action. As per a 2016 article in the Journal of Academic Medicine, a four step approach is recommended for physicians confronted with a patient's racism: 1) ignore such comments in an emergency; 2) focus the encounter on the shared goals of treatment; 3) depersonalize the event; and 4) foster a community of support within the hospital. (Whitgob, 2016)

5. Reflect on how this type of scenario can potentially be mitigated by addressing cultural competency in a standardized or educational manner.

Cultural competency of different educational backgrounds is necessary as every individual harbors with them their own beliefs based on their own life experiences and upbringing. Generalizing this education to health professions allows interprofessional understanding of the differences and similarities in training and education with respect to culture. Allowing space and time in the curriculum for students and educators to identify that they have biases and can learn from them, allows the field to move forward with an open mind. Education to all health professionals on how to handle such scenarios as above allows persons to approach similar instances with a preset of statements from which to respond so as to not have to come up with a response in real time.

6. Imagine that you are the provider for a patient with the following requests. Elaborate on how you would approach these various clinical scenarios with a mindset of clinical competency.

    a. You are a Dentist caring for a population who largely identifies as Haitian. Their cultural practices in chewing on chicken bones and cartilage has resulted in loss of tooth enamel for many of your patients. A dental hygienist passes by a patient room with such a patient case and remarks to another hygienist that 'she can't keep taking care of these people who keep chewing on bones and coming back with broken teeth.' How do you respond to such a passing comment?

A potential response of a bystander could be to address that cultural practices of various communities are deeply rooted in their history and that our job as healthcare professionals is not to judge and belittle these practices, but rather educate our patients on how these practices may be damaging to their oral health.

b. You are a physician in the hospital caring for a patient who has been diagnosed with encephalitis. Your patient is confused, altered, and mumbling to themselves. Your patient's parents strongly believe that their child has succumbed to 'the work of the devil' and they are requesting a bedside 'exorcism' to be executed by their Church members. How do you mitigate this patient request?

Many patients and families will look for answers to medical diagnoses in their faith or culture. If such a request is made, it would be appropriate to consult Pastoral services and the patient care coordinator to assess how the families' requests might be addressed in the hospital setting. Ignoring such a request could be harmful to the healing of the patient and the family.

c. You are a nurse caring for a patient in the hospital admitted for dehydration secondary to gastroenteritis. They identify as Hispanic and have been identified to have campylobacter on their stool culture as the etiology for their diarrheal illness. The patient does believe that their illness is from their process of butchering the chickens in their backyard as they eat from their own stock. The pharmacist releasing the antibiotic makes a statement about 'these Hispanic patients raising their own chickens and getting sick because of lack of hygiene.' How do you respond to your colleague regarding this statement?

A potential response to a statement such as this one could be to address the inappropriateness of the statement and recommend judgement of cultural practices be excluded from the care of this patient. It may be the norm for this patient and family to harvest their own food and education on best practices for handling raw meat would be a better approach in educating the family, rather patronizing them for their cultural practices.

Epilogue

Cultural competency has many definitions and takes many forms. It encompasses developing an understanding of the cultural practices and norms of those you serve and those you work with. Development of an intricate network of healthcare members entails hiring and working with people from backgrounds and cultures dissimilar to your own. This concoction of differences ultimately leads to the best care for the patient as it brings about medical decision making with a variety of cultural life experiences. Surface level acceptance of cultural practices of your patients as well as cultural backgrounds of your colleagues will not allow you to truly mitigate innate bias against that which we find different to what we know and learn; we must embrace these differences and understand them on a deeper level.

This case exemplifies the barriers to care that arise from potential incongruences between providers in a workplace. It follows a health care professional who is having difficulty assimilating to her new workplace with respect to the cultural practices of her colleague and boss who trained in a country outside of the United States. Her statements of dismay exemplify implicit and explicit bias towards persons of other cultural backgrounds and can potentially damage patient-provider trust and relationships as she is sharing such opinions and statements with a patient who is a close family friend of the colleague at hand.

We explored how a young nurse, Alana, encountered a difficult scenario at her routine annual dental check-up with her long-time Dentist Dr. Chavez (Dr. C). Alana grew up down the street from Dr. C and she was close friends with his two children. Dr. C was born and raised in Cuba, to which his deep accent can attest. Dr. C studied dental medicine in Cuba and practiced several years there before moving to the United States to seek better opportunities for his future family. His two children were born in Alana's small town and went to school with her. Dr. C is now a beloved and renowned Dentist in the community. On the morning of Alana's visit, she began to understand why openly addressing a person along with all that comes from their culture is so integral to every level of the healthcare system.

REFERENCES

Fischer, A., Conigliaro, J., Allicock, S., & Kim, E. J. (2021). Examination of social determinants of health among patients with limited English proficiency. *BMC Research Notes*, *14*(1), 299. doi:10.118613104-021-05720-7 PMID:34353369

Gozu, A., Kern, D. E., & Wright, S. M. (2009). Similarities and differences between international medical graduates and U.S. medical graduates at six Maryland community-based internal medicine residency training programs. *Academic Medicine*, *84*(3), 385–390. doi:10.1097/ACM.0b013e318197321b PMID:19240453

Green, A. R., & Nze, C. (2017). Language-Based Inequity in Health Care: Who Is the "Poor Historian"? *AMA Journal of Ethics*, *19*(3), 263–271. doi:10.1001/journalofethics.2017.19.3.medu1-1703 PMID:28323607

Hsieh, E. (2015). Not just "getting by": Factors influencing providers' choice of interpreters. *Journal of General Internal Medicine*, *30*(1), 75–82. doi:10.100711606-014-3066-8 PMID:25338731

Juckett, G., & Unger, K. (2014). Appropriate use of medical interpreters. *American Family Physician*, *90*(7), 476–480. PMID:25369625

Porter, J. L., Townley, T., Huggett, K., & Warrier, R. (2008). An acculturization curriculum: Orienting international medical graduates to an internal medicine residency program. *Teaching and Learning in Medicine*, *20*(1), 37–43. doi:10.1080/10401330701542644 PMID:18444184

Say, L., Chou, D., Gemmill, A., Tunçalp, Ö., Moller, A. B., Daniels, J., Gülmezoglu, A. M., Temmerman, M., & Alkema, L. (2014). Global causes of maternal death: A WHO systematic analysis. *The Lancet. Global Health*, *2*(6), e323–e333. doi:10.1016/S2214-109X(14)70227-X PMID:25103301

Swartz, M. S. (2006). "Conscience clauses" or "unconscionable clauses": Personal beliefs versus professional responsibilities. *Yale Journal of Health Policy, Law, and Ethics*, *6*(2), 269–350. PMID:17133969

Tonkin, E. (2017). *The Importance of Medical Interpreters*. The American Journal of Psychiatry Online Resident's Journal., doi:10.1176/appi.ajp-rj.2017.120806

Whitgob, E. E., Blankenburg, R. L., & Bogetz, A. L. (2016). The Discriminatory Patient and Family: Strategies to Address Discrimination Towards Trainees. *Academic medicine: journal of the Association of American Medical Colleges, 91*(11). 10.1097/ACM.0000000000001357

ENDNOTE

1 Acknowledgement: Dr. Samiksha Prasad contributed to the writing and research of this chapter. We acknowledge her contributions.

Chapter 7
Language Barriers in Healthcare

Jed Peter Mangal
https://orcid.org/0000-0002-7191-0090
Uniformed Services University of the Health Sciences, USA

Britney S. Farmer
Uniformed Services University of the Health Sciences, USA

EXECUTIVE SUMMARY

Communication errors in healthcare due to primary language discordance between patients and health-care staff are likely to increase in modern globalizing and linguistically diverse societies. In the existing literature, language barriers lead to miscommunications between healthcare professionals and patients, contributing to reduced satisfaction among both groups, decreased quality of care, and reduced patient safety. Language interpretation services are effective in improving care and are available in most large healthcare organizations, but may be absent in resource-limited settings and, when used, can increase the cost of care and the length of healthcare visits. Healthcare professionals may be tempted to forego interpreters in service of saving time; however, understanding the health impacts of suboptimal language and the ethical obligation of linguistic equity is central to providing competent healthcare.

BACKGROUND

Language barriers in healthcare occur when a clinician and a patient have a difference in fluency in their shared language. According to the 2020 United States Census, approximately 21.5% of respondents spoke a language other than English at home and 8.2% (increasing from an estimated 4.8% in 1980) of respondents reported speaking English less than "very well" (these patients can sometimes be labeled as having "Limited English Proficiency"; however, this moniker is controversial) (US Census Bureau, 2020). With an increasing number of patients reporting primary languages other than English and reduced English fluency accessing the US healthcare system, it is extremely important that healthcare staff are cognizant of the presence and impact of language barriers.

DOI: 10.4018/978-1-6684-5493-0.ch007

Effective patient-clinician communication is critical to quality healthcare delivery and the effects of language barriers have been well described to include a 50% increase in the likelihood of medical errors (such as misdiagnoses, medication errors, or adverse drug reactions) and increased risk of readmission (Al Shamsi et al., 2020; Cohen et al., 2005; de Bruijne et al., 2013; Stewart et al., 1995). Language barriers affect not only the quality of care but also increase the cost of providing care; for example, increased medical visit durations and increased health resource utilization have both been reported (Koff et al., 1999). Patients who were identified as having a language barrier also identified changes in the quality of care, reported poor satisfaction with care received, and reported barriers to seeking and receiving healthcare, with one study finding that 66.7% of these patients reported facing a barrier when accessing healthcare and 20% reported not seeking healthcare for fear of not understanding their healthcare provider (De Moissac et al., 2019; Wilson et al., 2005).

Efforts to determine the direct role of language barriers in safety events have been challenging due to frequent omissions from safety event reports (Benda et al., 2022). Additionally, several past studies have found inadequate detection, reporting, and attempts to bridge language barriers (Karliner et al., 2007). In part, this may result from a propensity of healthcare staff to overestimate a patient's English fluency, with studies estimating the misclassification of 25% of patients with a preferred language other than English as English preferring (Balakrishnan et al., 2016; Boscolo-Hightower et al., 2014). In a large survey study, medical providers reported trouble understanding patients that necessitated medical interpreter use in only 36% - 43% of patients who did not speak the same language as the provider (Kale et al., 2010).

The challenge of healthcare organizations to identify which patients may be most likely to benefit from language access services is a problem compounded by issues of access to interpretation. Although professional interpreters are considered the best strategy to address language barriers and are identified by the Institute of Medicine as both a quality measure and a patient safety imperative, 21% of medical providers in a large national study reported that poor access to interpreter services was the most common reason for not using an interpreter (Institute of Medicine., 2001; Kale et al., 2010). Nonprofessional or no medical interpretation was used often when language barriers were identified (estimated at 65% of encounters in one study) despite evidence that these practices increase medical errors (Flores et al., 2012). To address these gaps, in 2014 the Joint Commission International provided healthcare organizations with standards and guidance to address the presence of language barriers including stated instructions that 1. Patient education materials, follow-up instructions, and informed consent be given in a language the patient can understand; 2. Healthcare organizations should seek to reduce language barriers by offering competent language access services; and 3. Patients' preferred language to use when discussing healthcare should be collected and documented (Joint Commission, 2014). In 2016, section 1557 of the Affordable Care Act was officially adopted by the United States Department of Health and Human Services which included a legal requirement that healthcare providers must offer "qualified" interpreters (although medical interpreters are suggested, they are not required by law) and explicitly prohibits the use of non-professional third party interpreters. These protections for patients experiencing language barriers were reaffirmed in 2022 with language changes to strengthen protections (Nondiscrimination in Health Programs and Activities, 2022).

In addition to legal and policy changes to protect patients experiencing language barriers and improve the quality of care, it is important that health professions educators incorporate learning activities focusing on language barriers and linguistic equity as a facet of culturally competent care. Despite the large impact, relatively few published evidence-based practices for teaching communication practices exist in the literature (Drouin et al. 2003; Lie et al., 2006). This highlights the need for more educators to focus on these competencies and the cases that follow are intended to aid in bridging the gap presented by language barriers.

CASE 1: READING THE SIGNS

Goal

This case describes barriers to providing linguistically competent care during a healthcare encounter with a deaf patient.

Learning Outcomes

1. Identify the language-related barriers experienced by the patient in the case
2. Describe barriers to effective health care for individuals who are deaf or hard of hearing
3. Implement best practices in communicating with deaf or hard-of-hearing patients
4. Review an approach to communicating with patients using interpreters
5. Review legal protections and ethical considerations for patients experiencing language barriers

Case

Mr. O is a 26-year-old male who was born with congenital deafness caused by a presumed cytomegalovirus infection in utero. He attended college classes at a nearby school for the deaf and was brought to a large academic emergency department at approximately 2:00 AM on Sunday morning. Mr. O was transported by emergency medical services accompanied by 2 friends who communicated that Mr. O had been agitated and violent. One friend was deaf and communicated with the other hearing friend in American Sign Language (ASL).

The hearing friend communicated in spoken English to Emergency Department staff that the friends were at a party when Mr. O began acting strange, yelling at his friends and eventually striking them, causing the party to disperse. Emergency services were called and responded to the scene within a few minutes. Two paramedics arrived and attempted to approach Mr. O and calm him down by speaking to him loudly and slowly in English. Two Police officers also arrived on the scene and Mr. O only seemed to get increasingly agitated signing frantically in ASL and bellowing. Police also attempted to calm Mr. O by speaking loudly and slowly. Mr. O then attempted to strike an officer and police made an effort to subdue Mr. O, however, he became wildly combative. One paramedic administered a dose of ketamine intramuscularly into Mr. O's thigh and within one minute Mr. O was no longer actively combative. He was quickly placed on a stretcher and transported by ambulance on a monitor and an intravenous (IV) line infusing normal saline. The ambulance arrived and Mr. O was transported to an emergency department room bed from the stretcher.

The hearing friend then communicated to the emergency staff that Mr. O was deaf and preferred communicating with American Sign Language. The friend also said that as long as he had known Mr. O, this had never happened before and was very unlike him. The friends approached Mr. O, who appeared distressed and was frantically signing with his hands rapidly. They said goodbye and left the emergency department to return home and get some sleep.

Upon their departure, Mr. O remained in his room but was up pacing, signing, and had begun bellowing again. The assigned emergency department nurse notified the emergency physician, Dr. T, who instructed her to draw several doses of IV benzodiazepine medications. Dr. T asked the emergency clerk, "Are there any interpreters available?". The emergency clerk responded, "Yes doc, but at this hour you'll have to use the translation phone line." Frustrated, Dr. T reconvened with the nurse who had drawn the benzodiazepines as instructed. Dr. T said, "I think we are going to need those…" to which the nurse responded, "I'm ready, but he's pretty big…" referring to Mr. O's six-foot frame and estimating his weight at 250 pounds.

They requested staff assistance and entered Mr. O's room with several emergency department staff. Mr. O remained agitated and was out of bed but remained hooked to his IV line which trailed behind him. Dr. T said in a loud slow voice, "Mr. O, we are here to help you." Mr. O signed something that none in the room understood (as none of them understood ASL) and began to advance toward the group bellowing. Mr. O then motioned to strike Dr. T with his fist then 2 of the emergency staff members moved to subdue Mr. O under the arms and directed him back towards the bed. Dr. T said to the nurse, "Please give a dose now." The nurse administered one dose while the 2 staff holding Mr. O struggled to maintain control of his arms and legs. A few minutes later, Mr. O continued to attempt to free his arms and Dr. T asked for a second dose of benzodiazepine stating, "He is still pretty combative, let's increase the dose." The nurse administered double the first dose. In approximately 15 minutes, Mr. O appeared somnolent and was able to be repositioned in the bed. The nurse noted that Mr. O's respiratory rate was decreasing and said, "Dr. T, I think we may need to intubate him." Dr. T performed a rapid sequence intubation and placed Mr. O on a ventilator and continuous infusions of propofol, estimating the rate of infusion based on Mr. O's weight, and fentanyl. Vital signs, a full exam, and laboratory evaluations were collected, and a urinary catheter was placed. Mr. O's urine toxicology was positive for phencyclidine and cannabis. Dr. T called the intensive care unit resident for inpatient admission and Mr. O was transported to the ICU sedated without difficulty.

The ICU resident conducted an exam and verified the medical plan at approximately 4:00 AM. Mr. O was unable to communicate due to the continuing sedation but the resident planned to recommend to the day team that Mr. O be weaned off of sedation later in the day. Mr. O was placed in soft wrist restraints.

Several hours later at 9:00 AM, the day shift ICU resident, Dr. P, was called away from rounds to Mr. O's room by the ICU nurse. Mr. O was sitting up in bed, although the sedation was still infusing, and had removed his right wrist restraint and endotracheal tube. He appeared wide-eyed and appeared to be attempting to sign somewhat violently but his left wrist remained restrained. Dr. P said to the nurse, "Could you call for the ASL interpreter and tell them it is urgent?" The ICU resident entered the room and took care to articulate his lips so that they were easy to read and said, "I am your doctor in a hospital, but I don't know ASL. I will explain everything in a couple of minutes." Mr. O appeared to calm down and was no longer struggling with the restraints. Dr. P asked the nurse, "Could you remove his restraints and turn the sedation down some?" The nurse appeared somewhat skeptical, but he and Dr. P waited with Mr. O while the nurse did both. Mr. O remained calm although he continued to look afraid.

In 5 minutes, an ASL interpreter arrived at the bedside and introduced herself in ASL to Mr. O as a medical interpreter. Dr. P said, "Mr. O, you are in the intensive care unit at a hospital. You were brought to the hospital by an ambulance called by friends who told us you were acting strange and violent at a party. Do you remember any of this?" Dr. P paused to allow the interpreter to finish translating and waited for Mr. O to respond. Mr. O signed for a moment and the interpreter said, "I don't remember much, just smoking at a party with my friends. Am I in danger?" Dr. P said, "Actually, I don't think so.

The breathing tube was only to protect your breathing from the effects of the medicine that made you sleepy, since you don't look sleepy now, I don't think you need it anymore. I know it can be uncomfortable and scary to wake up with one of those tubes. I think the reason you were brought here and needed those things was the effect of drugs that must have been in whatever you smoked. At this moment, I think you are safe. How do you feel?" Mr. O signed calmly for another few moments and the interpreter said, "That's good. I still feel so sleepy. I've smoked weed before and nothing like this ever happened to me. Did I hurt anyone? What happens next?" Dr. P said, "We can talk about it more. Give me one minute." He then gestured to the nurse and the two stepped outside the room. Dr. P said, "I'm going to talk with Mr. O for a time while we've got the interpreter here. Can you stop the sedation and let the rest of the medical team know I'll be delayed? I think that he's been really scared and had no way to know what was going on or tell us what he was thinking. We probably need to talk about what happened last night with the night team."

QUESTIONS AND ANSWERS

1. In this case, what actions could have been considered missteps that limited communication with Mr. O and may have affected the quality of care?

There were several opportunities for improvement in the care of Mr. O. First, the initial mention of obtaining an interpreter was by his clinician, Dr. T, who quickly dismissed the idea after learning there would be barriers to obtaining an in-person translator (it should be noted, telephonic language interpretation services were available but would be inadequate for interpreting ASL). In a qualitative study of barriers to using interpreter services, disruptions to schedule and a lack of immediate availability were cited as common factors influencing a provider's choice to use or forgo an interpreter (Hsieh et al., 2015). As mentioned in the background, the quality of care for patients with language barriers increases tremendously with the use of medical interpreters (Al Shamsi et al., 2020).

Efforts to re-direct and de-escalate Mr. O were particularly problematic as several professionals who interacted with Mr. O adopted a strategy of increasing volume and speaking very slowly. An increase in volume would not be helpful for Mr. O, who was deaf. Speaking slightly slower might be helpful, however, speaking too slowly can actually reduce the ability to read lips (an ability that many people with hearing loss may depend on to understand speech). Although it is estimated that 40% of speech can be understood, lip-reading is not consistent between patients and requires the clinician to modify behavior to be optimal. It is recommended that patients be seen in well-lit rooms and that healthcare staff sit directly across from patients who are lip-reading, which was not necessarily the case for Mr. O (Smeijers et al., 2011). Dr. T or the emergency department clerk should have consulted with the hospital's interpreter service in order to determine if it was possible to obtain any language access services for a patient who prefers communicating in ASL. Contracts with translation services can (and should, as will be addressed later on) include video interpreters for ASL or on-call medical interpreters who could offer in-person services once engaged. It is important to note that no robust studies comparing the clinical effectiveness of remote (including video or telephonic) interpretation studies exist, however attitudinal studies have shown that patients and clinicians alike prefer in-person interpretation services (Locatis et al., 2010).

Partly because of the inability to communicate with Mr. O in the context of substance-related intoxication, efforts to de-escalate verbally were unsuccessful leading to the early and aggressive use of sedating medications (so much that Mr. O required intubation for the protection of his respiratory status). Although needed for safety, the care team should be aware that sedation decreases the patient's awareness of the situation and ability to communicate. Although the admitting resident did consider weaning, the decision should not have been delayed and sedation should be weaned as soon as it is not medically necessary. As in Mr. O's case, interventions that occur under sedation can include uncomfortable and mobility-limiting medical interventions like the placement of in-dwelling urinary catheters, intravenous lines, and mechanical ventilation which can be somewhat traumatic if the patient becomes more aware without any communication on the current circumstances. It was evident that Mr. O was fearful once he could communicate.

Although many patients who have hearing loss can speak, Mr. O did not speak and was indicated to have a preference for ASL almost immediately upon arrival at the hospital based on collateral obtained from his accompanying friend. One of the initial steps after admission to the hospital was to place Mr. O in bilateral soft wrist restraints which severely limits his ability to use his preferred expressive language. At the time this decision was made, Mr. O was receiving sedating medications and did not present a current threat of bodily harm to himself or others which are suggested by some guidelines as the ethical threshold for use of restraints in order to maximize patient dignity and autonomy (Lachance et al., 2019). The team should have considered Mr. O's ability to communicate when deciding to place wrist restraints and included the absence of a current threat in their ethical decision-making.

2. What are some other accessibility considerations for persons with hearing loss and limited speech in the healthcare setting?

As above, medical interpretation is the best intervention to improve the quality of care and linguistic equity for patients with hearing loss who prefer ASL. If using an in-person interpreter, discuss with patients what exposure to the interpreter they do and do not want. For example, establish with the patient whether the interpreter will remain present in the room for a physical exam or a medical procedure. If not, healthcare staff should make an effort to explain all planned actions while the interpreter is still present at the encounter. Additionally, in survey of ASL interpreters, the "teach back" method is an evidenced based incorporation that improves communication with deaf and hard of hearing patients that was rarely observed despite known efficacy (Hommes et al., 2018).

If in-person interpreters are not available, speech-to-text interpretations could be a useful option for patients who have hearing loss with the literacy skills to understand. It is important to note that patients who are deaf from an early age can develop low literacy skills and that speech-to-text services may not offer linguistic equity (Smeijers et al., 2011). In that case, video ASL interpretation would be the most ethically permissible language access service. The consideration of literacy skills should also be factored in when addressing language barriers in the absence of an interpreter by using translation apps or software that translate language into text.

Language barriers can also affect the ability to access care. Best practices to reduce barriers to access for patients with hearing loss include offering the ability to communicate the need for appointments or prescription refills via secure text messaging services and ensuring that the patient has a plan for communicating medical emergencies (for example, a teletypewriter telephone device or a service providing ASL/text to voice translation).

3. What resources are healthcare organizations legally required to provide deaf or hard of hearing patients?

Under the Americans with Disabilities Act (ADA), hospitals must provide effective means of communication for patients, family members, and hospital visitors who have communication barriers including hearing loss. Additionally, in patient rooms, hospitals must provide accessible equipment upon request (for example, teletypewriters, telephones that are hearing aid compatible, or televisions with closed captioning).

Interpreters are not required for all interactions in a hospital and written communication may suffice for low-complexity interactions (e.g., indicating a room number, completing a purchase at a vendor, or filling out insurance information forms). For most clinical encounters, hospitals and healthcare providers should consult with each individual with hearing loss to determine what services might be necessary. There can be no additional fees or charges for language access services for patients with hearing loss.

Any interpreters provided must be "qualified" which is defined as an ability to interpret competently, accurately, and impartially. Interpreters in medical settings must be familiar with the vocabulary needed to be able to interpret medical terms and concepts. Hospital personnel who have some familiarity with the language should be limited to emergency situations only and should seek to engage a qualified interpreter as soon as possible (Americans with Disabilities Act, 1990). In a large scoping review, bilingual nurses who found themselves acting as ad hoc interpreters highlighted concerns about workload and stress when asked to assume a dual role (Gerchow et al., 2024; Hsieh et al., 2015).

Friends and family members should not be asked to interpret by healthcare staff. In this case, seeking to engage Mr. O's hearing friend who seemed fluent in ASL as an interpreter would not have been the legal course of action. Although using friends or family members as interpreters for patients does not generate a greater number of errors than using medical interpreters, this practice increases the rate of interpreter errors with potential clinical consequences from 12% to 22% (Flores et al., 2012). It is important that interpreters in a healthcare setting strive to provide "mot à mot" (word-for-word) interpretation, ensuring the fidelity of the translated content. Medical interpreters are most likely to commit errors of omission (likely because of high content rapidly delivered by a party in the encounter) whereas ad hoc interpreters also commit omissions but additionally commit a much larger proportion of false-fluency errors (use of a word/phrase that does not exist or use of an incorrect word/phrase that substantially alters meaning) (Flores et al., 2012). Emotional context alters a friend or family member's ability to serve as an impartial interpreter and omissions (for example, withholding of a terminal diagnosis) may be culturally normal for some patients.

The ADA also specifies that hospitals should ensure that qualified interpreters should be available after hours with minimal delay, which should have been explored by Mr. O's healthcare team. Although the clerk indicated that they were aware of the telephonic interpreter, the hospital's local policy for after-hours interpreter consultation could be reviewed once it was identified that the telephonic translator would not be sufficient.

4. How did the communication strategies used by Dr. P improve upon the previous care provided?

Dr. P recognized Mr. O's emotional distress quickly and identified a barrier to communication evidenced by Mr. O's motions to sign in ASL with only one hand. Dr. P immediately called for a professional interpreter and attempted to communicate to Mr. O that language services were on the way using best practices for patients with hearing loss that are able to lip-read. Given the change in Mr. O's agitation, these practices were likely to have been successful. Dr. P also identified that limiting the physical barrier to communication posed by the limb restraints and reducing the sedation were also important changes to improve Mr. O's communication.

When the interpreter arrived, Dr. P communicated with Mr. O via the interpreter using best practices for interpretation including:

- Using the simplest language to communicate medical complexity
- Avoidance of stacking multiple questions in a single translated phrase
- Speaking directly to the patient and not to the interpreter
- Explaining his next actions using the interpreter (Lie, 2006)

The use of unnecessary medical jargon can result in inaccurate translation or miscommunication even with the use of professional interpreters who have an error rate of approximately 32.7 errors per encounter (Flores et al., 2012). Stacking questions can lead to confusion by the patient on which question to answer and lead to missed opportunities to collect information. Speaking to the interpreter instead of the patient reduces the perception of the relationship with the patient which can lead to both lower satisfaction and lower yield of information from the interaction. Dr. P explains that he will step out and return to the room through the interpreter which lowered Mr. O's need to wonder or worry about what was happening next in a situation where he was clearly afraid and had limited understanding before this conversation. It is important to note that while comparative studies regarding use of best communication practices when using interpreters are scant, there is evidence that efforts to train healthcare learners in appropriate interpreter etiquette, communication skills, and the role of interpreters increases the use of interpreters and the application of best practices (Silva et al., 2022). This is a strong argument for intentional inclusion in curricula.

Epilogue

This case provides an overview of a healthcare encounter in which barriers to effective communication were experienced by a patient with hearing loss in the hospital. The barriers identified could have been reduced by an understanding of the contextual legal and ethical considerations and employing best practices for communication with patients with a language barrier to hearing loss. Multiple healthcare staff missed opportunities to improve communication with Mr. O until Dr. P's interventions. Dr. P quickly was able to identify a language barrier and engage professional interpretation to address the emotional distress in Mr. O created by the barriers to receiving and transmitting information. The case also describes potential decreases in the quality of care received by Mr. O due to the failure to bridge a language barrier, a known effect of the presence of such barriers (Al Shamsi et al., 2020). It is for this reason that healthcare educators must incorporate the teaching of strategies to identify and approach language barriers of all kinds, including those experienced by patients with hearing loss.

CASE 2: THE QUIET ONES

Goal

This case describes barriers to providing linguistically competent care during a healthcare encounter if the patient declines language-assisted services

Learning Outcomes

1. Identify the language-related barriers experienced by the patient and parent in the case
2. Define the terms othering and understand interventions that can decrease its incidence
3. Develop techniques of how to elicit clinical information from a family member with a language barrier.
4. Identify resources other than medical interpretation to provide linguistically equitable care to family members and patients who are affected by a language barrier.

Case

Li was a 14-year-old male that presented to the outpatient child psychiatry clinic for "aggression at school." Li was referred by his primary care manager (PCM) after having his initial well-child check upon moving to the United States. During the PCM visit, Li's father, Mr. G, explained that Li is having school aversion and "does not want to be a part of anything dedicated to learning." The PCM noted that the patient was physically healthy but could not document the patient's perspective towards school as he did not speak to the PCM. The PCM wrote a referral to child psychiatry as they believed Li's past medical and dental care was questionable.

The patient presented for his psychiatry visit with Mr. G (native English speaker) and his biological mother, Mrs. N (native Mandarin speaking). Upon arrival in the lobby, Dr. B noted that the patient had poor eye contact, limited spontaneous speech, and an immature demeanor. Dr. B opened the encounter with small talk with the parents and attempted to gain Li's vitals sign. The patient was not cooperative with blood pressure assessment. Moving into her office, Dr. B started the interview asking the patient what brought him here and what he needs help with. Li did not answer the question and continued to avoid eye contact.

Mr. G commanded the interview and explained that Li is having difficulties adjusting to his American school. Li displayed defiance and unpredictable behavior at home. He explained that his wife doesn't speak English very well, so he was the only parent to enroll Li in school and receive feedback from Li's teachers regarding his behavior. The school that Li was enrolled in was the only school in his district with an ESL (English as a second language) track. Li remained silent during the interview, only occasionally laughing or smiling to himself and muttering under his breath. Mr. G reported that before moving to America with the family, Li was in a boarding school for "mentally handicapped children" in China where there was no structure, no rules, and no expectations. He explained that Mrs. N lived with Li as a baby and stayed with him until he was in elementary school when she moved to the states alone. He further explained that children who were born with intellectual disabilities in China are not expected to be contributing members of society and are not permitted formal education past elementary school. He stated that at Li's American school he would destroy property, hit teachers, and refuse to complete school tasks. Mr. G stated that it is very important for Li to learn English and that he and Mrs. N both believed that it was best accomplished with immersion in English while in school. Mr. G reported that he and his wife are concerned about Li's behavior because they want him to be able to absorb an "American education." Mrs. N stayed silent during much of the encounter. She would mostly nod in agreement. It was evident that she was not able to understand everything being mentioned, by the rate at which the stepfather was speaking and his word choices. Dr. B continued gathering as much history from Mr. G about Li's ongoing behavior.

Wanting to engage with the birth mother directly, Dr. B asked her a question directly, "What is she worried about for her son?" Mrs. N looked to Mr. G for clarification and Dr. B assumed he explained some keywords of the question in Mandarin. Mrs. N tried to articulate her concerns to Dr. B however Dr. B found it difficult to understand due to broken English and incomplete sentences. With Mr. G's information, it was understood that Li had only been living with Mr. G for the last year. Before that, Li and his mother lived together alone in China until he went to his boarding school. Dr. B then wanted to get more information about his birth history, early childhood, medical history, and boarding school. Dr. B had the language interpreter line on speed dial for language barrier cases and offered it to the family. Mrs. N declined by stating, "I understood enough." Mrs. N indicated that if she did not understand, her husband would translate for her. Dr. B respected the mother's decision and continued with the interview. Mr. G and Mrs. N explained that the patient had never been on medication management in the past due to not having academic expectations therefore limited defiant behavior. Mr. G described that the patient was a physically healthy child and only needed medical attention for his dental caries. Li's birth history was described as having no complications through the minimal language from Mrs. N to Dr. B. Dr. B understood that the history of the birth story was incomplete but continued to respect mother's decision to decline.

Dr. B explained that she did agree with Li's parents that she wanted Li to benefit from being in an American school. She further explained before initiating medication she would like to get more details about his childhood from his mother directly with a phone interpreter, written behavioral observations from the school, routine blood work, and a physical exam. Mr. G and Mrs. N agreed. Dr. B printed Mr. G information about medication for aggression and impulsivity. Dr. B acknowledged that the printed materials were in English and shared with Mr. G that it will be difficult to follow the standard informed consent process if Mrs. N continued to not want to utilize the interpreter line. Mr. G stated that he could be told the information and explain it to his wife after the visit. Dr. B offered the family techniques on how to communicate with Li the next steps of the evaluation and his behavioral expectations at school and home.

QUESTIONS AND ANSWERS

1. In this case, what may be some of the reasons the mother declined the use of a medical interpreter when offered?

In the above case, it was the patient who declined to use the interpreter. The parent's preferences should be taken into account in combination with evidence-based guidance regarding professional interpreters. Flores et al. stated that an ad hoc interpreter and the lack of any type of interpreter is suboptimal with limited English proficiency patients and should be avoided. Opting out of using a professional interpreter, in this case, can lead to significant medical errors (Flores et al., 2012). While there may be a multitude of reasons Li's mother declined, the following three salient objections will be explored. The ability to negate these barriers before they come up in clinical practice will also be discussed.

The first reason patients with language barriers may choose to decline an interpreter is the perception of financial constraints. Some patients may believe the misconception that having an interpreter would cost them an additional amount on top of the other care-related costs. Under the Americans with Disabilities Act (ADA), hospitals must provide effective means of communication for patients, family members, and hospital visitors free of charge (Americans with Disabilities Act, 1990). According to the HHS Guidance on LEP (limited English proficiency), the hospital or medical entity must absorb the cost of the interpreter as a part of business operating costs even if the interpreter costs more than their services.

The second reason may be due to having a bad experience with an interpreter in past clinical encounters. Medical errors have been reported at a statistically significant rate, even with the use of professional interpreters. The error rates were higher with ad hoc interpreters and without any interpreter however this does not put a patient's mind at ease when undergoing medical care in a foreign language (Flores et al, 2012). This would be to no fault of either party involved but may persist for the patient as a reason to not communicate through a third party. There may be an element of distrust with the interpreter due to not knowing them. There may be hesitancy to discuss a medical issue with a person outside of the family, or with incongruent identified gender, religion, or political views (Hadziabdic et al., 2014).

The third reason may be the inevitable power differential between physician and patient. In China, physician guidance and expertise are regarded over patient-centered treatment plans which were accepted with moderate enthusiasm (Ting et al., 2016). Chinese patients preferred for their physician to be caring and understanding but ultimately relied on the physician's judgment for the medical recommendation. For the patient (an entity with a perceived lack of power), asking for additional resources or accommodations from the experienced physician goes against the dynamic of the doctor-patient relationship. If the physician is to manage their power appropriately, they invite the patient to the shared decision-making process, therefore, providing space for a potentially reverent patient to be heard (Nimmon et al., 2016). In this particular case, Ms. N may have perceived that agreeing to have an interpreter would be insulting to Mr. G, therefore, covertly stated that his translation of the encounter was less than suitable for her child's needs.

2. Define the term "othering" and discuss how cultural competency is related to language barriers in healthcare.

The term othering as defined by Johnson et al. "is a process that identifies those that are thought to be different from oneself or the mainstream, and it can reinforce and reproduce positions of domination and subordination." Othering can lead to significant health complications such as decreased access to care, shorter life expectancy, increased infant mortality, and hypertension (Johnson et al., 2004).

In this case, Dr. B potentially increased Ms. N's perception of being othered by implying the need for an interpreter. Strategies to reduce the perception of inability and improve communication start with appropriate use of language when we are referring to others that are different from us. It can be assumed that Li's mother already felt significant guilt for Li's behavior in his new school and the daily calls home to the stepfather. She presented to the outpatient appointment looking for solutions and answers, not to feel even more isolated with the doctor implying that she couldn't understand the patient's history. Dr. B could have changed the tone in the room by highlighting the importance of Mrs. N's contribution and asking his mother how best that history could be obtained. Johnson continues to write that the burden lies with the healthcare professional to allow the patient to feel a part of the decision-making process and a sense of ownership in their care. The job of the healthcare professional is to "get curious, not furious", finding out more about the parents' rejection of an interpreter rather than being frustrated and giving up on delivering care to the patient.

Dr. B's approach goes beyond the concept of cultural competency and enters the realm of cultural sensitivity. Both of these concepts are paramount in avoiding othering during clinical encounters and therefore preventing negative outcomes. It is important that healthcare staff not regard their culture as the standard that all others are measured by and instead embrace the difference for what they are (Bhatt et al., 2021). Notably, although Ms. N declined a medical interpreter, many medical interpreters consider cultural interpretation and the delivery of culturally conscious language to be an essential part of their contribution to culturally competent care when addressing language barriers (Hsieh, 2008).

3. How do you collect clinically relevant data from a family member with a language barrier?

Bhatt and Gentile explain in their article about interviewing patients with developmental delays that being respectful is paramount when working with this patient population. Patients with developmental delays may already feel spoken at and talked around so when a clinician takes the time and addresses their needs, wants, and concerns instant trust and a partnership can be attained. Bhatt describes that using the following other techniques can be invaluable (Bhatt et al., 2021):

- Match questions and answers to the individual's level of expressive language.
- Ask permission to involve collateral data sources.
- Collect collateral information and manage the triangle
- Know what to expect. When possible, review all available medical records before the evaluation.
- Use simple language.
- Concretize the abstract.
- Use alternative ways to communicate when necessary (e.g., pictures, drawings).
- Ask the individual to repeat something if you did not understand what was said.
- Take responsibility for miscommunication.
- Eliminate distractions and unnecessary noise/ movements during the interview.
- Do not use slang or figurative speech.
- Allow more time and consider multiple meetings if needed.
- Recap and summarize what occurred during the evaluation.

It was evident that Dr. B tried to start the encounter by interviewing Li, therefore respecting his autonomy. She also had to "manage the triangle" of the patient and parent's input. This means truly listening and accounting for all decision-makers in the encounter and not prioritizing one that shared in her perspective of his treatment. It is not recommended to use jargon with patients of average to above-average intelligence therefore when working with a patient with developmental delays or an interpreter it is vital that jargon, slang, and idioms are avoided (Bhatt et al., 2021). Often in the clinical interview, these thoughts can be communicated more clearly in another way while saving time trying to explain this cryptic phrase to the family. For interviews with developmental delays or needing an interpreter, be sure to budget enough time or relay to the family that data collection may be broken up over subsequent clinical interviews. Ending the interview by explaining the next steps either verbally, in writing, and/or in a take-home fashion can be wildly impactful. This allows the family to understand the physician's expectations and prepare for the upcoming season leading to a more time-efficient and productive next encounter.

4. When a language barrier is present, what are some resources other than medical interpretation that can be used to educate patients and family members?

The Agency for Healthcare Research and Quality, in their topic on health literacy, described that matched language materials provide a common language for the provider and patient to communicate about their diagnosis and treatment. It is known that the production of matched language materials is limited in their existence and even rarer when a patient sees a subspecialist or is diagnosed with a low-prevalence condition or prescribed a newer medication (AHRQ, 2019). In the case above, Dr. B gave a patient educational material in a language other than the patient's primary language. Such a practice either provides no benefit to the patient or relies on a translating third party to serve as a conduit for this information. If Dr. B would have provided educational materials both in English for the stepfather and Mandarin for the patient and mother, the patient would have had better health outcomes, better compliance, and more equitable care for his presenting concerns.

Another resource that is available to the healthcare profession is a standard health literacy assessment. English literacy is distinct from spoken English fluency, and patients could benefit from patient education augmented by printed English materials. Underestimating a patient's health literacy is not common practice. Dickens and Lambert describe it is more common to overestimate a patient's health literacy which can lead to poor health care outcomes and higher readmission rates (Dickens et al., 2013). In this case, no assessment of health literacy was completed, and Dr. B and her patients did not have the opportunity to benefit. Sample questions from the Rapid Estimate of Adult Literacy in Medicine include being able to recognize and pronounce words in medical communication such as jaundice, menopause, and antibiotics (Cutilli, 2020). Additionally, the Short Assessment of Health Literacy the patient's task to identify the medication term that matches an interviewer's prompt. The number of correct pairings correlates with a measure of the patient's health literacy, either adequate or inadequate. Inadequate health literacy should prompt the provider to communicate more clearly to enable the shared decision-making process to happen successfully (AHRQ, 2019).

An additional resource that can aid in bridging language barriers is the use of pictographic instructions. This is widely used with patients that have language barriers and can be used with those that have low health literacy. This communication resource does need to be aligned with the patient's cultural representation of the picture that is included to not misinterpret the intention of the health information (Kassam, 2004). If Dr. B employed this method of patient education, she would have been able to more accurately describe the rationale for prescribing Li the medication for aggression while still honoring the patient's request to use her husband as a translator. In the 2007 study by Kripilani et al., use of a pill card to teach medication administration and indication showed that the patients that used the card found it helpful for remembering which medicines to take, as well as the medication name, indication, dosage, and time of administration. In 2014, the Joint Commission endorsed "I speak" cards that can be displayed in a practitioner's office to identify the native language used by the patient to facilitate effective communication (Joint Commission, 2014).

Epilogue

This case represents an instance in which there is inequity in decision making on the part of a vulnerable nonverbal patient due to the presence of a language barrier for one caregiver. With this layered complexity, it was important for the healthcare staff to create a culture of respect and seek to communicate in ways that promote equity among the caregivers. Healthcare staff should be mindful of the underlying considerations patients may have when considering the use of interpretation services, namely perceived financial burden, prior bad experiences, and power differentials. Members of the team should stand ready to meet the patient where they are in an effort to provide a shared decision-making experience. With the combined tools of cultural competency and cultural sensitivity, healthcare staff can avoid the pitfall of "othering" patients with cultures different from their own. This practice leads to better patient outcomes and less morbidity within the healthcare setting (Johnson et al., 2004). Finally, the charge in patient advocacy does not end with the closure of the encounter but continues wherever the patient spends their time and attention. Healthcare staff are critical in providing support and championing for their patients (particularly those with communication barriers) to sustain healthy and equitable existences.

REFERENCES

Agency for Healthcare Research and Quality (AHRQ). (2015). Health literacy universal precautions toolkit (2nd ed.).. AHRQ. https://www.ahrq.gov/professionals/quality-patient-safety/quality-resources/tools/literacy-toolkit/index.html

Al Shamsi, H., Almutairi, A. G., Al Mashrafi, S., & Al Kalbani, T. (2020). Implications of language barriers for healthcare: A systematic review. *Oman Medical Journal*, *35*(2), e122. doi:10.5001/omj.2020.40 PMID:32411417

Americans With Disabilities Act of 1990, Pub. L. No. 101-336, 104 Stat. 328 (1990).

Balakrishnan, V., Roper, J., Cossey, K., Roman, C., & Jeanmonod, R. (2016). Misidentification of English language proficiency in triage: Impact on satisfaction and door-to-room time. *Journal of Immigrant and Minority Health*, *18*(2), 369–373. doi:10.100710903-015-0174-4 PMID:25750135

Benda, N. C., Wesley, D. B., Nare, M., Fong, A., Ratwani, R. M., & Kellogg, K. M. (2022). Social determinants of health and patient safety: An analysis of patient safety event reports related to limited English-proficient patients. *Journal of Patient Safety*, *18*(1), e1–e9. doi:10.1097/PTS.0000000000000663 PMID:32168283

Bhatt, N., & Gentile, J. (2021). Interviewing Techniques for Patients with Intellectual Disability. *Journal of Mental Health Disorders*, *1*(1), 10–14.

Boscolo-Hightower, A., Rafton, S. A., Tolman, M., Zhou, C., & Ebel, B. E. (2014). Identifying families with limited English proficiency using a capture-recapture approach. *Hospital Pediatrics*, *4*(1), 16–22. doi:10.1542/hpeds.2013-0040 PMID:24435596

Cohen, A. L., Rivara, F., Marcuse, E. K., McPhillips, H., & Davis, R. (2005). Are language barriers associated with serious medical events in hospitalized pediatric patients? *Pediatrics*, *116*(3), 575–579. doi:10.1542/peds.2005-0521 PMID:16140695

Cutilli, C. C. (2020). Excellence in Patient Education: Evidence-Based Education that "Sticks" and Improves Patient Outcomes. *The Nursing Clinics of North America*, *55*(2), 267–282. doi:10.1016/j.cnur.2020.02.007 PMID:32389259

de Bruijne, M. C., van Rosse, F., Uiters, E., Droomers, M., Suurmond, J., Stronks, K., & Essink-Bot, M. L. (2013). Ethnic variations in unplanned readmissions and excess length of hospital stay: A nationwide record-linked cohort study. *European Journal of Public Health*, *23*(6), 964–971. doi:10.1093/eurpub/ckt005 PMID:23388242

De Moissac, D., & Bowen, S. (2019). Impact of language barriers on quality of care and patient safety for official language minority Francophones in Canada. *Journal of Patient Experience*, *6*(1), 24–32. doi:10.1177/2374373518769008 PMID:31236448

Dickens, C., Lambert, B. L., Cromwell, T., & Piano, M. R. (2013). Nurse overestimation of patients' health literacy. *Journal of Health Communication*, *18*(sup1), 62–69. doi:10.1080/10810730.2013.825670 PMID:24093346

Drouin, J., & Rivet, C. (2003). Training medical students to communicate with a linguistic minority group. *Academic Medicine*, *78*(6), 599–604. doi:10.1097/00001888-200306000-00009 PMID:12805039

Flores, G., Abreu, M., Barone, C. P., Bachur, R., & Lin, H. (2012). Errors of medical interpretation and their potential clinical consequences: A comparison of professional versus ad hoc versus no interpreters. *Annals of Emergency Medicine*, *60*(5), 545–553. doi:10.1016/j.annemergmed.2012.01.025 PMID:22424655

Foley, G. N., & Gentile, J. P. (2010). Nonverbal communication in psychotherapy. *Psychiatry (Edgmont (Pa.: Township))*, *7*(6), 38–44.

Gerchow, L., Burka, L. R., Miner, S., & Squires, A. (2021). Language barriers between nurses and patients: A scoping review. *Patient Education and Counseling*, *104*(3), 534–553. doi:10.1016/j.pec.2020.09.017 PMID:32994104

USFG. (2001) Guidance to Federal Financial Assistance Recipients Regarding Title VI Prohibition Against National Origin Discrimination Affecting Limited English Proficient Persons. 67 FR 4968

Hadziabdic, E., & Hjelm, K. (2014). Arabic-speaking migrants' experiences of the use of interpreters in healthcare: A qualitative explorative study. *International Journal for Equity in Health*, *13*(1), 49. doi:10.1186/1475-9276-13-49 PMID:24934755

Hommes, B., Borash, A. I., Hartwig, K., & DeGracia, D. (2018). American Sign Language Interpreters Perceptions of Barriers to Healthcare Communication in Deaf and Hard of Hearing Patients. *Journal of Community Health*, *43*(5), 956–961. doi:10.100710900-018-0511-3 PMID:29696596

Hsieh, E. (2008). "I am not a robot!" Interpreters' views of their roles in health care settings. *Qualitative Health Research*, *18*(10), 1367–1383. doi:10.1177/1049732308323840 PMID:18832768

Hsieh, E. (2015). Not just "getting by": Factors influencing providers' choice of interpreters. *Journal of General Internal Medicine, 30*(1), 75–82. doi:10.100711606-014-3066-8 PMID:25338731

Institute of Medicine. (2001). *Crossing the quality chasm: A new health care system for the 21st century*. National Academy Press.

Johnson, J. L., Bottorff, J. L., Browne, A. J., Grewal, S., Hilton, B. A., & Clarke, H. (2004). Othering and being othered in the context of health care services. *Health Communication, 16*(2), 255–271. doi:10.1207/S15327027HC1602_7 PMID:15090288

Joint Commission. (2014). International Accreditation Standards for Hospitals. *Joint Commission*.

Kale, E., & Syed, H. R. (2010). Language barriers and the use of interpreters in the public health services. A questionnaire-based survey. *Patient Education and Counseling, 81*(2), 187–191. doi:10.1016/j.pec.2010.05.002 PMID:20542656

Karliner, L. S., Jacobs, E. A., Chen, A. H., & Mutha, S. (2007). Do professional interpreters improve clinical care for patients with limited English proficiency? A systematic review of the literature. *Health Services Research, 42*(2), 727–754. doi:10.1111/j.1475-6773.2006.00629.x PMID:17362215

Kassam, R., Vaillancourt, L. R., & Collins, J. B. (2004). Pictographic instructions for medications: Do different cultures interpret them accurately? *International Journal of Pharmacy Practice, 12*(4), 199–209. doi:10.1211/0022357044698

Koff, M. D., & McGowan, J. J. (1999). MedSpanish: a language tool for the emergency department. In *Proceedings of the AMIA Symposium* (p. 565). American Medical Informatics Association.

Kripalani, S., Robertson, R., Love-Ghaffari, M. H., Henderson, L. E., Praska, J., Strawder, A., Katz, M. G., & Jacobson, T. A. (2007). Development of an illustrated medication schedule as a low-literacy patient education tool. *Patient Education and Counseling, 66*(3), 368–377. doi:10.1016/j.pec.2007.01.020 PMID:17344015

Lachance, C., & Wright, M. D. (2019). *Avoidance of physical restraint use among hospitalized older adults: a review of clinical effectiveness and guidelines*. CADTH.

Landrum, T. J., Tankersley, M., & Kauffman, J. M. (2003). What Is Special About Special Education for Students with Emotional or Behavioral Disorders? *The Journal of Special Education, 37*(3), 148–156. doi:10.1177/00224669030370030401

Lie, D. (2006). Interpreter cases for cultural competency instruction. *MedEdPORTAL: the Journal of Teaching and Learning Resources, 2*, 205. doi:10.15766/mep_2374-8265.205

Locatis, C., Williamson, D., Gould-Kabler, C., Zone-Smith, L., Detzler, I., Roberson, J., & Ackerman, M. (2010). Comparing in-person, video, and telephonic medical interpretation. *Journal of General Internal Medicine, 25*(4), 345–350. doi:10.100711606-009-1236-x PMID:20107916

Nimmon, L., & Stenfors-Hayes, T. (2016). The "Handling" of power in the physician-patient encounter: Perceptions from experienced physicians. *BMC Medical Education, 16*(1), 114. doi:10.118612909-016-0634-0 PMID:27091146

Nondiscrimination in Health Programs and Activities, 42 CFR Parts 438, 440, and 460; 45 CFR Parts 80, 84, 86, 91, 92, 147, 155, and 156 (2022)

Silva, A., Adelman, R. D., Singh, V., Gupta, R., Moxley, J., Sobota, R. M., Tsai, S., Abel, B. T., & Reid, M. C. (2022). Healthcare Provider Perspectives Regarding Use of Medical Interpreters During End-of-Life Conversations With Limited English Proficient Patients. *The American Journal of Hospice & Palliative Care*, *39*(2), 220–227. doi:10.1177/10499091211015916 PMID:34000817

Smeijers, A. S., Ens-Dokkum, M. H., van den Bogaerde, B., & Oudesluys-Murphy, A. M. (2011). Clinical practice: The approach to the deaf or hard-of-hearing paediatric patient. *European Journal of Pediatrics*, *170*(11), 1359–1363. doi:10.100700431-011-1530-6 PMID:21766166

Stewart, M. A. (1995). Effective physician-patient communication and health outcomes: A review. *CMAJ. Canadian Medical Association Journal*, *152*(9), 1423. PMID:7728691

Ting, X., Yong, B., Yin, L., & Mi, T. (2016). Patient perception and the barriers to practicing patient-centered communication: A survey and in-depth interview of Chinese patients and physicians. *Patient Education and Counseling*, *99*(3), 364–369. doi:10.1016/j.pec.2015.07.019 PMID:26776708

U.S. Census Bureau. (2020). Selected Social Characteristics in the United States [Retrieved from]. *Matrix (Stuttgart, Germany)*, DP02.

Wilson, E., Chen, A. H., Grumbach, K., Wang, F., & Fernandez, A. (2005). Effects of limited English proficiency and physician language on health care comprehension. *Journal of General Internal Medicine*, *20*(9), 800–806. doi:10.1111/j.1525-1497.2005.0174.x PMID:16117746

Chapter 8
Healthcare in Patients With Limited English Proficiency and Linguistic Diversity in Medicine

Taru Saigal
The Ohio State University Wexner Medical Center, USA

Kristen Lewis
https://orcid.org/0000-0001-9396-2652
The Ohio State University, USA

EXECUTIVE SUMMARY

Patients with limited English proficiency (LEP) are among healthcare's fastest growing and most vulnerable populations. They experience poor quality of care, worse clinical outcomes, higher medical error rates, and less patient satisfaction than English-proficient patients. Using medical interpreter services (MIS) does not fully mitigate the disparities in outcomes and inequities in healthcare and requires availability, longer provider times, and quality control. Hence, a multidimensional approach is warranted to provide culturally and linguistically appropriate services. This chapter will include three case discussions highlighting: 1) Appropriate use and loopholes in medical interpreter services, 2) Patient-provider language concordance to bypass language barriers, and 3) Relevance of medical translation to improve understanding of health, diseases, and medication adherence.

BACKGROUND

Limited English Proficiency (LEP) is a term used to refer to individuals who do not speak English as their primary language and have a limited ability to read, speak, write, or understand English. The US Census Bureau's operational definition for LEP is a patient's self-assessed ability to speak English less than "very well" at age five and older. This definition includes individuals with sensory impairments (SI), who are deaf or hard of hearing and communicate using American Sign Language (ASL), have speech impairments, or are blind or have visual impairments("Empire Justice Center," 2009). In 2015, the US

DOI: 10.4018/978-1-6684-5493-0.ch008

Census Bureau American Community Survey (ACS) indicated that more than 25 million people had limited English Proficiency (LEP), which accounts for about 9% of the US population aged five years and older. In the past ten years, most communities across the US experienced growth in their immigrant population and an increase in languages spoken. Although most LEP individuals are foreign-born, a sizable share (about 19 percent, or 4.8 million) of this population is native-born("Access and Functional Needs Toolkit: Integrating a Community Partner Network to Inform Risk Communication Strategies. Atlanta, GA: U.S. Department of Health and Human Services (HHS).", 2021). People with LEP make up a large and growing population that needs to overcome language barriers for safe, equitable, quality, and cost-effective health care. Although LEP is an independent determinant of health outcomes, it is a social determinant of health and can be a source of disparities in health care access and health outcomes.

Healthcare providers bear both legal and ethical responsibilities for utilizing medical interpreter services (MIS) when caring for patients with LEP. From a legal perspective, in the United States, Executive Order 13166, "Improving Access to Services for Persons with Limited English Proficiency" builds on the principals established in the Civil rights Act of 1964. In sum, recipients of federal funding must utilize oral interpretation and written translation services in order to avoid discrimination on the basis of language. From an ethical perspective, patient autonomy to make informed decisions requires communication between patients and their providers. For patients with LEP, without incorporation of a qualified medical interpreter, this autonomy is undermined (Gaurab, 2017). Physicians and hospitals have been held liable for failing to adequately obtain informed consent when they have not appropriately incorporated MIS into their informed consent processes. Despite the laws, regulations, and recommendations, MIS remain unpopular and underused. LEP patients and clients continue to have challenges and concerns regarding disparities in access, utilization, and healthcare outcomes. For all of these reasons, deliberate instruction regarding best practices when caring for patients with LEP must be incorporated into health professions education.

CASE 1: "IT'S A RIGHT, NOT A PRIVILEGE"

Goal

This case educates about the barriers to using and different mediums of MIS.

Learning Outcomes

1. Summarize existing laws and recommendations regarding for the care of patients with limited English proficiency.
2. Identify benefits and limitations of various types of medical interpreter services.
3. Describe barriers to the appropriate use of medical interpreter services.
4. Recognize the risks associated with using ad-hoc interpreters and implement strategies to promote patient acceptance of medical interpreter services.
5. Examine the importance using medical interpreter services when obtaining informed consent from patients with limited English proficiency.

Case

A sixty-eight-year-old Nepali-speaking Bhutanese refugee patient, Mr. P, was brought to the emergency room by his family with fever, shortness of breath, and confusion. The hospitalist, Dr. H, admitted Mr. P to the progressive care unit for treatment of sepsis due to bacterial pneumonia. During a conversation with Dr. H, Mr. P's family requested that Hindu vegetarian meals be provided. They also noted that he is "hard of hearing" and exclusively speaks Nepali. The family planned to return to the hospital the next day.

After Mr. P's family left, Nurse R, came to assess her new patient. She asked, "Sir, what language do you speak?" Mr. P stared at her and used some incomprehensible words. Nurse R flipped through the emergency room papers in haste and noticed the status of LEP and Nepali as the "preferred language." She then tried to explain to Mr. P how to use the interpreter phone but noticed that he seemed distracted. Soon, Nurse R was pulled away to attend to another ill patient. While she was away, the hospital food service delivered the Hindu vegetarian meal tray in the room, gave a warm smile to Mr. P, uncovered the food, which included eggs, and made a quick exit.

Next morning, Mr. P's son came in early to check on him. The day shift nurse, Nurse N met Mr. P, and noticed that he appeared alert and was talking to his son in Nepali. Using the phone interpreter, Nurse N asked Mr. P, "How are you today?" Mr. P nodded and said, "I don't know why I am here." After asking multiple questions which Mr. P did not answer appropriately, she hung up the call. Frustrated, Nurse N asked Mr. P's son to help with interpretation in the future.

During rounds with the medical team, Nurse N mentioned, "I suspect he may have undiagnosed dementia; he has been confused, has not been able to follow instructions despite using an interpreter, and has not eaten at all. The patient's son overheard the conversation and grew upset. He expressed, "We requested a Hindu vegetarian meal, but they gave him eggs to eat. We will need to bring him food from home." He also expressed frustration with the nurse's insensitive and inaccurate remark about his father having dementia. He clarified that his father had only been confused for the past day while ill.

Later that day, after Mr. P's son had left the hospital to go to work, Mr. P's intravenous access (IV) malfunctioned and needed to be replaced. Nurse N told the patient, "We are going to place another IV access," while showing the needle with a syringe. After two failed attempts, the unit's charge nurse moved to the other arm and started looking for a vein. However, the patient soon became restless and swung his arm. The nurse aborted the procedure and recommended trying again in the presence of the family. The nurse discussed this with Dr. H and documented in the chart - "Patient was agitated, failed three attempts to place IV access. Plan to attempt under ultrasound guidance in the presence of family. Physician notified." Mr. P missed two doses of IV antibiotics before IV access was re-established with family present that evening.

The following morning, Mr. P's son contacted the hospital patient experience department. He complained that IV access had been attempted without informed consent or explaining the procedure and that his father had unnecessarily missed important antibiotic doses. He also expressed concern that his father had been discriminated against, with a lack of adequate interpreter service use, and a lack of accommodation for his father's hearing impairment.

QUESTIONS AND ANSWERS

1. What are some laws and guidance on the use of MIS?

Title VI of the 1964 Civil Rights Act provides LEP individuals a legal right to access language assistance services and prohibits recipients of federal financial assistance from discriminating based on LEP, among other things.

The protections of the Americans with Disabilities Act of 1990 and Section 504 of the Rehabilitation Act of 1973 apply equally to LEP individuals with disabilities or those who are hard of hearing.

In August 2000, President Clinton issued Executive Order (EO) 13166, *Improving Access to Services for Persons with Limited English Proficiency*. EO 13166 reiterates Title VI requirements for federal fund recipients and directs all federal agencies to ensure that their programs provide equal access to LEP individuals.

Under Section 1557 of the Affordable Care Act (ACA), covered entities, including hospitals, clinics, physician practices, and home health care agencies, must post notices of nondiscrimination and taglines that alert individuals with LEP to the availability of language assistance services.

The National Standards for Culturally and Linguistically Appropriate Services (CLAS) in Health and Health Care describe a framework to deliver culturally and linguistically appropriate services.("CMS," 2016). CLAS mandates are current Federal requirements for all recipients of Federal funds.

In 2011, the Joint Commission published Patient-Centered Communication standards in the *Comprehensive Accreditation Manual for Hospitals*. These standards emphasize effective communication, cultural competence, and patient-centered care as essential elements of safe quality of care.

The Agency for Healthcare Research and Quality (AHRQ) recommends fostering a supportive culture, identifying, reporting, and preventing medical errors among LEP Patients.

2. What are the different mediums of interpretation? In this case, should one have been preferred over another?

The available mediums of interpretation include on-site and in-person interpreting (OSI), over the phone interpreting (OPI), and video remote interpreting (VRI). Over the years, even more so during the pandemic, in-person interpretation has transitioned to telephonic or video interpretation due to availability, safety, and cost issues. The current body of evidence does not indicate a superior interpreting method(Joseph, Garruba, & Melder, 2018). The most significant advantage of telephone interpreting is accessibility, cost, and availability of interpretation in uncommon languages. One study showed that encounters with in-person interpretation were rated significantly higher by providers and interpreters, while patients rated all methods the same. There were no significant differences in provider and interpreter ratings of remote methods. Providers and interpreters also showed a distinct preference for video over the phone (Locatis et al., 2010). Organizations should allocate language service resources efficiently and effectively. Hospitals should develop policies and procedures for requesting an interpreter service and choosing a specific modality of interpretation. Procedures like placing OSI or VRI requests in advance can aid with planning. Many assistive technical devices are available to LEP individuals with disabilities. In this case, attempts to utilize interpreter services should not have stopped due to initial struggles using OPI. The initial challenges likely related more to Mr. P's delirium as well as lack of accommodation for his impaired hearing. In this case a visual aid, such as through VRI or OSI could have been good next options.

3. What are some common barriers to the use of MIS illustrated in this case?

Despite the requirements and availability of qualified MIS, there are multiple potential barriers to the use of interpreter services. The most commonly cited barrier is time constraints. Busy healthcare professionals with multiple competing responsibilities may wish to avoid the time required to call an OPI or connect with a VRI services. Additionally, conversations completed utilizing an interpreter naturally require more time. Limited availability of OSI, and the need to plan ahead for interpreter presence can also inhibit its use. The frequent periodic communication between healthcare providers and patients in the hospital setting also makes the utilization of OSI less practical. These barriers were all exemplified in this case.

In this case, as commonly occurs, Mr. P's son ultimately served as an ad-hoc interpreter to overcome the above barriers to MIS use. An ad-hoc interpreter is an untrained person called upon to interpret, such as a family member, friend, or nonqualified staff interpreter. It is common for patients or providers to use ad hoc interpreters, to use their basic or limited linguistic skills to "get by" or to "make do," or to falsely deny LEP. A person who does not have formal training in medical interpreting can be a source of miscommunication between patient and provider and can lead to potential harm. In fact, the use of ad-hoc interpreters remains among the most reported cause of errors by frontline staff and leaders. A 2011 study found that 43% of LEP patients communicated without an interpreter during admission, and 40% communicated without an interpreter after admission (Schenker, Pérez-Stable, Nickleach, & Karliner, 2011). Research confirms that hospital staff often serve as interpreters for LEP patients, despite evidence that hospital staff who serve as interpreters on an ad hoc basis are more likely to make clinically significant mistakes than qualified medical interpreters (Diamond et al., 2009; Flores et al., 2016).

While not illustrated in this case, an additional potential barrier to MIS use is patients' self-assessed linguistic ability perception. A patient's English proficiency may differ from moment to moment and from situation to situation. It may be easier to understand words in English when the situation is simple and less stressful than when things are complicated and stressful. This can sometimes lead to denial of LEP and refusal of language interpreter services in scenarios where they would be valuable. Telling a patient or family that they may have a "limited English proficiency" when they have believed otherwise and feel confident about their skills may pose a challenge. Some patients may also pretend to understand English to avoid embarrassment or fear of poor treatment based on their linguistic abilities.

In-language collateral may help reluctant patients understand how medical interpretation can contribute to a better patient experience and outcome. A short factsheet in different languages on qualified interpreters' expected benefits, including meaning-for-meaning communication, impartiality, medical privacy, and improved patient safety and satisfaction, can be useful to explain the benefits of MIS use. However, if a patient still declines, providers should document the offer of free language services, the name of the interpreter designated by the patient, the interpreter's relationship to the LEP person, and the time or portions of the patient encounter that used the ad hoc interpreter. Organizations and hospitals should invest in robust and accessible MIS, as studies have shown that utilization of MIS reduces readmissions and hospital expenditures, and improves patient satisfaction (Jacobs, Sadowski, & Rathouz, 2007; Karliner, Pérez-Stable, & Gregorich, 2017)

4. Did this patient provide informed consent for IV placement?

The American Medical Association describes the process of informed consent as communication between a patient and physician resulting in the patient's authorization or agreement to undergo a specific medical intervention. Expressed consent is typically done in writing, while implied consent is generally conveyed through a patient's actions or conduct, like while placing an IV access.

In this case, the nurse used limited words in a language the patient did not understand, without utilizing MIS. Hence effective communication regarding the planned intervention did not occur. The patient's actions specifically indicated lack of consent to proceed with the IV placement.

Legally, many states have codified informed medical consent into statutory law, and lack of adherence to the statute can lead to per se negligence for the physician. Hospitals have been found guilty of medical malpractice in cases where failure to employ interpreter or translation services resulted in poor patient comprehension of their medical conditions and inadequate informed consent. A study to determine the impact of language barriers on documentation of informed consent among patients showed that hospitalized patients who do not speak English are less likely to have documentation of informed consent for common invasive procedures despite on-site professional interpreter services (Schenker, Wang, Selig, Ng, & Fernandez, 2007)

Besides clinical work, clinical research is another crucial area where informed consent is vital, and MIS should be incorporated. Underrepresentation of LEP patients in clinical research limits research's generalizability and exacerbates healthcare inequities. Through systematic incorporation of MIS into clinical research protocols, participation of LEP patients can increase, and the benefits of the research to society can expand.

5. Who should use interpreter services in health care settings?

Not just clinicians, but all ancillary services staff who contact patients should use interpreter service with LEP patients. This includes clerical staff, registration and scheduling staff, laboratory personnel, and pharmacies. Patient transport and food delivery services should also use interpreter services when they come in direct patient contact. Many cultures and religions have certain prohibited foods that should be respected. As illustrated in this case, difficulties are compounded by an inability to understand the native language spoken or to ask questions about the meals unless an interpreter service is used.

Epilogue

In this case, the healthcare team acknowledged the miscommunication after a team meeting with Mr. P, Mr. P's son, Dr. H, Nurse N, and a patient experience advocate. The team apologized for miscommunication, not using a consistent interpreter, and the delay in treatment. It should be noted that despite the availability and an attempt to use MIS, ultimately Mr. P's son was used as an ad-hoc interpreter. Using OPI was not a good option for this patient. Since the patient had a hearing impairment and delirium, visual and nonverbal cues with facial expressions, gestures, and body language became even more critical. Clinical encounters that require complex conversations or high-risk conditions like admission, discharge, obtaining informed consent for procedures, discussing goals of life, etc., should preferentially use OSI or VRI. To prevent such incidents, hospitals can develop policies and procedures for requesting an interpreter service and choosing a specific modality of interpretation. The staff attempted to place an IV access on Mr. P without obtaining informed consent. Informed consent to medical treatment is fundamental in ethics and law, and organizations should educate their healthcare providers regarding their states' statutory laws. It is also of utmost importance to use translated consent forms to indeed be "informed consent".

Hospital systems should reinforce the easy availability of the documents, educate staff on their use, and conduct internal auditing to assess use. When using translations in research, translation processes need to be made explicit in research protocols and reports, and translation experts need to be part of the research team.

The case emphasizes that besides educating patients and staff on MIS, cultural competence training, balancing patient loads, and staffing can be instrumental in improving the use of MIS.

CASE 2: "IT TAKES MORE THAN TWO TO TANGO"

Goal

This case portrays how communication barriers can lead to poor outcomes in patients with LEP and how providing Language Concordant Care and using other MIS can offset patient safety risks.

Learning Outcomes

1. Discuss the impact of entering and utilizing Race/ Ethnicity/ Language (REL) data in the electronic health record.
2. Analyze how and why patients with limited English proficiency experience worse health outcomes.
3. Define back-channeling and identify the role non-verbal communication plays during patient-provider communication.
4. Examine the impact of increased rates of restraint use on the autonomy of patients with limited English proficiency.
5. Describe the positive impact language concordance between patients and providers can have on patient outcomes.
6. Implement best practices for communicating with patients while using medical interpreter services.

Case

An emergency department nurse evaluated a 40-year-old Hindi-speaking patient with LEP, Mrs. K, who presented with three weeks of low-grade fever, generalized rash, anasarca, and shortness of breath. Nurse J asked the patient, "Do you speak English?" Mrs. K said, "Yes." Nurse J replied, "Please let me know if you do not understand English and want me to use a medical interpreter." Mrs. K said, "Ok, thank you." Neither the nurse nor registration staff entered LEP in the patient's chart. The ED physician evaluated the patient without the use the interpreter service and documented that the patient was a poor historian. Family was not present at the bedside to provide collateral information.

Mrs. K was started on intravenous furosemide and empiric antibiotics prior to transfer to the medical floor. Her working diagnoses included acute heart failure and pneumonia. Overnight, Mrs. K had a fall and was subsequently placed in soft restraints. When the hospitalist physician, Dr. T, who happened to be fluent in the patient's language, Hindi, discussed the patient with her nurse on morning rounds, the nurse expressed concern that Mrs. K had also declined the ordered intravenous furosemide overnight. As a result, she had a significant net positive fluid balance. The nurse reported that Mrs. K had said "No" to intravenous furosemide repeatedly. The restraints had been placed because despite multiple reminders to use her call button, Mrs. K kept on leaving the bed. Soft restraints had been ordered as a patient safety measure following her fall.

Upon meeting Dr. T, Mrs. K expressed relief in having a Hindi-speaking physician. She tearily said, "I am happy to see you, but I want to go home." Mrs. K's daughter expressed to Dr. T that she was upset for not having been notified of the fall or the application of restraints overnight. On further discussion with Dr. T, it became clear that Mrs. K had never intended to convey a refusal of intravenous furosemide. Dr. T realized that the nurse's observations of Mrs. K shaking her head side to side and saying "NO" had been mis-interpreted. In reality, Dr. T suspected the patient had been displaying a relatively common gesture in South Asian cultures, a head bobble or shake, while indicating that she had "No" problem with the medication being given. In addition, Mrs. K said she felt ashamed and anxious about using the bedpan. Because she couldn't figure out how to use the call button, she had resorted to frequently going to the restroom to avoid incontinence. That is when she became dizzy and fell.

Dr. T submitted a patient safety event report indicating concerns regarding the lack of appropriate use of MIS as well as a lack of appropriate communication with the patient's family regarding the decision to apply restraints.

In this case, Mrs. K's "some English" was indeed "enough English" to put her at risk for medical error. This is when patients or providers can speak or understand a language to "get by" or to "make do." Mrs. K's chart was updated to include limited English proficiency (LEP), and restraints were discontinued. The nurse placed a video interpreter in the room. Dr. T educated the patient and healthcare team to use MIS during all interactions except with hospital-approved Hindi-speaking staff. The patient and staff followed and enforced the recommendations during the remainder of her inpatient stay.

QUESTIONS AND ANSWERS

1. How might the presence of REL documentation in this patient's chart have impacted her care?

In this case, early identification of Mrs. K's LEP could have alerted providers to access MIS early in her care. While Mrs. K did not initially ask for an interpreter, recognition of the limited history should have prompted Dr. T to suggest an interpreter be used. With use of MIS, Mrs. K likely would not have been labeled a "poor historian." In addition, utilization of MIS at the bedside would have prevented the nurse's misunderstanding of Mrs. K's head nods, and also would have allowed Mrs. K to more easily express her concerns regarding the use of the call light and apprehension about the bedpan.

Reliable language and English proficiency data are supposed to be entered at the patient's point of entry to the hospitals or clinics with documentation of the language services required during the patient-provider encounter. Office for Civil Rights defines primary language as the language that a Limited English Proficient individual identifies as the language they use to communicate effectively and would prefer to use to communicate. Although the terms "preferred" and "primary" language differ slightly, the intention is to find out the language that the patient would like to communicate with while with healthcare providers. Organizations can assess their language needs using an interactive mapping tool, the Civil Rights Division's Language Map App, to plan services and allocate resources. The tool determines the concentration of languages spoken by LEP individuals in a community.("LEP.gov," 2020). A study from 2012 suggested that despite the attempts to improve of REL data there seems to be variability in the ways in which primary and preferred language data was entered. (Duong, Singh, Buchanan, Phillips, & Gerlach, 2012)

2. In what ways did this patient's LEP result in a worse outcome than would have been experienced by an English-speaking (ES) patient?

In this case, the assumption of refusal of treatment (intravenous furosemide) led to withholding treatment from the patient that would not have occurred in the absence of a language barrier. The Joint Commission's Sentinel Event Database reveals that communication problems are among the root causes of 59% of serious adverse events reported(Wasserman et al., 2014). Research suggests that LEP patients are more likely than ES patients to experience safety events caused by communication errors. Specifically, LEP patients who experienced an adverse event were found more likely to be harmed. Additionally, when compared with ES patients, communication errors more frequently caused the adverse events, and the harm was more likely to be serious(Divi, Koss, Schmaltz, & Loeb, 2007).

In this case, the delayed administration of iv furosemide may have contributed to a prolonged hospitalization. Additionally, Mrs. K experienced a fall and forced physical restraint, both of which would likely not have occurred in the absence of a language barrier. One study showed that LEP patients had longer hospital stays when professional interpreters were not used compared to ES patients with the same clinical condition. Patients with LEP had higher rates of hospital-acquired conditions such as infections, surgical infections, falls, and pressure ulcers. The risk of surgical delays and readmissions is also higher ("Improving Patient Safety Systems for Patients With Limited English

Proficiency: A Guide for Hospitals," 2012). Quality of care is lowered when patients do not understand their health care providers, when patients and providers do not speak the same language, and when a provider's approach is not linguistically competent, such as when a provider does not effectively utilize MIS when indicated.("Office of Disease Prevention and Health Promotion,").

LEP status is an independent determinant of health outcomes during illnesses. It is also a social determinant of health and impacts access to and utilization of healthcare. It can be a source of disparities in health care access and health outcomes. Patients with LEP often have other disadvantages, including limited financial resources, limited health literacy, vulnerability due to uncertain immigration status, and mental health issues like anxiety and stress. Language barriers make it even more difficult for patients to advocate for themselves, ask questions, and navigate the nuances of health care systems. They are often less satisfied with their care than others and experience more diagnostic errors (Bell et al., 2022). According to one study, patients with (LEP) are often excluded from patient-reported outcome measures due to language barriers. However, their exclusion reduces opportunities for access to better cancer treatment and outcomes (Garcia Farina et al., 2022).

Mrs. K's care also suffered due to misinterpretation of her non-verbal communication, specifically head shaking. Gestures are movements of the head, hands, arms, and other parts of the body that convey meaning and serve interactive functions. When an individual conveys signals of attention to a conversation, this is referred to as "Back-channeling". Examples of back-channeling include utterances such as "uh-huh," "oh, really," and head nodding, among others. Head nods are a relatively common gesture in many cultures yet can indicate very different things. Mis-understood back-channeling potentially impacted care in this case. Due to cultural variation in the meaning of such signals, reliance on back-channeling alone as a means of communication can contribute further to errors and should be avoided.

3. In what ways was this patient's autonomy undermined?

In this case, the use of restraints was inappropriate and unlawfully undermined Mrs. K's autonomy. In a medical setting, mechanical and chemical restraints limit a patient's movement to prevent harm to the patient or others, including caregivers. Examples of physical restraints range from applying a wrist, ankle, waist, or abdominal restraints, tucking in a sheet very tightly so the patient can't move, keeping all side rails up to prevent the patient from getting out of bed, or using an enclosure bed. Even though considered less invasive, methods such as using video, mechanical (e.g., seat exit alarms), or acoustic surveillance are also types of as restraint. Pharmacological, also called chemical restraints, are a form of restraint in which medications are used to restrain patients. Due to the limits restraints place on patient autonomy, they must only be used when absolutely necessary. A patient should never be restrained solely for the convenience of the hospital staff or as punishment. Most state laws, Medicare regulations, and Joint Commission standards prohibit such punitive or convenience restraint use. A study on intensive care unit (ICU) patients with LEP showed patients with LEP were more likely to have restraints used (Barwise et al., 2018). Another study to assess determinants of mechanical restraint in an acute psychiatric care unit showed that the presence of a language barrier was associated with a significantly higher risk of mechanical restraints (El-Abidi et al., 2021). Appropriate utilization of MIS services is one strategy to reduce the unnecessary use of restraints.

4. How did access to a language concordant provider impact the care of this patient with LEP? How might care by language concordant providers impact patients?

In this case, once a physician who spoke the same language as Mrs. K became involved in her care, the previous misunderstandings were quickly identified, and her care improved. Dr. T's awareness of cross-cultural nonverbal communication also contributed to improved care.

One way to bypass language barriers is to recognize the value added to hiring and training bilingual healthcare providers. Language concordant care (LCC) enhances physician-patient trust, optimizes health outcomes, and advances health equity for diverse populations. Studies have shown that LEP patient outcomes, the education and counseling patients receive, and patient satisfaction all improve in the context of LCC. Some of the effects can be mitigated with the use of an interpreter. However, in one study, patients with language-discordant providers also reported worse interpersonal care and were more likely to give their providers low ratings. Using an interpreter did not mitigate these effects. A systematic review published in 2019, demonstrated that language concordant care is associated with improved patient ratings of provider interpersonal style, communication/information quality, listening skills and feeling understood, and risk factor control. In this review, where the outcome measures were quality of care, satisfaction with care/communication, medical understanding, and mental health, seventy-six percent of the studies demonstrated that at least one of the outcomes assessed was better for patients receiving LCC (Diamond et al., 2019). The presence of bilingual providers means more effective and timelier communication and improved patient satisfaction. Evidence supports better medication adherence and fewer emergency room visits when language-concordant clinicians provide care (Cano-Ibáñez, Zolfaghari, Amezcua-Prieto, & Khan, 2021; Hsueh, Hirsh, Maupomé, & Stewart, 2021; Ngo-Metzger et al., 2007).

Unfortunately, a significant "language gap" exists between those languages spoken by physicians and their patients ("Language Barriers in U.S. Health Care Understanding communication trends between U.S. physicians and patients," 2017). Overcoming this gap will require careful leadership attention to training and hiring practices moving forward.

5. What communication strategies can staff use with LEP patients while using MIS?

In hospitals or nursing homes, the nurse call button is a button or cord used by patients to ask for assistance. In a study, nurses perceived that patients with LEP use the call lights less frequently than their English-speaking counterparts. According to the nurses, patients with LEP may be discouraged from using the call light due to difficulty communicating. Staff revealed that they have difficulty explaining how to use the call light system to patients with LEP. Patients with LEP might also have a diminished sense of control and safety that the call light button provides (Galinato et al., 2016).

Physicians, staff, and interpreters should be trained in the process of communication and interpretation to minimize conversational loss and maximize the information and relational exchange with interpreted patients. Below are some best practices to implement:

- Always face and speak directly to the patient, not the interpreter. Use first-person language (e.g., you, your, you're) and avoid precursory instructions like "ask the patient" or "tell her/him."
- Use short sentences and phrases while insisting on sentence-by-sentence interpretation. Avoid wordy and complex sentences.
- Make eye contact and speak clearly, audibly, and slowly rather than loudly.
- Use plain and non-medical language.
- Pause often and allow the interpreter to finish before speaking
- Remain mindful of cultural and linguistic communication variances.
- Pay attention to nonverbal communication, such as facial expressions and gestures.
- Show graphics and demonstrate when possible.
- Invite patient participation and encourage questions
- Apply teach-back when applicable
- Respect an interpreter's judgment that a question is culturally inappropriate and either rephrase or ask the interpreter's help in eliciting the information more appropriately.
- Some evidence shows that having the interpreter beside or slightly behind the patient may facilitate better communication.

Epilogue

In this case, Mrs. K improved clinically at discharge and expressed gratitude for the excellent care from the Hindi-speaking physician. But it wasn't a classic "all's *well that ends well.*" On the patient satisfaction survey, she indicated *"sometimes"* for "courtesy and respect from the nurse" and *"never"* for "the nurse listened carefully." However, the nurse ought not be singled out as solely responsible for this patient's poor experience. From the beginning, the patient, physician, and staff all failed to recognize her LEP, leading to the failure to enter REL data at admission. This case highlights that policies, procedures, and tools are essential for collecting language-need data. The Health Research and Education Trust (HRET) has published best practices and training materials for REL data collection.("Improving

Health Equity Through Data Collection and Use: A Guide For Hospital Leaders," 2011). This case also highlights the potential value of having more than one checkpoint to assess language barriers and the need for interpreter services.

This case is another example of a preventable medical error where failure to recognize the patient's LEP led to the false perception of the patient's refusal of furosemide. Additionally, because interpreter services were not used to explain the call button's use, the patient was not able to use this tool. Additionally, the patient's autonomy was undermined through the unlawful use of physical restraints. These types of errors occur frequently and are preventable. should ensure a safe environment, organizations must encourage the reporting of medical errors due to language barriers. Strategies to monitor and prevent medical errors or near-miss events due to language barriers should also be implemented. Hospitals can adopt the AHRQ guide to identify use, report, monitor, and prevent medical errors in patients with LEP. The TeamSTEPPS LEP module can be utilized to help develop and implement a customized plan to improve.("Patients With Limited English Proficiency. Content last reviewed July 2017. Agency for Healthcare Research and Quality, Rockville, MD.,")

Finally, this case is an example where the availability of LCC resulted in the discovery of miscommunication and medication error and improved patient satisfaction. Data supports that LCC improves outcomes and patient satisfaction. Hence, organizations should offer patients options for LCC by recruiting, incentivizing, and training bilingual staff.

CASE 3: "YOU DON'T READ MORSE CODE?"

Goal

This case illustrates the essential role of translation service in medical interpretation as well as its impact on patient care and outcomes.

Learning Outcomes

1. Identify how access to documents written in one's own language can impact health outcomes.
2. Discuss laws and recommendations regarding the use of translation services in healthcare settings.
3. Differentiate between the services provided by translators and interpreters.
4. Summarize current guidelines regarding documentation of and reimbursement for interpreter and translation services.
5. Reflect on the challenges posed to patients with LEP in accessing digital health technologies.

Case

Mrs. P, a fifty-eight-year-old Cantonese-speaking patient with LEP, presented to the primary care clinic for management of diabetes mellitus. Despite trying her best, Mrs. P struggled with brittle diabetes and frequently experienced both hypoglycemia and hyperglycemia. In the last 12 months, she has required three emergency department visits and one hospitalization, all related to uncontrolled diabetes. Mrs. P lived alone and was independent with all activities of daily living.

After bringing Mrs. P to an exam room, the medical assistant set up video remote interpreting (VRI). Then, the primary care provider Dr. D came in the room and said, 'Hello Mrs. P, how have you been? Did you bring all your medications? I want to check them myself." Mrs. P smiled and pointed to the bag full of medications. Dr. D started going through the medication bottles one-by-one while asking questions. Mrs. P had seventeen bottles, including prescription, supplements, and over-the-counter medications. Dr. D could also tell that the bag included both current medications and medications she had asked the patient to discontinue at the last visit.

Dr. D held up two bottles, one with Atorvastatin 40 mg and one with Atorvastatin 80 mg. Dr. D asked, "Which one of these are you taking?" Mrs. P looked anxious, took the bottles in her hands, tried to look at something, and said, "I take both." Next, Dr. D separated the supplements from the prescription medications and asked, "Are you taking all of these supplements? Mrs. P replied hesitantly, "I don't know; I take them as needed." She added, "I get confused. I can't read the labels." Dr. D muttered, "Here we go again."

During Mrs. P's last visit, Dr. D and the pharmacist had sorted through her medications and suggested her daughter help with a pill organizer. Dr. D asked about the pill organizer, and Mrs. P stated, "The pill organizer doesn't work for me. I can't read the English medication names, dosages, and instructions. My daughter helps when she can but is also busy with her job and kids."

Blood testing that day revealed a glycosylated hemoglobin of 9.8, unchanged from the last visit. When asked about her diet, Mrs. P said, "I am doing the best I can. I don't even eat my favorite candies". During a visit with the dietician, she had trouble recollecting details of dietary and lifestyle education instructions given to her previously.

Dr. D noted that Mrs. P often failed to respond to electronic health record (EHR) messages and had previously missed appointments and follow-up labs. Dr. D then added the diagnosis code, Z 91.1 (medication noncompliance), to the patient chart and counseled the patient again.

The clinic's pharmacist suggested to Dr. D that the hospital translation service might be able to assist with printing medication labels in Cantonese. Dr. D agreed that would be helpful and requested the pharmacist to take the lead on it. Fortunately, the translation service agreed to provide the medication list and labels. However, they then commented, "We can do this once, but we can't provide translation service for all patients. We don't have the time, money or staff."

QUESTIONS AND ANSWERS

1. How might access to prescription labels and educational materials in her own language have improved the patient's health outcomes?

In this case, Mrs. P was able to perform all of her activities of daily living independently. This suggests that the primary barrier to her ability to follow medical instructions was related to LEP. Providing her with medication labels in her own language likely would have enabled her to read the instructions and take all of the medications as recommended, including recognizing those medications that should be discontinued. Additionally, dietary and lifestyle counseling regarding diabetes is complex. Given Mrs. P's inability to utilize information written in English, she needed to rely entirely on her memory of verbal instructions. Through providing her with information in her own language, Mrs. P would have been able to access more tools to effectively implement the recommended lifestyle changes.

Professional translation of medical documents enhances patients' understanding of their care plans and improves their outcomes. Medical translation is a complex process and emphasizes conceptual accuracy over a word-for-word rendition. The use of computer translation of scientific and medical documents is controversial. It is not accepted as the standard of qualified translation service and can lead to dangerous mistakes. A study that used a popular general-purpose machine translation tool to translate 213 medical record sentences from English into Spanish, Chinese, Russian and Korean showed that in each language, the majority of the translations were incomprehensible (76% to 92%) and incorrect (77% to 89%). The leading causes were vocabulary difficulty and syntactical complexity (Zeng-Treitler, Kim, Rosemblat, & Keselman, 2010). AHRQ provides translated documents for some common conditions through internet resources ("Improving Patient Safety Systems for Patients With Limited English Proficiency: A Guide for Hospitals," 2012). This artificial intelligence-based technology is expected to improve in the future.

A study showed that people with LEP struggle to understand the English information provided on dispensing prescription labels, and a substantial proportion of participants rarely or never read the labels. After receiving the bilingual dispensing labels, participants reported a marked increase in reading the dispensing labels with an associated reduction in further explanation required by someone. It was also noteworthy that 62% of people had identified instances where they took their medication inappropriately (Herrera, Alsaif, Khan, Barnes, & Rutter, 2019). A few state legislatures have passed laws requiring pharmacies to print prescription labels in languages other than English when the patient requests. The significant potential benefits of such laws are clear: fewer patient medication-related errors and greater adherence to treatment plans due to a better understanding of instructions. New York and California multilingual prescription label laws and Oregon's dual-language prescription drug labeling law are steps towards enhancing understanding of medication directions for patients with LEP and caregivers.

Large corporate chain pharmacies have significantly greater resources and are more likely to provide multilingual prescription labels than independent pharmacies due to cost issues. Centers for Medicare & Medicaid Services provides Toolkit Part 11, Understanding and using the "Toolkit Guidelines for Culturally Appropriate Translation," which has guidelines to help produce culturally appropriate translations ("CMS," 2016). The translation may have an integral role in communicating and engaging with patients of LEP in their healthcare and research.

2. What written information must be translated for patients? What written information should be translated for patients?

Understanding how LEP patients consume the information that clinicians share is crucial. A systematic review confirmed that providing written and verbal health information is more effective in improving knowledge and satisfaction than providing verbal information only (Johnson & Sandford, 2005). In the case of LEP patients, using interpreter service or language concordant care for verbal communication but providing information and instructions in a language they can't decipher could practically mean these patients have only verbal health information to reply on. The US Department of Health and Human Services (HHS) defines vital documents as "documents that affect access to, retention in or termination or exclusion from a recipient's program services or benefits. There are six types of documents that must be translated according to Title IV of the Civil Rights Act of 1964. These are considered vital medical translation projects and include:

- Notices of free language assistance
- Notices of eligibility criteria for services
- Informed consent documents
- Intake forms that have clinical consequences
- Discharge instructions
- Complaint forms

However, organizations should consider translating additional medical documents that can be beneficial for patients to understand instructions fully, like

- Prescription labeling and drug usage Information
- Health and lifestyle education material
- Patient & doctor manuals
- Patient Rights and responsibilities
- intake forms with clinical consequences
- Waiver forms

3. What is the difference between an interpreter and a translator?

The terms "interpreter" and "translator" are often incorrectly used interchangeably. A translator converts written information from one language to another; an interpreter is a specialist in converting oral information from one language to another. These individuals have significantly different training and skill sets. Organizations and medical providers should understand that medical interpretation and translation are two distinctive services, each required by law and not optional.

Healthcare organizations should assess and decide what documents they should translate depending on the needs of LEP patients and clients and allocate resources accordingly.

Written translation is the rendering of a written text in one language in a comparable written text in another language. Most professional translators provide only unidirectional translations, working into their dominant language. Sight translation is the oral rendition of text written in one language into another language and is usually done at the moment

4. How should one document, code, and bill communication need and use of interpreter and translation services in LEP patients?

"If it wasn't documented, it wasn't done" holds true in the case of MIS use. It is vital to document the use of interpretation by providers. Staff should report both the use and refusal of interpreter service. Registering refusal of interpretive services in the medical record protects providers and practices and ensures consistency for monitoring. The patient should be aware that interpreter service is available without additional costs. Staff should use smart phrases for documentation for tracking and monitoring purposes to optimize use.

Significant time and personnel efforts go into interpretation and translation services. Although the patient cannot be billed for the actual service provided by the interpreter, one may be able to bill a prolonged service code (99354-99357) in addition to the appropriate E/M code. Longstanding CMS policy permits reimbursement for translation/interpretation activities, so long as they are not included and paid for as part of the rate for direct service.

5. Why might this patient not have utilized the patient portal or have missed follow-up appointments and lab draws

A patient portal is a secure online website that gives patients convenient, 24-hour access to personal health information from anywhere with an internet connection. Patients can view health information such as recent doctor visits, discharge summaries, medications, immunizations, allergies, and lab results. Some patient portals also allow patients to secure message doctors, request prescription refills, schedule non-urgent appointments, make payments, and receive educational materials. Patient portals have revolutionized how patients and providers communicate outside of clinical encounters. Patient portals can also save time, support care between visits, and keep patients abreast with development. However, one can reap those benefits only if one understands the patient portal's use and information. While most hospital systems utilize patient portals, few portals are friendly for LEP patients. The patient in this case likely was not able to access and read the information in the patient portal as would have an English-speaking patient. National data show that underserved populations are substantially less likely to access patient portals, especially those with limited English proficiency.("United States Census Bureau," 2022). This can exacerbate disparities in utilization of healthcare and health outcomes. To meet the needs of LEP patients, portals and messaging must be multilingual. Some patient portals have developed systems to be multilingual. Many portal systems can send text messages to patients in multiple languages, alerting them to changes in their portal account or notifying them of upcoming appointments.

With the recent expansion of telehealth, the Justice Department and the US Department of Health & Human Services recently issued guidance on nondiscrimination in telehealth. The guidance provided clarity on how federal nondiscrimination laws require accessibility for people with disabilities and LEP persons in health care provided by telehealth.("United States Department of Justice," 2022)

Healthcare advocacy should make policymakers aware of the great divide in digital health and develop strategies to make digital health more accessible and user-friendly for patients with LEP.

Epilogue

Looking at her medication prescription labels in Cantonese, Mrs. P smiled like she had seen her favorite candies. She read the prescription labels to the pharmacist and demonstrated an understanding of instructions. Her adherence to treatment, fluctuations in blood glucose levels, and incidents of ED visits and hospitalization all improved significantly over the next six months. In this case, while the patient had access to MIS during the visit, she did not have access to a medical translation service. She was not able to take her medications as prescribed due to her inability to read discharge instructions and was not able to understand or follow health education and lifestyle interventions fully. Hospitals and pharmacies should consider a patient-centered prescription drug label by providing labels in the language that a patient understands to reduce medication errors and improve patient self-efficacy. A formal policy requiring written information for LEP patients should be in place. When using translations in research, translation processes need to be made explicit in research protocols and reports, and translation experts need to be part of the research team.

The patient in this case was unable to use the patient portal. Messages, reminders for appointments, and labs orders were all inaccessible to her. The case highlights how patients' portals and digital health need to be more inclusive and friendly for LEP patients. A physician should selectively use patient portals to engage with patients depending on access and usability. Several portal vendors (product makers) offer language accessibility options. Healthcare advocates and policymakers must be aware of the great divide between digital patient portals and the LEP population.

CONCLUSION

The healthcare systems need to catch up with the needs of a large and growing LEP population. This requires resource allocation and budget development to promote availability and access to MIS, translated documents, patient center prescription labels, hiring bilingual staff, and ensuring adequate staffing. Key priorities include patient and staff education, reporting and monitoring of use and errors, and research and advocacy. The key stakeholders, administrators, staff, healthcare providers, purchasers and portal vendors, insurance companies, and policymakers must join efforts for the LEP population to thrive.

REFERENCES

AHA. (2011). *Improving Health Equity Through Data Collection and Use: A Guide For Hospital Leaders.* AHA.

AHRQ. (2012). *Improving Patient Safety Systems for Patients with Limited English Proficiency. A Guide for Hospitals.* AHRQ. https://www.ahrq.gov/sites/default/files/publications/files/lepguide.pdf

AHRQ. (2017). *Patients With Limited English Proficiency.* Agency for Healthcare Research and Quality. https://www.ahrq.gov/teamstepps/lep/index.html

Barwise, A., Jaramillo, C., Novotny, P., Wieland, M. L., Thongprayoon, C., Gajic, O., & Wilson, M. E. (2018). Differences in Code Status and End-of-Life Decision Making in Patients With Limited English Proficiency in the Intensive Care Unit. *Mayo Clinic Proceedings, 93*(9), 1271–1281. doi:10.1016/j.mayocp.2018.04.021 PMID:30100192

Bell, S. K., Dong, J., Ngo, L., McGaffigan, P., Thomas, E. J., & Bourgeois, F. (2022). Diagnostic error experiences of patients and families with limited English-language health literacy or disadvantaged socioeconomic position in a cross-sectional US population-based survey. *BMJ Quality & Safety*, bmjqs-2021-013937. Advance online publication. doi:10.1136/bmjqs-2021-013937 PMID:35121653

Cano-Ibáñez, N., Zolfaghari, Y., Amezcua-Prieto, C., & Khan, K. S. (2021). Physician-Patient Language Discordance and Poor Health Outcomes: A Systematic Scoping Review. *Frontiers in Public Health, 9*, 629041. doi:10.3389/fpubh.2021.629041 PMID:33816420

CMS. (2016). *A practical Guide to Implementing the National CLAS Standards.* National Committee for Quality Assurance. https://www.cms.gov/About-CMS/Agency-Information/OMH/Downloads/CLAS-Toolkit-12-7-16.pdf

Diamond, L., Izquierdo, K., Canfield, D., Matsoukas, K., & Gany, F. (2019). A Systematic Review of the Impact of Patient-Physician Non-English Language Concordance on Quality of Care and Outcomes. *Journal of General Internal Medicine, 34*(8), 1591–1606. doi:10.100711606-019-04847-5 PMID:31147980

Diamond, L. C., Schenker, Y., Curry, L., Bradley, E. H., & Fernandez, A. (2009). Getting by: Underuse of interpreters by resident physicians. *Journal of General Internal Medicine*, *24*(2), 256–262. doi:10.100711606-008-0875-7 PMID:19089503

Divi, C., Koss, R. G., Schmaltz, S. P., & Loeb, J. M. (2007). Language proficiency and adverse events in US hospitals: A pilot study. *International Journal for Quality in Health Care*, *19*(2), 60–67. doi:10.1093/intqhc/mzl069 PMID:17277013

Doximity. (2017). *Language Barriers in U.S. Health Care: Understanding communication trends between U.S. physicians and patients.* Doximity. https://s3.amazonaws.com/s3.doximity.com/press/Doximity%20Language%20in%20U.S.%20Health%20Care%20Report.pdf

Duong, L. M., Singh, S. D., Buchanan, N., Phillips, J. L., & Gerlach, K. (2012). Evaluation of primary/preferred language data collection. *Journal of Registry Management*, *39*(3), 121–132. PMID:23443456

El-Abidi, K., Moreno-Poyato, A. R., Toll Privat, A., Corcoles Martinez, D., Aceña-Domínguez, R., Pérez-Solà, V., & Mané, A. (2021). Determinants of mechanical restraint in an acute psychiatric care unit. *World Journal of Psychiatry*, *11*(10), 854–863. doi:10.5498/wjp.v11.i10.854 PMID:34733647

Flores, O., Seminario, S. S., Contreras, E., & Perez, P. (2016). Actitud terapéutica de los tutores y residentes de cuarto año de Medicina Familiar y Comunitaria de Girona frente a las infiltraciones periarticulares. *Atencion Primaria*, *48*(6), 421–422. doi:10.1016/j.aprim.2015.09.007 PMID:26817805

Galinato, J., Montie, M., Shuman, C., Patak, L., & Titler, M. (2016). Perspectives of Nurses on Patients With Limited English Proficiency and Their Call Light Use. *Global Qualitative Nursing Research*, *3*. doi:10.1177/2333393616637764 PMID:28393085

Garcia Farina, E., Rowell, J., Revette, A., Haakenstad, E. K., Cleveland, J. L. F., Allende, R., Hassett, M., Schrag, D., & McCleary, N. J. (2022). Barriers to Electronic Patient-Reported Outcome Measurement Among Patients with Cancer and Limited English Proficiency. *JAMA Network Open*, *5*(7), e2223898. doi:10.1001/jamanetworkopen.2022.23898 PMID:35867056

Herrera, H., Alsaif, M., Khan, G., Barnes, N., & Rutter, P. (2019). Provision of Bilingual Dispensing Labels to Non-Native English Speakers: An Exploratory Study. *Pharmacy (Basel, Switzerland)*, *7*(1), 32. doi:10.3390/pharmacy7010032 PMID:30934609

HHS. (2021). Access and Functional Needs Toolkit: Integrating a Community Partner Network to Inform Risk Communication Strategies. U.S. Department of Health and Human Services (HHS), CDC.

Hsueh, L., Hirsh, A. T., Maupomé, G., & Stewart, J. C. (2021). Patient-Provider Language Concordance and Health Outcomes: A Systematic Review, Evidence Map, and Research Agenda. *Medical Care Research and Review: MCRR*, *78*(1), 3–23. doi:10.1177/1077558719860708 PMID:31291823

Jacobs, E. A., Sadowski, L. S., & Rathouz, P. J. (2007). The impact of an enhanced interpreter service intervention on hospital costs and patient satisfaction. *Journal of General Internal Medicine*, *22*(S2, Suppl 2), 306–311. doi:10.100711606-007-0357-3 PMID:17957416

Johnson, A., & Sandford, J. (2005). Written and verbal information versus verbal information only for patients being discharged from acute hospital settings to home: Systematic review. *Health Education Research*, *20*(4), 423–429. doi:10.1093/her/cyg141 PMID:15572437

Joseph, C., Garruba, M., & Melder, A. (2018). Patient satisfaction of telephone or video interpreter services compared with in-person services: A systematic review. *Australian Health Review*, *42*(2), 168–177. doi:10.1071/AH16195 PMID:30021688

Karliner, L. S., Pérez-Stable, E. J., & Gregorich, S. E. (2017). Convenient Access to Professional Interpreters in the Hospital Decreases Readmission Rates and Estimated Hospital Expenditures for Patients With Limited English Proficiency. *Medical Care*, *55*(3), 199–206. doi:10.1097/MLR.0000000000000643 PMID:27579909

LEP.gov. (2020). *Source and Methodology*. Limited English Proficiency gov. https://www.lep.gov/source-and-methodology

Locatis, C., Williamson, D., Gould-Kabler, C., Zone-Smith, L., Detzler, I., Roberson, J., & Ackerman, M. (2010). Comparing in-person, video, and telephonic medical interpretation. *Journal of General Internal Medicine*, *25*(4), 345–350. doi:10.100711606-009-1236-x PMID:20107916

Ngo-Metzger, Q., Sorkin, D. H., Phillips, R. S., Greenfield, S., Massagli, M. P., Clarridge, B., & Kaplan, S. H. (2007). Providing high-quality care for limited English proficient patients: The importance of language concordance and interpreter use. *Journal of General Internal Medicine*, *22*(S2, Suppl 2), 324–330. doi:10.100711606-007-0340-z PMID:17957419

Schenker, Y., Pérez-Stable, E. J., Nickleach, D., & Karliner, L. S. (2011). Patterns of interpreter use for hospitalized patients with limited English proficiency. *Journal of General Internal Medicine*, *26*(7), 712–717. doi:10.100711606-010-1619-z PMID:21336672

Schenker, Y., Wang, F., Selig, S. J., Ng, R., & Fernandez, A. (2007). The impact of language barriers on documentation of informed consent at a hospital with on-site interpreter services. *Journal of General Internal Medicine*, *22*(S2, Suppl 2), 294–299. doi:10.100711606-007-0359-1 PMID:17957414

United States Census Bureau. (2022). *CS 5-Year Estimates Public Use Microdata Sample*. USCB. https://data.census.gov/mdat/#/search?ds=ACSPUMS5Y2018&cv=ENG%282,3,4%29&wt=PWGTP

United States Department of Justice. (2022). *Justice Department and HHS Issue Guidance on Nondiscrimination in Telehealth the Week of the 32nd Anniversay of the Americans with Disabilities Act*. USDJ. https://www.justice.gov/opa/pr/justice-department-and-hhs-issue-guidance-nondiscrimination-telehealth-week-32nd-anniversary

Wasserman, M., Renfrew, M. R., Green, A. R., Lopez, L., Tan-McGrory, A., Brach, C., & Betancourt, J. R. (2014). Identifying and preventing medical errors in patients with limited English proficiency: Key findings and tools for the field. *Journal for Healthcare Quality*, *36*(3), 5–16. doi:10.1111/jhq.12065 PMID:24629098

Zeng-Treitler, Q., Kim, H., Rosemblat, G., & Keselman, A. (2010). Can multilingual machine translation help make medical record content more comprehensible to patients? *Studies in Health Technology and Informatics*, *160*(Pt 1), 73–77. PMID:20841653

Chapter 9
Classism:
Navigating the Hierarchy

Kate J. F. Carnevale
https://orcid.org/0000-0001-6898-0381
Nova Southeastern University Dr. Kiran C. Patel College of Allopathic Medicine, USA

Melissa Armas
https://orcid.org/0000-0002-4202-2764
Nova Southeastern University Dr. Kiran C. Patel College of Allopathic Medicine, USA

Vijay Kumar Rajput
Nova Southeastern University Dr. Kiran C. Patel College of Allopathic Medicine, USA

EXECUTIVE SUMMARY

Social class and classism can be traced back to the beginning of written history when social standing was based on nobility and family rank. In modern-day society, social standing is based on wealth and socioeconomic status. Classism refers to the marginalization of an individual or a group based on social class or perceived social class. It can be intentional or unintentional and is classified as individual or institutional. Institutional classism relates to policies and practices within an institution that present barriers and increase the difficulty of accessing resources for individuals in a particular social class. These cases highlight examples of unintentional institutional classism in healthcare that provide learners and practitioners with the tools to identify institutional classism or procedural blind spots in the healthcare setting and its implications. It is important for healthcare learners and institutions to be educated on actions, procedures, and strategies to mitigate classism in healthcare.

DOI: 10.4018/978-1-6684-5493-0.ch009

BACKGROUND

Class is a social construct used to apportion individuals into categories based on financial or economic status, geographical location of habitation, and/or social affiliations and connectedness to individuals in authority (Dos Santos, 1970). Class can be interpreted as the differences in the relative social rank in terms of income, wealth, education, status and/or power (classaction.org). Wilkerson defines classism as "granting or withholding of respect, status, honor, attention, privileges, resources, benefit of the doubt, and human kindness to someone on the basis of their perceived rank or standing in the hierarchy" (Wilkerson, 2020). Thus, classism can lead to systematic assignment of worth based on social class, and affect policies and practices both at the level of individuals and institutions. It is important to note that classism can lead to class privilege, that is the tangible or intangible unearned advantages of "higher-class" status. The differential treatment based on social class or perceived social class typically benefits more class-privileged people at the expense of the individuals or groups that are considered less class-privileged (classaction.org). Class privilege may be displayed through diverse channels, for example, personal contacts with employers, good childhood health care and education, inherited money, and/or speaking with the same dialect/accent as people with institutional power (Adams *et al.,* 2007). This often results in stark differences in income, wealth inequality, and unmet basic human needs (Wilkerson, 2020).

Historically, the family line a person was born into determined the economic and social power available to that person. Ancient models throughout the world granted power and authority to landowners at the expense of the working-class group (i.e. serfs, peasants, servants, slaves, etc.). Three major instances of caste systems that appear in history are found in India, Nazi Germany, and the modern society of developed countries (Dumont, 1981). Firstly, the Indian caste system (based on location and origins of birth) ascribed the lowest caste members as the "Untouchables"/Dalits. They were historically poorer and had more limited resources, and were relegated to undesirable and dangerous jobs in society. Parallels have been drawn between the Indian caste system and how poor, immigrant, and minority race and ethnicity individuals have been treated as "untouchable" in US culture (Wilkerson, 2020). In India, this system was intricately supported by Hinduism beliefs in reincarnation of the soul, based on the idea that a lower caste was deserved due to wrong doings in the previous life, but that by obeying caste rules individuals could be rewarded in the next life. This mirrors a pervasive implicit bias held in American society, that individuals of low socioeconomic status deserve their circumstances and should work harder to achieve higher status, by following the "American Dream" (Chomsky 2017). This myopic view fails to consider the barriers that prevent individuals, families, and communities from upward mobility (Bates 1997). These societal views result in various forms of marginalization and exploitation of the lower castes in India. Despite the formal laws being established to ban caste system in India in the 1940s, the system persists (Wilkerson, 2020).

A second prominent instance of a caste system was observed in Nazi Germany which displayed bias between individuals of Aryan and Jewish roots. Nazi elites drew inspiration for laws to create and enforce their caste system by looking at race legislation passed in America, such as miscegenation laws and rules for segregation (Ezzell, 2002). These laws created the legal basis for the Aryan Nation, which evolved into the Nuremberg Laws that stripped the "lower-status" social class of their basic human rights (Wilkerson, 2020). And it can be inferred that, at its most extreme, unchecked classism contributed to the mass exterminations of those perceived as "different" and therefore "lesser" due to ethnicity, religion, political beliefs, behavior and/or sexual orientation, during the holocaust. (US Holocaust Memorial Museum, 2020).

Classism

In modern day society, the social construct of class has been shifted from birthright or legal designations, to personal wealth and socioeconomic status, such as is seen in the United States of America's system of social stratifications (Boone, 2020). Complex factors may weave the unique tapestry of an individual's perceived class. In American society, social classes encompass large groups of people who share a similar economic position in society, with groups of people in America commonly being stratified as working class, middle class, and affluent (Lott, 2012). However, aspects of individuals' lived experiences such as race, gender, family composition, marital status, sexual orientation, education, employment, and community resources can affect which class a person may be designated by society to belong. These individual factors can intersect, creating unique and additive effects on individuals under the various systems of power at play in society (Hankivsky, 2022). With this, the marginalization of individuals or groups on the basis of social class or perceived social class, is pervasive in the US (Limbert and Williams, 2014). In general, individuals of lower socioeconomic status are more likely to experience classism. Studies have shown that individuals who are perceived to be of lower socioeconomic status are more likely to experience feelings of being negatively judged, degraded, devalued, blamed, and looked down on by others in the society (Simons *et. al.*, 2017).

Classism can be individual or institutional, and is systemic in the US (Sivashanker, 2020). Individual classism refers to an individual's negative attitudes, actions, or beliefs regarding others in a particular social class. As an example, a person may view individuals of lower socioeconomic status as lazy or unintelligent. Institutional classism refers to the ways in which intentional and unintentional classism manifests in the various institutions of our society. Classism may be perpetuated by the policies and practices at institutions that present barriers and increase the difficulty of accessing resources for individuals in a particular social class, leading to systems that disproportionately affect member of that class (Scambler, 2019). Institutional classism can be exemplified in such instances as when a hospital encourages physicians to adjust the clinical management of patients based on health insurance status, or healthcare service providers choose to locate their clinics in affluent parts of town rather than in lower socioeconomic status areas (Lott, 2012). Current scholarship and practice include documentation of institutional classism and its effects, critical analyses that situate classism within power relations, and proposals for incorporating class awareness into clinicians' training and practice (Limbert and Williams, 2014). It is important to note that classism is intersectional in nature, meaning that individuals experiencing classism may also be experiencing discrimination in other areas of their lives in addition to their experience with classism (Green *et. al.*, 2017). For instance, a Black woman who is of lower socioeconomic status may also be experiencing discrimination on the basis of class, gender, and race -- compounding and exacerbating observed health disparities (Evans, 2018).

Many individuals of lower socioeconomic status struggle with receiving adequate and equitable healthcare due to the numerous systemic and interpersonal hurdles they face, with the end result being a statistical difference between individuals of lower socioeconomic status and education having lower life expectancy than their better educated and affluent counterparts (Thompson, 2018). Geographic regions with lower socioeconomic status also typically represent higher rates of under- and uninsured persons, and higher rates of preventable chronic illness (Shrider, 2021 & Minkler, 2006).

Potentially the most vulnerable populations, with little recourse to migrate away from their assigned social class or advocate for themselves, are children living in poverty and children who have been entered into the government's child welfare system, often referred to as foster care. Children in foster care are typically more likely to be removed from low socioeconomic homes (Pelton, 2015). This may be due to compounding factors of food and housing insecurity, limited opportunities for parents, along with the added stress that parents living in poverty experience leading to adverse outcomes. Additionally, there may be lacking social and logistical support for parents in poverty, potentially also contributing to neglect, substance abuse and domestic violence (Fong, 2020).

Children and adolescents in foster care experience healthcare inequity due to various factors related to gaps in healthcare support. They often lack primary care providers or necessary medical homes and tend to be reliant on the emergency department for care. Additionally, they may come into foster care with missing or incomplete medical records. (Bright *et. al.*, 2018). These factors may lead to discontinuity of health care providers who could contribute insights on and monitoring of chronic or persistent medical concerns. Caregivers are vital to meeting the healthcare needs of foster children by ensuring children are seen by medical providers and communicating their medical needs (Schneiderman *et. al.*, 2012). This requires collaboration between caregivers, healthcare providers, and administrators of child welfare to fill in knowledge gaps and provide the highest quality of care for vulnerable children.

Whether the classism experienced is unintentional or overt, undoubtedly, classism can create barriers in access to equitable healthcare. Failure of healthcare providers to take sociocultural factors into account may lead to stereotyping and in worst case scenarios bias or discriminatory treatment of patients based on race, culture or social status (Smedley *et. al.*, 2003). Evidence suggests that people from lower socioeconomic backgrounds experience discrimination and marginalization within the healthcare system (Becker and Newsom, 2003). Additionally, negative healthcare experiences can deter patients from seeking and utilizing health services in the future (Tang *et. al.*, 2015).

Providing health professional learners and practitioners, and potential caregivers, with educational tools to orient them to the special considerations for children in foster care in the healthcare setting is important. It is imperative that health care professionals are trained to recognize their biases, conscious and unconscious, as well as quickly identify their gaps in knowledge and are further directed on ways to mitigate them. The cases discussed in this chapter highlight unintentional instances of institutional classism and aims to provide knowledge, skills and awareness regarding institutional classism and strategies to mitigate it in the healthcare setting.

CASE 1: V.I.P. - VARYING IMPORTANCE OF PATIENTS

Goal

This case exemplifies institutional classism within a hospital system.

Learning Outcomes

1. Define classism and analyze it in the health care setting and how it impacts health care disparities.
2. Appraise classism in the clinical care and clarify instances of classism affecting patient care.
3. Examine the impact of institutional classism on health professional learners, educators, and patients.
4. Assess the nature of classism and its intersectionality with other systems of discrimination.
5. Develop strategies to mitigate classism in the clinical setting and restore equity in patient care.

Case

Dr. Williams, a resident physician, is part of a large residency program in a free clinic run by a not-for-profit academic safety net hospital. The free clinic and hospital are located downtown, near an underserved area of the city. The free clinic primarily serves disadvantaged minority and/or uninsured undocumented immigrant patients. The clinic has a full schedule of patients daily and the attending physicians rotate between the free clinic and the community based academic hospital. Many of the patients are regulars who have come to rely on the clinic for their medical needs. Other members of the medical team in the free clinic include nurse practitioners, medical students, medical assistants, and front desk managerial staff.

On Monday morning, as Dr. Williams and the team are getting ready to see the first few patients of the day, a call comes in from hospital administration requesting that the attending physician, Dr. Alvarez, see a patient that has been admitted to the hospital. The patient, Mr. Wells, is a known benefactor to the hospital and was admitted to the hospital after complaining of chest pains and shortness of breath. He has specifically requested Dr. Alvarez, as she is well known in her field.

Dr. Alvarez is informed that hospital administration has asked that she see Mr. Wells. Dr. Alvarez is not pleased with this news, as she had follow-up appointments scheduled with her patients in the free clinic. She remarks that "All of our patients are VIP patients! Mr. Wells is not more important than our patients in the free clinic."

Dr. Alvarez asks if Dr. Williams and Mr. Chen, the nurse practitioner scheduled for the day, can see her patients that require simple follow-up to avoid cancelling all her appointments for the day. The other appointments will need to be cancelled and rescheduled.

The next morning at the team meeting, the team discusses yesterday's patient appointments:

Dr. Williams: "I met with Ms. West for her follow-up appointment. She is doing well after finishing her antibiotics for pneumonia but seems to be having some mild side effects from her high blood pressure medication. I told her I would discuss it with you and not to stop the medication without hearing from you, but I am not sure she will listen. She seemed disappointed that you weren't present for her appointment."

Mr. Chen: "I had a similar experience with Mr. Gutierrez. He is still struggling with smoking cessation. He wouldn't even discuss the topic with me. He only wanted to discuss it with you. He expressed frustration at seeing someone else when he was expecting you."

Dr. Alvarez: "I am frustrated with the whole situation. This isn't the first time this has happened. I shouldn't have to bump my patients for someone else who the board deems more important. Why do they get to decide who I am allowed to provide care for?"

Dr. Williams: "Also, we have multiple voicemails from the patients that had to be cancelled and rescheduled. We had to inconvenience our patients when there were other capable physicians who were on call and could have care for Mr. Wells' health concerns."

Dr. Alvarez: "Other patients do not have the ability to choose their physicians when admitted into the hospital."

Following the team meeting, the team feels helpless and frustrated regarding the situation. They are unsure how to address this problem with the administration.

QUESTIONS AND ANSWERS

1. Describe how classism is occurring and discuss whether it is individual or institutionalized.

In the above case, patients at the free clinic lost their scheduled appointments with their medical provider because a benefactor to the hospital, Mr. Wells, was admitted to the hospital and specifically requested the medical provider, Dr. Alvarez, to care for him. Mr. Wells was given priority over the patients in the free clinic due to his status as a wealthy benefactor to the hospital. He was also granted his medical provider of choice, solely due to his status as a wealthy benefactor to the hospital. The patients at the free clinic were most likely uninsured with many likely residing in underserved areas of the city nearby. This is clearly a case of classism as Mr. Wells, the wealthy benefactor is given priority over the patients in free clinic. This is a case of institutionalized classism as the hospital administration is the entity removing the physician from scheduled appointments in the free clinic and sent to the hospital to provide care for Mr. Wells, until he is discharged.

2. Discuss how patient care is being affected as a result of classism in the above case. How does Dr. Alvarez suddenly being called away impact patient care in the free clinic?

Some of her patient appointments had to be cancelled and rescheduled, as a result of Dr. Alvarez being called away at the last minute to care for Mr. Wells. Those patients that were not cancelled were surprised and frustrated at having to see another provider, with whom they had not developed a rapport, and they were not receptive to discussing certain aspects of their care with a new provider. As a result, the patients at the free clinic were not receiving high quality uninterrupted care. Instead, their care was disrupted, and the quality decreased. This may contribute to downstream issues such as non-adherence or patient distrust in the healthcare system, due to feeling undervalued by it.

3. How does this case reflect the intersectional nature of classism regarding other forms of discrimination?

Patients at the free clinic are from underserved areas near the hospital and many belong to minority groups. As a result, minority groups are being disproportionately affected by the institutional classism that is occurring at the hospital and free clinic. Additionally, patient gender and/or sexual orientation may further amplify the disadvantages faced by these patients. While not necessarily intentional, the decision of the hospital administration to prioritize wealthy patients, like Mr. Wells, causes the minority population that frequents the free clinic to experience discontinuity in their healthcare and reduced quality of care they receive. As a result, they may feel that the hospital administration does not value them as patients and that they are viewed as less worthy of high-quality care than other patients. Impressions of lower value and worth can be felt by minority groups who are consistently marginalized, these feelings are often and reinforced by experiences where individuals and institutions provide individuals from minority groups with limited or poor options, and can be compounded by intuitional classism, as observed in this case.

4. How does institutionalized classism create potential conflicts for team members? Why does the team feel helpless and frustrated with the situation?

The potential conflict for team members lies in the fact that, while they do not agree with the hospital administration's decisions, they are still employed by the hospital. As employees, they may feel that they have little recourse available to change the system, especially when the patient in question is a benefactor to the hospital and the hospital relies on donations from benefactors to manage its day-to-day operation expenses. The team members feel their duty is to their patients but, at the same time, they realize that they are subordinates of the hospital and if they lose their employment, they will no longer be able to help their patients in the free clinic or the hospital.

5. Discuss how Dr. Alvarez should address this issue individually.

Dr. Alvarez can attend national/international conferences and seminars relating to classism and how it affects patients and the health care system. Additionally, she can research data regarding healthcare and classism. She can then take the information and knowledge she has gained from attending the conferences and her research and use it to develop seminars at her institution to spread awareness among her colleagues. Dr. Alvarez can also take the information and knowledge she learned and use it to advocate for a full-time attending physician position at the clinic.

6. Develop potential strategies that the team can bring to hospital administration to help mitigate classism in the hospital system and increase patient equity.

It is important to address institutional classism and the inequities in healthcare it creates. Additionally, the concerns of the team members regarding patient care need to be addressed as they are pivotal to providing excellent care for the patients at the free clinic. Potential strategies can be developed and brought to the attention of the medical director who can address it with hospital administration. Potential strategies include:

- Having Dr. Alvarez identify other capable physicians that could care for Mr. Wells, and similar patients, when she is scheduled in the free clinic. This can be facilitated by introducing Mr. Wells, and similar patients, to the alternative providers, so that the patients will be comfortable with all the physicians rotating the care responsibilities of the patients.
- Requesting additional providers who can follow up on Dr. Alvarez's previously scheduled free clinic appointments and similar procedures to be put in place to avoid needing to cancel patient appointments. If multiple physicians are in rotation, this can be implemented in a practical and feasible manner.
- Introducing patients in the free clinic to other providers that may fill in for Dr. Alvarez, allowing her patients to establish relationships with the providers prior to unforeseen circumstances that takes Dr. Alvarez away from the free clinic. These providers can be the established substitutes so that the patients will not be caught off guard. Additionally, this will reduce cancellations in the event of an unforeseen circumstance. It will also be essential to make hospital administration aware of how the current policy is causing health care inequities and further disadvantages for minority groups.

Epilogue

Several months later, Dr. Alvarez has attended a conference about classism and has collected information and data regarding institutional classism and its effects on healthcare. She is scheduled to present a seminar on institutional classism and its impacts on healthcare at her institution later in the month. Dr. Alvarez is hopeful that by spreading awareness amongst her colleagues, the first steps can be made toward changes in policy.

Due to Dr. Alvarez' efforts, a workgroup is organized by the hospital administration to handle on-call physicians for any last-minute schedule changes to the clinic. This includes organizing substitute attending physicians in the case of emergencies and rearranging appointments should the need arise. It is the hope of Dr. Alvarez and the clinic members that this workgroup will help minimize the impact of last-minute schedule changes on the clinic patients by reducing interruptions in their care and increasing patient trust in the system.

Institutional classism provides patients of a certain social standing or social class priority over others of a lower social standing or social class. This often intersects with other forms of discrimination based on gender, sexual orientation, or minority status. As a result, it is important for healthcare providers and administrators to self-educate through consulting reputable resources, and attending conferences and seminars, as well as spread awareness through the development of seminars and by sharing the information with others. The initiative and passionate dedication of a few individuals along with an institutional culture that values self-improvement can help identify and correct instances of institutional classism to promote more equitable and better health outcomes for all.

CASE 2: ONE SIZE DOESN'T FIT ALL

Goal

This case exemplifies the influence of socioeconomic status and education level of patients and their caregivers on the quality of healthcare they receive.

Learning Outcomes

1. Discuss the unique social class of children in foster care (under child welfare protective custody).
2. Describe how continuity of care and access to health records can impact foster children in health crises.
3. Explore how clinicians and caregivers can improve patient care outcomes for children in foster care.
4. Elucidate the role of communication between health care providers, foster parents, and the child welfare agency.

Case

Jose is a 20-month-old boy who is brought to the emergency department (ED) for trouble breathing, following a cold. He is accompanied by his foster mother, who has had the boy in her care for approximately two weeks. Jose has a prescription for an albuterol nebulizer that the foster mother says she has been giving to Jose according to the instructions while he has been sick, but it has not provided lasting relief, especially when the child is laying down to sleep. The ED they arrived at was not equipped with a pediatric unit, but it was the closest facility to their home. The hospital staff assures the foster mother that they can transfer them to a pediatric hospital if Jose needs to be admitted.

After the initial screening, where the foster mother is unable to provide any medical history for Jose, the ED physician on staff, Dr. A, admits to the foster mother that while he is not a pediatrician, he is concerned about Jose's low oxygen saturation and wants to get to the bottom of the underlying cause by running some tests. The foster mother agrees. Being in foster care, Jose's medical expenses are covered by the state, so the foster mother does not question what tests will be administered. Similarly, Dr. A does not feel obligated to be selective about which tests to subject Jose to, since there is not a financial consideration for the family. Over the next six hours Jose undergoes a chest x-ray, urine and blood draws with equipment that is sized for adults, a course of broad-spectrum IV antibiotics, and is placed on supplemental oxygen with a mask that is too big for his face, since the hospital does not have pediatric nasal cannulas. There are also long periods of time between test administrations where no one enters the room to check on Jose. No food or water are offered. The extensive poking and prodding with inefficient adult-sized equipment has left Jose traumatized, combative, and exhausted. With further tests still pending and his condition not improving, transportation is arranged, and Jose and his foster mother are taken by ambulance to a pediatric hospital on the other side of the county.

At the pediatric hospital, Jose is evaluated in the ED. The pediatric hospitalist, Dr. X, asks the foster mother some questions, including how many treatments Jose received at the previous hospital. She is surprised to hear that Jose was only given oxygen and not albuterol, and frowns when she hears how many tests Jose was subjected to. When the foster mother asks if that was appropriate, Dr. X responds only with "We'll take care of you here." Afterwards, a new IV line with a pediatric sized wrist board is fitted, Jose is swabbed with a pediatric test kit for several of the most typical viral respiratory infections, and he is started on a triple dose of albuterol via nebulizer. The respiratory therapist, Mr. Y, makes polite conversation with the foster mother while setting up Jose's treatment, telling her that he used to be a foster kid. Mr. Y kindly reassures Jose that everything will turn out all right. The nurse provides some juice and snacks before Jose is admitted to a room in the respiratory wing. The hospital also has electronic records of Jose being previously admitted for a similar episode of reactive airway disease, of which the foster mother was unaware and remarks, "That would have been helpful to know!" After several days on steroids, albuterol, and a new inhaler, Jose is weaned off supplemental oxygen and is returned to his foster family.

QUESTIONS AND ANSWERS

1. Discuss the unique social class of children in foster care.

Children in foster care are statistically more likely to come from environments where poverty is a compounding factor in removal from their home (Rostad et. al. 2020). While in care they are usually afforded state benefits for medical care, educational assistance, food and clothing stipends, and other services, that may cause individuals to have implicit biases for or against children in foster care (Puzzanchera *et al.*, 2022). Foster children can also suffer from traumatic stress, either caused by the circumstances that led to their removal, or solely from being separated from their biological families (Greeson *et. al.*, 2011). These factors may also make it more difficult for children in foster care to connect with others and/or lead to delays in typical development and communication skills necessary for helping others to effectively meet their needs. All of this is often compounded by incomplete or missing health records being available for children in foster care.

2. Discuss how classism (institutional and individual) impacted Jose's quality of care. Consider the role of the hospital and child welfare systems, the attitudes of the healthcare teams, and access to medical records and appropriate medical resources.

Institutional classism is occurring within the child welfare system as the system should have ensured that the foster mother had all of Jose's necessary medical records so that she could properly advocate for Jose when he required medical care. As the foster mother was unfamiliar with his health condition, she was not able to immediately differentiate appropriate from inappropriate therapeutic action for Jose. This lack of knowledge and experience of the caretaker led to the foster mother failing to appropriately advocate for Jose, who could not advocate for himself. An example of institutional classism can be seen in the first ED. The first ED lacked the appropriate medical resources and tools to care for a 20-month-old child undergoing an episode of reactive airway disease. The healthcare staff at the first ED were fully aware of this fact. Better quality of care would have been to limit the number of unnecessary invasive tests and to expedite appropriate treatment at a facility equipped with the expertise and equipment to care for a 20-month-old undergoing an episode of reactive airway disease. Individual classism can be seen both in the actions of the staff at the first ED and Dr. A. The staff were inattentive to Jose, which may infer implicit bias against a patient they see as "poor" or, due to his age, unlikely to complain about neglectful treatment. While Dr. A may have had good intentions in wanting to treat Jose, Dr. A subjected Jose to a battery of tests that were unnecessary and invasive. He was also not selective about which tests to perform on Jose as the state was covering the costs. Dr. A also delayed transfer to a pediatric hospital that would have been better equipped to help Jose. On the other hand, the doctor and staff at the pediatric hospital were attentive, compassionate, and quickly met the needs of Jose and his foster mother. Additionally, the serendipitous discovery of Jose's past admission records at the pediatric hospital, to which Jose had been transferred, assisted the medical staff in creating a directed and efficient plan of action to rehabilitate Jose.

3. Discuss how this situation might have been different for a child, similar to Jose, who was not in foster care (i.e., living with biological or adoptive parents, or long-term guardians).

Likely a child in the continuous care of biological or adoptive parents or guardians would have caretakers with insights into the child's chronic medical conditions due to past experiences. Children who are not placed in foster care may also have more complete health records with their caregivers and/or continuity of care with the same physicians and healthcare institutions that they regularly visit, which could expedite accurate diagnosis and appropriate treatment.

Children from low socioeconomic backgrounds who rely on public assistance for medical insurance may experience similar haphazard or excessive testing; or they may have the opposite experience where hospitals and clinicians are reluctant to order necessary tests or procedures that are more expensive, out of concern that a government-based insurance company might be less likely to be fully reimburse the costs.

4. Discuss what potential alternative actions from the healthcare team at the first ED might have mitigated the delay in critical care for Jose.

The staff at the first ED were aware of their facility's limitations for treating pediatric patients and could have immediately requested a transfer to a pediatric ED or directed the foster mother to a more appropriate facility. The ED physician, Dr. A, and medical staff also could have been more selective and timely with the tests and procedures they chose to administer. Upon hearing that Jose was in foster care, Dr. A should have asked for Jose's Child Resource Record (CRR) to gain a better understanding of Jose's medical history. This could have been facilitated by the hospital having standardized protocol or providing training to their physicians about special considerations for children in foster care. While Dr. A was aware of his gaps in knowledge in treating pediatric patients, and there was limited advocacy from the child's foster mother due to lack of experience with the condition, the physician should have taken the initiative to consult resources or colleagues to determine appropriate protocols for treating a child presenting with asthmatic symptoms. More input from the interdisciplinary medical team at the hospital might have yielded insights and experiences that may have led to more informed decision-making for the patient's treatment course.

5. Discuss the role of communication between health care providers, foster parents and child welfare agency and how breaks in these communication channels can affect potential outcomes for children in foster care.

The communication role of the child welfare agency in this scenario would have been to ensure that the foster mother had all of Jose's current medical records both within a well-organized Child Resource Record binder, as well as providing a verbal debriefing on the state of the child's health and important signs to look out for and/or appropriate steps to manage his health. The communication role of the caregiver in this scenario should have been to advocate for the best possible quality of care for Jose by asking the doctor and hospital staff more in-depth questions, and ideally calling the hospital ahead of the visit to ensure they were equipped to care for a pediatric patient. The communication role of the healthcare provider and staff ideally would be to ask more question of the caregiver, request to see Jose's Child Resource Record binder, and refer to other resources to fill in their own knowledge gaps when dealing with an unfamiliar condition in a pediatric patient. These breaks in communication can lead to problematic medical care and delays to appropriate treatment, as seen in Jose's case with his reactive airway disease episode. Without the transfer to the pediatric hospital and discovery of Jose's past medical records, his outcome may have been much worse.

Epilogue

On follow up, Jose and his foster mother meet with Jose's new primary care pediatrician, Dr. Z, who comes up with an asthma plan for Jose's reactive airway disease. Jose is managed with a twice daily inhaler and experiences no further incidences of reactive airway flare ups requiring medical intervention. Following this incident, the foster mother organizes and updates Jose's Child Resource Record binder with his current medical documentation to be able to better provide an accurate medical history for Jose in the future. She also chooses to write a letter to the first emergency department administration recommending training for physicians on the Child Resource Record (CRR) and how they should be routinely requested and used to take a more complete medical history for children in foster care.

This case highlighted several factors that can interplay to affect the quality of healthcare for children in the foster care system. The caregiver must be properly equipped by the child welfare agency with knowledge about the child's medical condition(s) and needs, so they will be able to satisfactorily advocate for appropriate healthcare. Similarly, the healthcare team needs appropriate training to know what questions to ask and what materials to request from caregivers of children in foster care. In this case, Dr. A, was not properly qualified to manage a pediatric patient and did not appear to have training on the special considerations for children in foster care, such as asking for the Child Resource Record binder, nor did Dr. A chose to consult with other physicians or medical resources to attempt to fill in his knowledge gaps regarding pediatric presentation of reactive airway disease. This led to performing unnecessary diagnostics and treatments that were ineffective. While this example of poor-quality healthcare for a child in foster care was successfully resolved, it becomes clear that not all children in foster care may be so fortunate. Therefore, there is a pressing need to equip healthcare providers and caregivers with the tools and know-how to provide outstanding care, especially for children in the foster care system, to generate better health equity for this vulnerable population.

CASE 3: NO CARD, NO SERVICE

Goal

This case exemplifies the influence of health insurance status and the impact it may have on the quality of healthcare that may be received.

Learning Outcomes

1. Discuss the financial burden of uninsured patients on hospital systems and resultant biases that may arise.
2. Describe potential differences in the quality and timeliness of care for uninsured versus insured patients.
3. Explore the healthcare and psychosocial outcomes for individuals who are (or are perceived to be) unable to pay for medical services.
4. Elucidate individual and institutional practices that can mitigate classism biases against uninsured or underinsured patients.

Case

John is a 20-year-old male who is brought to the emergency department (ED) by emergency medical services (EMS) in the middle of the night, following an automobile collision. During the accident the vehicle flipped over, and the windshield fell into the vehicle and severed all four extensor tendons in John's left hand. When John regained consciousness, while under the care of the EMS team, he was asked about his health insurance. John was not aware that he had any health insurance and told EMS that he had none. According to local EMS protocol, uninsured patients should be taken to the local teaching hospital, to mitigate healthcare costs to the patient. At the teaching hospital, John also tells the hospital staff that he does not have health insurance. After multiple hours of waiting in the busy ED, holding blood-soaked gauze to cover his lacerated hand, John is finally admitted to the ED and receives care. Since EDs in the United States are required to stabilize patients regardless of insurance status or ability to pay, John's hand is sutured to stop the bleeding, but the severed tendons are not repaired.

When John's mother, Marion, arrives at the hospital several hours later, she corrects the hospital records with John's current health insurance information. John is still considered a dependent under Marion's employee health plan, of which John was unaware. John is discharged from the teaching hospital by the end of the day with instructions to follow up with a surgeon to repair his severed tendons.

Marion and John search online to find the contact information for the only hand surgeon in their area healthcare network, Dr. Aven. When they call to schedule the tendon repair surgery, they are distressed to discover that Dr. Aven's calendar is booked, and he will not be able to schedule the surgery until three months later. The office staff offer Marion and John information about an elite concierge medical service, in efforts to help them move up sooner in the waitlist, but Marion finds the monthly fee to be unaffordable. During the intervening three months, John has no use of the four fingers of his left hand and needs assistance with daily living tasks, such as washing and getting dressed. He also experiences a loss of wages from to being scheduled for fewer hours at his restaurant job due to his employer finding him less helpful without the use of his left hand. John's mother is upset with the whole situation and wonders if John would have gotten better and more complete care immediately after the accident if John would have told the EMS or hospital that he did have health insurance.

QUESTIONS AND ANSWERS

1. How did John's perceived lack of health insurance influence the type of care he received? Discuss any potential differences in the quality or timeliness of care that may have occurred.

Since US EDs are only required to stabilize patients regardless of insurance status or ability to pay (Fields et. al., 2001), John's hand was sutured to stop the bleeding, but his severed tendons were not repaired. His insurance status is updated hours later, and he is discharged with instructions to follow up with a surgeon to repair his severed tendons. When he and his mother call the surgeon, they are unable to get an appointment for 3 months. If his insurance status had been known earlier, it is possible that he would have been referred to Dr. Aven from the hospital and been able to make an appointment to get surgery to repair his tendons sooner. Another possibility is that the hospital would have repaired would have performed the surgery immediately.

2. Describe the potential financial impacts to a hospital system when it is required to care for an uninsured patient. How might this create unintentional biases against uninsured patients?

Hospital systems rely on financial reimbursements from insurance companies to remain financially stable. The more uncompensated care a hospital system provides, the more likely a hospital system is to acquire unrecoverable debt. Safety net hospitals like academic teaching hospitals rely on disproportionate share payments (DSH) provided by those able to pay. These factors lead to more financially vulnerable hospital systems, and they are more likely to experience financial pressure or losses (Neuhausen *et. al.*,

2014) This might create unintentional bias in the sense that the hospital system may be more likely to discharge uninsured patients, sooner than insured payments, in order to limit the amount of unrecoverable debt they acquire. They may also provide the minimum necessary care required by law to uninsured patients in order to maintain financial stability within the hospital system. While unintentional, these biases may constitute institutional classism and can affect the quality and equity of healthcare across populations.

3. Expound upon the health outcomes of patients that are uninsured or perceived to be uninsured. What psychosocial outcomes might also occur in these patients?

Uninsured patients or patients perceived to be uninsured may receive lower quality care and it may take longer to receive appropriate care (Bell and Zarzaur, 2013). Since uninsured patients tend to seek care at the ED and are more likely to delay seeking care, uninsured patients are more likely to be diagnosed with a later stage of disease (Cerisier, 2019). Uninsured patients or patients perceived to be uninsured may only receive treatment to stabilize their illness or injury but not complete treatment, depending on cost. This may result in delay of healing the injury or deficient treatment of disease. This delay in treatment and healing may lead to increased negative psychosocial outcomes such as increased anxiety and stress in the patient if they are unable to return to work due to prolonged injury or illness, which would in turn put extra financial strain on the patient, from lost wages. Depression may also occur if the patient is unable to completely heal from injury or illness, and subsequently feels that their life may never improve or return to some form of a normal functional level. Substance use disorder may also result if the injury or illness causes a lasting chronic pain syndrome that is not addressed medically.

4. Discuss the role of access to care and the availability of healthcare providers in the outcomes of patients with disadvantages in social and economic class. How could institutional systems help mitigate poor health outcomes due to these factors?

Access to care and the availability of healthcare providers plays a significant role in the health outcomes of patients in lower social and economic class. (Begley *et. al,* 2011) Patients of lower socioeconomic status tend to be uninsured or have partial insurance thus reducing their access to healthcare providers. This results in a higher reliance on the ED or local community clinics that offer health services at reduced cost. Institutional systems can help mitigate poor health outcomes by partnering with other community health care systems, as well as local government, to find ways to improve the quality and access of care. For example, the policy of taking all uninsured patients to the local teaching hospital may lead to an increased burden on the teaching hospital since all uninsured patients are sent there. Instead, the local teaching hospital can partner with other community health care systems and local governments to create a more effective policy for care of uninsured patients that will reduce the burden on the local teaching hospital and its resources.

5. Elucidate the role of healthcare networks in patient choice and quality of care.

Healthcare networks provide a reliable system of insurance coverage for healthcare providers and patients with specific health insurance plans. Patients with insurance rely on health care networks that are part of insurance carrier plans. Remaining in the healthcare network results in reduced cost to the insured patient (Rose *et. al*, 2021). However, the insured patient may end up waiting longer to see a physician within their healthcare network or having limited options for healthcare providers due to a small number of participating physicians in a particular specialty. Patients who are not pleased with their options for in-network healthcare providers may or may not be able to afford the financial or travel burden to seek providers outside of their healthcare network. Despite the illusion of patient choice through private insurance, healthcare networks effectively confine subscribers to more limited options when the patient subscribers are unable to overcome the pay-wall involved in seeking alternative care.

6. Describe how concierge medical services might drive preferential treatment of patients.

A typical concierge medical practice limits the number of patients and provides highly personalized attention that includes comprehensive annual physicals, same-day appointments, preventive and wellness care, and fast, around the clock response time (Paul and Skiba, 2016). The concierge model for practicing medicine relies on an annual fee that may vary by patient age and other parameters. For practicing physicians, switching to this model means a steady, predictable income from membership fees and no longer being dependent on shrinking fee-for-service reimbursements (Serna, 2019). Concierge medicine has become popular in the last decade among both the physicians as well as patients who might be inconvenienced by the limitations associated with scheduling and other such logistics in healthcare organizations. Health care policy makers and experts have shed light on how concierge medicine can encourage an elitist practice of medicine and its widespread implementation may increase the shortage of an already scarce availability of primary care physicians (Paul and Skiba, 2016). These services, if implemented without appropriate forethought, may perpetuate the impact, bias and disparity towards access to healthcare the socio-economic "class" that an individual may encounter.

Epilogue

After John is finally able to have his hand surgery, he undergoes physical therapy and regains 80-90% of the mobility he once had. The physical therapist, Dr. Byrd, informs John that if the tendons had been repaired at the time of the accident, he would have had a much easier time with physical therapy and would have fully regained his mobility with less residual pain. Marion considers taking legal action against the hospital, but eventually decides against it. Marion and John are physically, emotionally, and financially drained from the dealing with expenses from the car accident, medical copays, and lost wages from John's drawn-out recovery period, and they don't think they can afford the lawyer fees or to take any more time off from work.

This case highlighted factors that can interplay to affect the quality and timeliness of healthcare for individuals who are deemed incapable of paying for their healthcare services, such as the uninsured. While federal laws protect individuals from being turned away from emergency departments based on their ability to pay, these laws do not prescribe the quality of care that a patient must receive beyond stabilization.

ACKNOWLEDGMENT

Dr. Samiksha Prasad contributed to the writing and research of this chapter. We acknowledge her contributions.

REFERENCES

Adams, M., Bell, L. A., & Griffin, P. (Eds.). (2007). Teaching for diversity and social justice (2nd ed.). Routledge/Taylor & Francis Group. doi:10.4324/9780203940822

Bates, T. (1997). *Race, Self-Employment, and Upward Mobility: An Illusive American Dream*. The Johns Hopkins University Press.

Becker, G., & Newsom, E. (2003). Socioeconomic Status and Dissatisfaction with Health Care Among Chronically Ill African Americans. *American Journal of Public Health*, *93*(5), 742–748. doi:10.2105/AJPH.93.5.742 PMID:12721135

Begley, C., Basu, R., Lairson, D., Reynolds, T., Dubinsky, S., Newmark, M., Barnwell, F., Hauser, A., & Hesdorffer, D. (2011). Socioeconomic status, health care use, and outcomes: Persistence of disparities over time. *Epilepsia*, *52*(5), 957–964. doi:10.1111/j.1528-1167.2010.02968.x PMID:21320113

Bell, T., & Zarzaur, B. (2013). Insurance status is a predictor of failure to rescue in trauma patients at both safety net and non-safety net hospitals. *The Journal of Trauma and Acute Care Surgery*, *75*(4), 728–733. doi:10.1097/TA.0b013e3182a53aaa PMID:24064890

Boone, L. (2020). *Classism*. Salem Press Encyclopedia.

Bright, M. A., Kleinman, L., Vogel, B., & Shenkman, E. (2018). Visits to Primary Care and Emergency Department Reliance for Foster Youth: Impact of Medicaid Managed Care. *Academic Pediatrics*, *18*(4), 397–404. doi:10.1016/j.acap.2017.10.005 PMID:29081362

Cerisier, K. (2019). Connecting Chronically Ill, Uninsured Patients Who Use the Emergency Department as a Medical Home: A Process Improvement Project. *Journal of Emergency Nursing: JEN*, *45*(3), 249–253. doi:10.1016/j.jen.2018.08.011 PMID:30293814

Children's Bureau. (2020). *The AFCARS report: Preliminary FY 2019 estimates as of June 23, 2020 -No. 27*. U.S. Department of Health and Human Services, Administration for Children and Families. https://www.acf.hhs.gov/cb/resource/afcars-report-27

Chomsky, N. (2017). *Requiem for the American Dream: The 10 Principles of Concentration of Wealth & Power. Seven Stories Press.*

Dos Santos, T. (1970). The Concept of Social Classes. *Science and Society*, *34*(2), 166–193.

Dumont, L. (1981). Homo Hierarchicus: The Caste System and Its Implications (2nd ed.). University of Chicago Press.

Evans, C. R., Williams, D. R., Onnela, J. P., & Subramanian, S. V. (2018) A multilevel approach to modeling health inequalities at the intersection of multiple social identities. *Social Science & Medicine*, *203*, 64-73. doi:10.1016/j.socscimed.2017.11.011

Ezzell, B. (2002). Laws of Racial Identification and Racial Purity in Nazi Germany and the United States: Did Jim Crow Write the Laws That Spawned the Holocaust. Southern University Law Review, 30, 1-14.

Fields, W. W., Asplin, B. R., Larkin, G. L., Marco, C. A., Johnson, L. A., Yeh, C., Ghezzi, K. T., & Rapp, M. (2001). The Emergency Medical Treatment and Labor Act as a Federal Health Care Safety Net Program. *Academic Emergency Medicine*, *8*(11), 1064–1069. doi:10.1111/j.1553-2712.2001.tb01116.x PMID:11691669

Fong, K. (2020). Getting Eyes in the Home: Child Protective Services Investigations and State Surveillance of Family Life. *American Sociological Review*, *85*(4), 610–638. doi:10.1177/0003122420938460

Green, M. A., Evans, C. R., & Subramanian, S. V. (2017). Can intersectionality theory enrich population health research? *Social Science & Medicine*, *178*, 217–219. doi:10.1016/j.socscimed.2017.02.029 PMID:28238539

Greeson, J. K. P., Briggs, E. C., Kisiel, C. L., Layne, C. M., Ake, G. S., Ko, S. J., Gerrity, E. T., Steinberg, A. M., Howard, M. L., Pynoos, R. S., & Fairbank, J. A. (2011). Complex Trauma and Mental Health in Children and Adolescents Placed in Foster Care: Findings from the National Child Traumatic Stress Network. *Child Welfare*, *90*(6), 91–108. https://www.jstor.org/stable/48625371 PMID:22533044

Hankivsky, O. (2022). *Intersectionality 101*. Institute for Intersectionality Research and Policy. https://resources.equityinitiative.org/handle/ei/433

Limbert, W., & Williams, W. R. (2014). Classism. In T. Teo (Ed.), *Encyclopedia of Critical Psychology*. Springer. doi:10.1007/978-1-4614-5583-7_43

Lott, B. (2012). The Social Psychology of Class and Classism. *The American Psychologist*, *67*(8), 650–658. doi:10.1037/a0029369 PMID:23163450

Minkler, M., Fuller-Thomson, E., & Guralnik, J. M. (2006). Gradient of disability across the socioeconomic spectrum in the United States. *The New England Journal of Medicine*, *355*(7), 695–703. doi:10.1056/NEJMsa044316 PMID:16914705

Neuhausen, K., Davis, A. C., Needleman, J., Brook, R. H., Zingmond, D., & Roby, D. H. (2014). Disproportionate-share hospital payment reductions may threaten the financial stability of safety-net hospitals. *Health Affairs (Project Hope)*, *33*(6), 988–996. doi:10.1377/hlthaff.2013.1222 PMID:24889948

Paul, D. P. III, & Skiba, M. (2016). Concierge Medicine: A Viable Business Model for (Some) Physicians of the Future? *The Health Care Manager*, *35*(1), 3–8. doi:10.1097/HCM.0000000000000088 PMID:27892907

Pelton, L. H. (2015). The continuing role of material factors in child maltreatment and placement. *Child Abuse & Neglect*, *41*, 30–39. doi:10.1016/j.chiabu.2014.08.001 PMID:25169149

Puzzanchera, C., Taylor, M., Kang, W., & Smith, J. (2022). *Disproportionality Rates for Children of Color in Foster Care Dashboard.* National Council of Juvenile and Family Court Judges. http://ncjj.org/AFCARS/Disproportionality_Dashboard.aspx

Rose, L., Aouad, M., Graham, L., Schoemaker, L., & Wagner, T. (2021). Association of Expanded Health Care Networks With Utilization Among Veterans Affairs Enrollees. *JAMA Network Open, 4*(10), e2131141. doi:10.1001/jamanetworkopen.2021.31141 PMID:34698845

Rostad, W. L., Ports, K. A., Tang, S., & Kelvins, J. (2020). Reducing the Number of Children Entering Foster Care: Effects of State Earned Income Tax Credits. *Child Maltreatment, 25*(4), 393–397. doi:10.1177/1077559519900922 PMID:31973550

Scambler, G. (2019). Sociology, Social Class, Health Inequalities, and the Avoidance of "Classism". *Front Sociol., 4*, 56. doi:10.3389/fsoc.2019.00056 PMID:33869379

Schneiderman, J. U., Smith, C., & Palinkas, L. A. (2012). The caregiver as gatekeeper for accessing health care for children in foster care: A qualitative study of kinship and unrelated caregivers. *Children and Youth Services Review, 34*(10), 2123–2130. doi:10.1016/j.childyouth.2012.07.009 PMID:23139436

Serna, D. C. (2019). Lifestyle Medicine in a Concierge Practice: My Journey. *American Journal of Lifestyle Medicine, 13*(4), 367–370. doi:10.1177/1559827618821865 PMID:31285719

Shrider, E. A., Kollar, M., Chen, F., & Semega, J. (2021). *Income and poverty in the United States: 2020.* U.S. Census Bureau. https://www.census.gov/library/publications/2021/demo/p60-273.html

Simons, A. M., Koster, A., Groffen, D. A., & Bosma, H. (2017). Perceived classism and its relation with socioeconomic status, health, health behaviours and perceived inferiority: The Dutch Longitudinal Internet Studies for the Social Sciences (LISS) panel. *International Journal of Public Health, 62*(4), 433–440. doi:10.100700038-016-0880-2 PMID:27572684

Sivashanker, K., Couillard, C., Goldsmith, J., Walker, N., & Eappen, S. (2020). Addressing the caste system in U.S. healthcare in the era of COVID-19. *International Journal for Equity in Health, 19*(1), 184. doi:10.118612939-020-01298-x PMID:33076929

Smedley, B. D., Stith, A. Y., & Nelson, A. R. (2003) Institute of Medicine (US) Committee on Understanding and Eliminating Racial and Ethnic Disparities in Health Care. In *Unequal Treatment: Confronting Racial and Ethnic Disparities in Health Care.* National Academies Press (US). https://www.ncbi.nlm.nih.gov/books/NBK220364/

Tang, S. Y., Browne, A. J., Mussell, B., Smye, V. L., & Rodney, P. (2015). 'Underclassism' and access to healthcare in urban centres. *Sociology of Health & Illness, 37*(5), 698–714. doi:10.1111/1467-9566.12236 PMID:25720520

United States Holocaust Memorial Museum. (2020). *Documenting Numbers Of Victims Of The Holocaust And Nazi Persecution.* https://encyclopedia.ushmm.org/content/en/article/documenting-numbers-of-victims-of-the-holocaust-and-nazi-persecution

Villegas, S., Rosenthal, J. A., O'Brien, K., & Pecora, P. (2011). Health outcomes for adults in family foster care as children: An analysis by ethnicity. *Children and Youth Services Review*, *33*(1), 110–117. doi:10.1016/j.childyouth.2010.08.020

Wilkerson, I. (2020). *Caste: The Origins of Our Discontents*. Random House.

Chapter 10
Gender Bias and Performativity

Algevis Wrench
Nova Southeastern University Dr. Kiran C. Patel College of Allopathic Medicine, USA

Jocelyn Mitchell-Williams
https://orcid.org/0000-0002-6007-6598
Cooper Medical School of Rowan University, USA

Vijay Rajput
Nova Southeastern University Dr. Kiran C. Patel College of Allopathic Medicine, USA

EXECUTIVE SUMMARY

This chapter addresses gender bias, gender performativity, and sexual harassment in the clinical setting. The prevalence of gender disparities and bias is well documented in fields such as orthopedic surgery, urology, radiology, neurosurgery, and plastic surgery. Marginalized groups are more frequently impacted by these negative behaviors. Notably, in the field of urology, female residents comprise less than 30% of the demographic and often face bias. Gender performativity may play a role in the stereotyping seen for males in the nursing profession. Traditional views of masculinity and femininity may limit a supervisor's ability to see the potential in clinical staff members and cause conscious or unconscious limitations for professional growth. The interactions represented in these cases offer an opportunity for discussion of the prevalence and impact of gender bias and associated microaggressions in medicine. Various strategies to effectively mitigate gender bias in the clinical and academic environment are also discussed.

BACKGROUND

Gender Bias and Microaggressions

Gender bias is defined as any one of a variety of stereotypical beliefs about individuals based on their gender, particularly as related to the differential treatment of females and males. Gender biases are conveyed verbally and/or nonverbally through facial expression, gaze, and other gestures. They can be subtle, but often are expressed directly, and can cause psychological harm or discomfort (Capodilupo et al., 2010). Examples of gender based microaggressions include the improper use of gender-based lan-

DOI: 10.4018/978-1-6684-5493-0.ch010

guage, denial that gender bias exists, assumptions of traditional gender roles, assumptions of inferiority, and institutional factors such as pay gap.

Gender-based bias in the medical field has been well documented (McKinley et al., 2019). The most well-known theory is implicit gender bias, which assumes that women are less capable than men in certain medical fields or they do not follow social gender norms. In the United States, women continue to be underrepresented in fields that are historically considered to be male dominated specialties. These fields include plastic surgery, urology, radiology, neurosurgery, and orthopedic surgery where female residents only comprise 31%, 27%, 26%, 18% and 15% respectively (AAMC, 2020). Additionally, several studies have indicated that the prevalence of gender bias can negatively influence intent and motivation to pursue an education in a career that does not meet societal expectations (Brown et al., 2020).

The effects of gender bias and microaggressions are vast. They can affect the physical and mental health of the recipients. Reasons for this impact include their chronic and cumulative nature, and pervasiveness in many aspects of a recipient's life (education, work, social situations). Factors such as depression, low quality of life, job dissatisfaction, burnout, imposter syndrome and suicidality can occur in those who experience gender bias and microaggressions (Capodilupo et al., 2010; Shanafelt et al., 2011; Hu et al., 2019; Nadal et al., 2021). This can lead to suboptimal care practices, major medical and medication errors, and decreased patient satisfaction with medical care (West et al., 2011).

It is of primary importance to integrate diverse content and programming into health profession's school curricula that will equip learners with strategies and skills to recognize, mitigate and navigate gender biases within the clinical and academic environment. Curricular interventions such as case-based learning and implicit bias training have been shown to improve students' knowledge and confidence around gender bias (Gill et al., 2022).

Institutional action plays a vital role in moving forward in preventing gender bias. Organizations could develop gender equality or affirmative action policies, engage in awareness raising and information sharing, serve in advocacy and accountability functions, conduct gender sensitization workshops, offer mentoring, faculty career development, and leadership programs to women, require sexual harassment policy training, and clearly outline reporting procedures (Newman et al., 2016).

Gender Performativity

Racial, ethnic, and gender diversity are important in all areas of healthcare. Having a diverse medical workforce provides the opportunity to deliver more culturally sensitive and respectful care, which can improve patient satisfaction and outcomes (Gomez & Bernet, 2019). Gender performativity is largely socially constructed. It is a theory that gender, and gender roles are complex performances of popular perceptions of what males or females can or cannot do, and that these roles are then reinforced by repetition over time (Butler, 1999). Gender performativity issues and gender discrimination are not uncommon in the clinical environment.

While there has been a push to increase female representation in male dominated disciplines of medicine, the paucity of male nurses and the gender bias they experience has not been adequately addressed. Although nursing began as a profession solely for males, female dominance has been in place since the feminist reform work of Florence Nightingale. She pushed the idea that only women could possess the traits needed to provide nursing care due to their nature as mother and nurturer (Harrison, 2021). Nurses are often described as kind, caring, nurturing, and compassionate. Socially these are characteristics that are reinforced and are more often associated with females (Christov-Moore, et al 2014). Gender performativity has contributed to males being less hands on and more knowledge focused. This unfortunately leaves them as being stigmatized as less gentle and uncaring in the field of nursing (LeBlanc, 2017). In fact, male nurses reported feeling the need to "act" in a more caring, feminine, softer, or even "gay" manner to fit in while at work (LeBlanc, 2017). These characterizations and stigmas have become barriers to males entering the nursing profession. In times when nursing shortages are great, work needs to be done to overcome these hurdles. Effort is needed to mitigate gender bias in the workplace to enhance equality of experiences, treatment, and care.

CASE 1: DR. LOPEZ'S CHALLENGES

Goal

The primary goal of the scenario is to highlight how gender bias and gender related microaggressions can emerge in the clinical learning environment and to stimulate discussion about strategies to recognize and address these types of behaviors.

Learning Outcomes

1. Define the concept of gender bias and gender based microaggressions.
2. Describe common challenges experienced by female trainees in the medical profession.
3. Discuss strategies to recognize and mitigate gender biases in the learning environment.
4. Reflect on personal biases surrounding gender.

Case

After 12 years of marriage with two daughters and a son, Jeff and his wife Michelle decided it was time for him to undergo a vasectomy. Jeff is a 42-year-old high school teacher with no medical issues except seasonal allergies. Michelle is a 40-year-old chemical engineer who works for a local company. They have been discussing a vasectomy for a while, but finally made the decision when Michelle no longer wanted to take oral contraception. They present for a consultation to the office of Dr. Barry Walker, a male urologist. Dr. Lopez, a 29-year-old, Hispanic female and first-year urology resident joins Dr. Walker during the consultation. Dr. Walker requests that Dr. Lopez take the patient's reproductive, medical, and surgical history and then perform the physical exam. Before Dr. Lopez begins the history taking, she explains the vasectomy procedure in detail, the risks associated with it, and post-operative expectations. She also discusses the permanent sterility intent of the procedure and asks Jeff and Michelle if they have any questions. Jeff smiles and says, "*No questions at all, thank you for that very clear explanation.*"

Dr. Walker suddenly interrupts and says to Jeff,"*Don't worry, I will be performing the physical exam as the male doctor here.*" Jeff glances at his wife Michelle with a confused look. Dr. Lopez is perplexed and feels awkward and embarrassed by this situation as she thought she was doing a good job during the consultation. She does not speak for the remainder of the consultation.

Later that day, during a debrief Dr. Walker says to Dr. Lopez, "*You acted like you weren't even engaged in the care of this patient. If you are going to be a woman in this field you're going to need to know how to connect with male patients*". Dr. Lopez feels very uncomfortable responding openly to Dr.

Walker about her feelings as he is her supervisor. She looks down and says, "*I am sorry.*" She does not share with Dr. Walker that she felt undermined when he decided to perform the physical exam and is now insulted by his derogatory comment about females in urology. Dr. Lopez goes to the break room to reflect on the interaction and begins to contemplate that maybe she should reconsider her choice of urology, as it appears to be a specialty for men.

This interaction typifies a classic instance of gender bias in a discipline of medicine where females are underrepresented and often feel marginalized. The male attending urologist undermines the role of the female resident during a patient consultation and makes further statements that insult her competency as a physician based on her gender. Gender bias and associated microaggressions, as well as strategies to address and mitigate bias in the context of gender will be discussed.

QUESTIONS AND ANSWERS

1. Identify instances where the interactions between Dr. Walker and Dr. Lopez were inappropriate during and after the patient consultation: The first instance is when Dr. Walker interrupts Dr. Lopez and overrides his initial decision to have her perform the physical exam. The reason he provides is that he is the male physician in the room and his statement infers that women are not as capable as males in conducting such a physical exam on a male patient. Dr. Walker's statement invalidates Dr. Lopez's skills, competency, and training. This is a classic example of gender bias. It is also a gender based microaggression. Although his statement was not made directly to Dr. Lopez, it still undermined and invalidated her role in the patient interaction.

Another instance is later in the day during a debrief where Dr. Walker says to Dr. Lopez, "*You acted like you weren't even engaged in the care of this patient. If you are going to be a woman in this field you're going to need to know how to connect with male patients.*" This is also a microaggression, specifically a microinsult. Microinsults are a subtype of microaggression characterized by communications that convey rudeness and insensitivity and demean a person's identity. Microinsults often occur as subtle snubs, frequently unknown to the perpetrator, but clearly convey a hidden insulting message to the recipient. Dr. Lopez felt insulted but did not vocalize this to her attending physician, Dr. Walker. This is not uncommon for residents who often fear repercussions from their supervisors. When Dr. Lopez says "*I am sorry*" to Dr. Walker without sharing her true feelings, this might have been an opportunity to be open and honest about feeling insulted. Think about ways in which you would have handled this if you were in Dr. Lopez's shoes.

2. Consider the interaction between Dr. Walker and Dr. Lopez and how this may have impacted the experience of the patient Jeff and his spouse. How do you think the statements by Dr. Walker could have been perceived by Jeff's wife, Michelle, or Jeff himself?: After Dr. Lopez gives her detailed explanation of the procedure, Jeff appears to be satisfied with the information provided based on his response to Dr. Lopez. He is also smiling which indicates that he is comfortable. However, when Dr. Walker decides to take over to perform the physical exam, Jeff's facial expression indicates that he is confused as to the reason for this change. Both Jeff and Michelle might have perceived that there was a problem with the information they were given or their health care due to a sudden change in the roles of Dr. Walker and Dr. Lopez. They might start having second thoughts about

the procedure itself or their choice of providers. The couple might even be thinking how this might affect Jeff's care moving forward. It is important for members of a healthcare team to be mindful of how communication between each other both verbally and non-verbally can affect the patient experience.

3. How prevalent is gender bias in the field of medicine and what are some other challenges that female physicians might face?: Gender bias in medicine, both in academia and the clinical environment, is well established (Carr et al., 2000; Carr et al., 2015; Fnais et al., 2014). In a recent study of residents at a large academic medical center, 61% reported experiencing some form of gender bias during their training. The prevalence of gender bias was higher in females (98%) than males (19%) and most instances of bias manifested as role misidentification and a difficult working environment (Chatterjee et al., 2021). Often these biases are grounded in thoughts that "women are not equal to men". This also manifests in other ways such as lower salaries for female versus male physicians, under-representation of women in senior roles and sexual harassment. Fewer women are given the opportunity to present at certain events such as grand rounds, with men even being more likely to be referred to by their official titles than women. (Carr et al., 2000; Carr et al., 2015; Chatterjee et al., 2021; Fnais et al., 2014).

In medical education gender bias is also common. Among medical students, female students are more affected by these biases than their male peers. For example, there are biases in how students are evaluated based on gender. One study evaluated gender bias in Medical Student Performance Evaluations (MSPEs) and found that women were more likely than men to be described as ''compassionate,'' ''sensitive,'' and ''enthusiastic'' and men were more likely than women to be seen as ''quick learners.'' (Axelson et al., 2010). This is believed to negatively impact female student proficiency evaluations as the rate of increase in male student proficiency has been shown to be twice that of women.

4. What are some strategies that could be used to mitigate gender bias in the clinical learning environment?

The strategies listed below can aid in the recognition and mitigation of gender bias and can also generally help to create an equitable environment in healthcare.

- Bias training for clinicians, especially males in supervisory roles
- Health systems implementing reporting systems that are anonymous, and that enable tracking of instances of bias so that targeted interventions can occur.
- Training for Underrepresented in Medicine (URiM) clinicians on how to handle bias and microaggressions from other co-workers and patients.
- Mentorship for female clinicians and equitable job requirements and clear promotion guidelines for women.
- Development and implementation of a gender bias curriculum in medical schools.

5. What would have been an effective way for Dr. Lopez to address her concerns regarding Dr. Walker's statements?: Depending on the level of comfortability of the resident, different approaches might be used to address this sensitive issue, especially considering the concern that Dr. Lopez has regarding her reaction being perceived as insubordination.

Dr. Lopez could have respectfully responded to Dr. Walker and said, "Thanks for that insight, Dr. Walker. I do feel comfortable and capable of doing the physical exam." She could have brought it up later with Dr. Walker during the debrief by asking him if there was a particular reason he did not want her to do the physical exam. She could have asked him, "was it because you thought I was not ready?"

Dr. Lopez could have also addressed the gender issue by saying: "Dr. Walker, when you said you would complete the exam because you were male, it made me feel like you did not think I was capable of doing a good job because I was a female. I don't mean to put you on the spot or undermine your role as my superior, I am just trying to understand where you are coming from."

If Dr. Lopez does not feel comfortable enough to address Dr. Walker directly, she can also discuss the issue with the residency program director or department chair.

6. What tools can you use to identify and reflect on your own biases around gender?: Biases can be implicit (unconscious) or explicit. Gender biases are another common form of implicit biases which are unintentional cognitive effects of our thoughts about a particular gender or gender minority group. Oftentimes one's unconscious beliefs about gender might differ from their explicit actions. A great tool to identify or measure gender bias is the Harvard Implicit Association Tests (IATs). This tool was developed in 1998 and can be accessed here: https://implicit.harvard.edu/implicit/. The IATs helps you to be aware of your own biases and to reflect on them from an individual perspective.

Practicing awareness or mindfulness also helps us be more cognizant of our prejudices or behaviors. Mindfulness is implemented through meditation. When we meditate, we increase awareness of our thought patterns and feelings.

Epilogue

Gender bias is prevalent in many specialties in medicine and other health professions. It is important to discuss the implications of gender bias in clinical interactions between providers, patients, supervisors, and medical trainees, as this can negatively impact motivation and performance of trainees and their superiors, as well the patient experience. Integrating curricular content into health profession's programs is a good place to start discussions about gender bias and to orient learners to how to handle gender bias and gender related microaggressions in the academic and clinical setting. Dr. Lopez is a resident who was subjected to gender bias and microaggressions at the hands of her supervising attending while in the presence of a patient. As a resident in a discipline where females are underrepresented, Dr. Lopez is in a uniquely challenging situation where she is forced to deal with bias about her gender and how to discuss it with her superior who is the aggressor, but also the attending who evaluates her performance as a resident. Furthermore, Dr. Lopez identifies as a person of color, she also might be struggling with how to acclimate into the dominant culture where Hispanic females are underrepresented. Her reluctance to address Dr. Walker about the incident, as well her thoughts of doubt regarding continuing in the field of Urology, is evidence of her internal struggles. Dr. Lopez could benefit from mentoring and training about how to recognize and address bias. Dr. Walker could benefit from implicit bias and cultural sensitivity training to help him recognize that he has an implicit bias against females. Although he might not have made his statements with negative intent, Dr. Lopez's feelings demonstrate the far-reaching effects of

Dr. Walker's actions. Equipped with the ability to recognize and mitigate bias, Dr. Lopez might have reacted and felt differently about Dr. Walker's statements.

CASE 2: STEREOTYPING IN NURSING - AWARENESS AND MITIGATION OF BIAS

Goal

This case scenario aims to highlight the prevalence of stereotyping, bias, gender performativity issues, patient initiated sexual harassment, and discrimination in the field of nursing, especially as it relates to male nurses and their superiors. The case also provides examples of bystander response as well as strategies and resources for supporting colleagues in the clinical environment.

Learning Outcomes

1. Define the concept of gender performativity.
2. Evaluate the impact of supervisor-initiated gender bias on employees in the clinical environment.
3. Analyze common challenges and microaggressions experienced by male nurses in the workplace.
4. Appraise the various forms of patient-initiated sexual harassment.
5. Discuss strategies to mitigate gender biases and harassment in the clinical environment.

Case

It is the change in shift for nurses on a busy medical/surgical floor in an academic teaching hospital. As the charge nurse, Karen, begins assigning patients to the on-coming staff, she says, "There were three new admissions overnight. Two of them are fairly 'challenging' (she uses her fingers to illustrate quotations when she says challenging), so I am going to assign them to Joe."

Joe is a 35-year-old male nurse who has been working in the field for 5 years, but he is relatively new to this hospital. Joe is taken back by Karen's comments because from previous interactions with her, he is fairly certain that she is making an offensive dig about the patients and is not being complimentary of his nursing skills. One of the other staff nurses, Julie, says,"So you don't think the rest of us are capable of taking care of challenging patients?" To which Karen replies, "Trust me you don't want those assignments. They are going to require some physical strength and one patient could even be dangerous."

Joe is the only male nurse on the team and as he reflects on his assignments over the last several months, he realizes that he is disproportionately assigned to patients with significant mobility, weight, and mental health issues. Joe is a skilled nurse who enjoys caring for all his patients regardless of their demographics, body habitus, or social circumstances but he does feel that Karen's assignment pattern has been unbalanced since she became evening charge nurse.

Karen takes Joe in to meet one of his new patients, Mrs. Johnson. Two medical students are at her bedside taking her history. As Joe enters the room, he sees the sign on her door that says, "fall risk" and also notices that Mrs. Johnson is morbidly obese and having difficulty positioning herself in the hospital bed. Mrs. Johnson perks up when she sees them coming and comments that she is happy that Karen has finally brought the doctor in to see her. Karen rolls her eyes in annoyance and then states, "Joe is not your doctor. Your doctor is Jane Fowler and 'she' will be in to see you shortly." Karen put strong emphasis on the word 'she'. Quite frankly, she is tired of people always assuming that Joe is a doctor. Joe looks at Karen feeling somewhat embarrassed about the situation and wonders if this might be why she doesn't seem to like him or provide him with the same type of mentorship that some of his female colleagues seem to be receiving from her. Joe goes over to help Mrs. Johnson at her bedside and introduces himself as the nurse who will be taking care of her today. Mrs. Johnson looks very surprised and says, "What, I have a male nurse? I didn't know there was such a thing?" After giving Joe the head-to-toe glance over, she adds, "Well, I won't complain because look at those muscles. You certainly are the right choice to help me get to the bathroom and tuck me into bed." Dr. Fowler is now at the door and hears this exchange. The two medical students move to exit the patient's room and chuckle when they pass by Joe. Joe forces a smile and continues over to take the patient's vitals. In his head, he says to himself, "here we go again." Karen and Dr. Fowler say nothing. This is not the first time Joe has had inappropriate comments of this nature from patients. Later at the nurse's station, Joe expresses his frustration about this to another colleague. His colleague tells him that he is being too sensitive and that the patient meant no harm, which makes Joe feel invalidated in his role as a nurse. He begins to seriously consider changing departments or even applying to another hospital since nothing seems to be changing.

QUESTIONS AND ANSWERS

1. What assumptions are being made by assigning Joe to the noted patients?: Karen is assuming that because Joe is a man that he is able to handle any patient regardless of their weight or mental status. This suggests that he must in some way be stronger and tougher than his female colleagues or that it is appropriate for a male nurse to handle what she considers to be more "difficult" or "challenging" patients. Nurses have a primary commitment to the patient. Their code of ethics calls for a practice of compassionate and respectful care for all. They have a responsibility to maintain integrity and continue professional growth. They pledge to advocate for the rights, safety, and health of their patients, and to work to decrease health disparities. Karen assumes that her female staff nurses would prefer not to have these "challenging" assignments and/or that they are not capable of handling them in the same manner as Joe, which goes against these principles of nursing and gender equality.
2. How might Karen's gender biases towards nursing assignments for patients impact Joe's growth as a professional?: As a new nurse, Joe needs to have the opportunity to care for patients with a broad variety of medical conditions. Loading his assignments to patients who are difficult to move or who may require one-on-one nursing may limit the experiences he needs to grow as compared to his female counterparts. A balance of patient experiences allows the development of skills and likely prevents burnout. Limiting female nursing staff from working with such patients also stifles their professional development. All nurses need to know how to care for patients that have weight related mobility issues or patients who are simply at risk of falling. Similarly, learning to help people cope with different emotional and psychological states, no matter how difficult, is core to the practice of medicine.
3. How appropriate are Mrs. Johnson's comments regarding having a male nurse?: While Mrs. Johnson may believe that she is being complimentary, her comments to Joe are a prime example of sexual harassment and create a hostile environment. The incidence of sexual harassment among nurses

reported in the literature ranges from 10% - 90% (Papantoniou, 2021; Spector et al., 2014). A common misconception is that males in general do not experience sexual harassment. Papantonoiu reported 4 in 10 male nurses experienced some sort of sexual harassment on varying levels of frequency. They were more likely to experience sexual harassment in the first 1-5 years of their careers with the most common type being gender harassment (62%), followed by unwanted sexual attention (48%) and sexual coercion (24%). The offenders in this study were more likely to be male physicians (38.4%) or other male nurses (24%), however, female physicians (18%), patients (11%), and family members (9%) also served as perpetrators. Another study similarly found the 34% of male nurses reported sexual harassment with patients and physicians as the most common perpetrators (Cogin & Fish, 2009).

Sexual harassment like that expressed in this case example can have a profound impact on the victim, especially if there are recurrent instances of this type of behavior. Victims often report an increase in stress, mental health issues, and sleep disturbances. Some have difficulty concentrating and carrying out their job functions effectively. Many do not report the harassment because they fear not being believed or that they will be labeled negatively. Others feel that no action would be taken if they did report (Papantoniou, 2021). It is important to acknowledge the high incidence of sexual harassment that is also experienced by female nurses. In a systematic review, a prevalence rate of 43% was noted with the highest percentage of offenses coming from patients and doctors (Kahsay, et al., 2020). Patient initiated harassment can come in a variety of forms from inappropriate comments (as seen in this case) to groping, to intentional exposure of body parts, to asking for a date. If the offender is a supervisor, the power dynamic can make it increasingly difficult to report the behavior.

4. How could Joe or other team members effectively address Karen's comments about the patients? About the assignments?: Team members should be empowered to speak up and interrupt these types of conversations in the real time. An example might be, "Excuse me Karen, I'd like to call a timeout and have us start over. I'm sure you meant no harm, but our newly admitted patients deserve the best care we can offer them and if we start out by attaching labels to them, we may introduce bias in their care by our team."

Although not specifically designed for this type of situation, the **SBAR** communication tool could be utilized here. SBAR stands for Situation, Background, Assessment, and Recommendation (Thomas et al., 2009). It could be suggested that Karen utilize this method to better convey the needs for the admitted patients to her team. An example of how this might be verbalized is provided below:

S: We had a challenging admission overnight. Patient X was a recent surgical discharge but was readmitted secondary to a fever and wound infection. She is also experiencing significant diarrhea. Intravenous antibiotics were started. She will need imaging today.

B: We have had difficulty assisting her to the bathroom and moving her in the bed secondary to her weight challenges and pain with ambulation. She was not happy about having to use disposable underpants but became tearful when she could not make it to the bathroom in time.

A: My assessment is that a bedside commode would be a good alternative until we get her pain better controlled. She will still need assistance with getting out of the bed.

R: I believe it would be best to have a two-person team assigned to patient X during her stay. This will help us assure her safe ambulation and movement while in our care.

5. What actions might be appropriate for Karen? How could Mrs. Johnson's behavior/comments be addressed?: Karen's language and behavior at times were inappropriate and unprofessional. Her biased comments may influence the workplace culture, so that "complicated" patients are seen as undesirable. She not only uses a tone that may be offensive to the patient as she corrects her about the assumption of Joe being the doctor, but she also belittles Joe in the process. Depending on the comfort level of her co-workers, someone could pull her aside and talk to her privately about her behavior and allow her the opportunity to apologize. This may be more appropriate for a first-time offense. For repetitive acts, team members should report Karen's behavior to her supervisor or through an anonymous reporting method if they fear retribution. Her supervisor should review her behavior and outline the impact this has on staff and patient care. Karen should at minimum have to complete unconscious bias training and be monitored for further breaches. She could be mandated to enroll in a professionalism program to reinforce the principles of the nursing profession and/or a communications program to address her inability to be empathetic and sensitive when talking to staff about patients. Repeat behavior of this nature on Karen's part would warrant dismissal from her position of authority and/or job at the institution.

Addressing patients who make inappropriate, biased, sexist, or racist remarks can be extremely challenging. Depending on the recipient's comfort level, they may want to directly address the patient in the moment. Ideally, by-standers should intervene, when possible, to minimize any additional emotional trauma and to alert the offender that harassment of healthcare providers will not be tolerated. A mechanism to report incidents of bias and/or sexual harassment should be in place. Reporting options should include an anonymous method. Possible responses for this case might include:

Joe: "Yes - I am your nurse today. Your comments made me uncomfortable but perhaps, I misunderstood you. Could you clarify what you mean by that?"

or

"Excuse me. I'm not sure how to interpret your statement/question. Could you clarify it for me, so I understand exactly what you are inferring or suggesting?"

Physician in the room: "Yes, Joe is your nurse. He is an excellent member of our team, and we are lucky to have him. Being of a specific gender does not exclude anyone at our hospital from any particular job, in fact we actively pursue diversity. Also, just as we expect patients to be respectful to our female nurses and not comment on their physical attributes, we expect the same treatment for our male colleagues. What you just said is not really appropriate." The physician should also address the unprofessional snickering made by the medical students.

Any bystander (including students): complete an incident report so that the comments and frequency of these kinds of events can be tracked. Debriefs with staff members could be done later to review appropriate ways to handle offensive patients and follow up should be done to assess the well-being of the victim (Joe).

Institution: Healthcare organizations should have a system in place for reporting incidents of racial, gender, religious, and other bias. Regular review and tracking of these incidents can help identify areas and/or individuals that need intervention. Policies prohibiting patient and employee harassment of healthcare employees should be developed if not already in place.

6. What other discriminatory assumptions are often made about male nurses?: Nursing is portrayed as a career that is more suitable for females. Males pursuing the profession are often considered

less masculine (Harrison, 2021) or assumed to be gay (Stanley et al., 2016). Assumptions are made that males who decide to apply for nursing school are unable to get into medical school or are failed doctors. Male nurses are also unfairly considered to be less caring or compassionate to their patients (Wociechowski, 2015). Results of some studies indicate that male nurses are more likely to be thought of as lazy, disorganized, and unhappy in the profession (Rabie et al., 2020).

Epilogue

Stereotyping in the healthcare environment can have a negative impact on both providers and patients. When judgements are made about individuals or groups of people based on social norms or physical appearance, there can be a risk of making decisions that may cause emotional and/or physical harm. There are many stereotypes that male nurses have been challenged with over the years. In this case, Joe is seen as the go-to nurse when "muscle" is deemed necessary to care for a given patient. This is one of the most common issues faced by male nurses, with one study reporting 58.2% of males experiencing this kind of inappropriate job assignment (Stanley et al., 2016). Healthcare professionals should be cognizant of personal biases and work to treat colleagues equally and with respect. The healthcare environment should be a place where employees feel comfortable speaking up when inappropriate comments are made based on stereotyped gender roles and bias. Failure to prevent or interrupt these kinds of behavior can lead to job dissatisfaction, poor mental health, and may impact patient outcomes.

REFERENCES

Association of American Medical Colleges. (2020). *The state of women in academic medicine: The pipeline and pathways to leadership*. https://store.aamc.org/the-state-of-women-in-academic-medicine-2018-2019-exploring-pathways-to-equity.html

Axelson, R. D., Solow, C. M., Ferguson, K. J., & Cohen, M. B. (2010). Assessing implicit gender bias in Medical Student Performance Evaluations. *Evaluation & the Health Professions*, *33*(3), 365–385. doi:10.1177/0163278710375097 PMID:20801977

Brown, M. E. L., Hunt, G. E. G., Hughes, F., & Finn, G. M. (2020). 'Too male, too pale, too stale': A qualitative exploration of student experiences of gender bias within medical education. *BMJ Open*, *10*(8), e039092. doi:10.1136/bmjopen-2020-039092 PMID:32792453

Butler, J. (1999). *Gender Trouble: Feminism and the Subversion of Identity*. Routledge.

Capodilupo, C. M., Nadal, K. L., Corman, L., Hamit, S., Lyons, O. B., & Weinberg, A. (2010). The manifestation of gender microaggressions. In *Microaggressions and marginality: Manifestation, dynamics, and impact* (pp. 193–216). John Wiley & Sons Inc.

Carr, P. L., Ash, A. S., Friedman, R. H., Szalacha, L., Barnett, R. C., Palepu, A., & Moskowitz, M. M. (2000). Faculty perceptions of gender discrimination and sexual harassment in academic medicine. *Annals of Internal Medicine*, *132*(11), 889–896. doi:10.7326/0003-4819-132-11-200006060-00007 PMID:10836916

Carr, P. L., Gunn, C. M., Kaplan, S. A., Raj, A., & Freund, K. M. (2015). Inadequate progress for women in academic medicine: Findings from the National Faculty Study. *Journal of Women's Health, 24*(3), 190–199. doi:10.1089/jwh.2014.4848 PMID:25658907

Chatterjee, P., Warner, L. N., Basil, M. C., Christopher, M., Manning, K., Fisher, H. N., Rexrode, K. M., Solomon, S. R., Kakoza, R. M., & Yialamas, M. A. (2021). "Make the Implicit Explicit": Measuring Perceptions of Gender Bias and Creating a Gender Bias Curriculum for Internal Medicine Residents. *Advances in Medical Education and Practice*, *12*, 49–52. doi:10.2147/AMEP.S292166 PMID:33488136

Christov-Moore, L., Simpson, E. A., Coude, G., Grigaityte, K., Iacoboni, M., & Ferrari, P. F. (2014). Empathy: gender effects in brain and behavior. *Neurosci Biobehav Rev, 46*(Pt 4), 604-627. doi:10.1016/j.neubiorev.2014.09.001

Cogin, J., & Fish, A. (2009). Sexual harassment—A touchy subject for nurses. *Journal of Health Organization and Management*, *23*(4), 442–462. doi:10.1108/14777260910979326 PMID:19862867

Fnais, N., Soobiah, C., Chen, M. H., Lillie, E., Perrier, L., Tashkhandi, M., Straus, S. E., Mamdani, M., Al-Omran, M., & Tricco, A. C. (2014). Harassment and discrimination in medical training: A systematic review and meta-analysis. *Academic Medicine*, *89*(5), 817–827. doi:10.1097/ACM.0000000000000200 PMID:24667512

Gill, A. C., Zhou, Y., Greely, J. T., Beasley, A. D., Purkiss, J., & Juneja, M. (2022). Longitudinal outcomes one year following implicit bias training in medical students. *Medical Teacher*, *44*(7), 744–751. doi:10.1080/0142159X.2021.2023120 PMID:35021935

Gomez, L. E., & Bernet, P. (2019). Diversity improves performance and outcomes. *Journal of the National Medical Association*, *111*(4), 383–392. doi:10.1016/j.jnma.2019.01.006 PMID:30765101

Harrison, T. (2021). Florence Nightingale's legacy on the role of men in community nursing. *British Journal of Community Nursing*, *26*(6), 302–306. doi:10.12968/bjcn.2021.26.6.302 PMID:34105367

Hu, Y. Y., Ellis, R. J., Hewitt, D. B., Yang, A. D., Cheung, E. O., Moskowitz, J. T., Potts, J. R. III, Buyske, J., Hoyt, D. B., Nasca, T. J., & Bilimoria, K. Y. (2019). Discrimination, Abuse, Harassment, and Burnout in Surgical Residency Training. *The New England Journal of Medicine*, *381*(18), 1741–1752. doi:10.1056/NEJMsa1903759 PMID:31657887

Kahsay, W. G., Negarandeh, R., Dehghan Nayeri, N., & Hasanpour, M. (2020). Sexual harassment against female nurses: A systematic review. *BMC Nursing*, *19*(1), 58. doi:10.118612912-020-00450-w PMID:32612455

LeBlanc, B. (2017). *Gender Performativity in Nursing: Men, Power, and the Construction of the Ideal Nurse* [Unpublished doctoral dissertation]. University of Ottawa, Ontario, Canada.

McKinley, S. K., Wang, L. J., Gartland, R. M., Westfal, M. L., Costantino, C. L., Schwartz, D., Merrill, A. L., Petrusa, E., Lillemoe, K., & Phitayakorn, R. (2019). "Yes, I'm the Doctor": One Department's Approach to Assessing and Addressing Gender-Based Discrimination in the Modern Medical Training Era. *Academic Medicine*, *94*(11), 1691–1698. doi:10.1097/ACM.0000000000002845 PMID:31274522

Nadal, K. L. K. R., Sissoko, G., Floyd, N., & Hines, D. (2021). The legacies of systemic and internalized oppression: Experiences of microaggressions, imposter phenomenon, and stereotype threat on historically marginalized groups. *New Ideas in Psychology, 63*.

Newman, C., Ng, C., Pacque-Margolis, S., & Frymus, D. (2016). Integration of gender-transformative interventions into health professional education reform for the 21st century: Implications of an expert review. *Human Resources for Health*, *14*(1), 14. doi:10.118612960-016-0109-8 PMID:27067144

Papantoniou, P. (2021). Are male nurses sexually harassed? A cross-sectional study in the Greek Health System. *BMC Nursing*, *20*(1), 137. doi:10.118612912-021-00656-6 PMID:34372829

Rabie, T., Rossouw, L., & Machobane, B. F. (2020). Exploring occupational gender-role stereotypes of male nurses: A South African study. *International Journal of Nursing Practice*, *12890*. Advance online publication. doi:10.1111/ijn.12890 PMID:32964584

Shanafelt, T. D., Balch, C. M., Dyrbye, L., Bechamps, G., Russell, T., Satele, D., Rummans, T., Swartz, K., Novotny, P. J., Sloan, J., & Oreskovich, M. R. (2011). Special report: Suicidal ideation among American surgeons. *Archives of Surgery (Chicago, Ill.)*, *146*(1), 54–62. doi:10.1001/archsurg.2010.292 PMID:21242446

Spector, P. E., Zhou, Z. E., & Che, X. X. (2014). Nurse exposure to physical and nonphysical violence, bullying, and sexual harassment: A quantitative review. *International Journal of Nursing Studies*, *51*(1), 72–84. doi:10.1016/j.ijnurstu.2013.01.010 PMID:23433725

Stanley, D., Beament, T., Falconer, D., Haigh, M., Saunders, R., Stanley, K., Wall, P., & Nielson, S. (2016). The male of the species: A profile of men in nursing. *Journal of Advanced Nursing*, *72*(5), 1155–1168. doi:10.1111/jan.12905 PMID:26799533

Thomas, C. M., Bertram, E., & Johnson, D. (2009). The SBAR communication technique: Teaching nursing students professional communication skills. *Nurse Educator*, *34*(4), 176–180. doi:10.1097/NNE.0b013e3181aaba54 PMID:19574858

West, C. P., Shanafelt, T. D., & Kolars, J. C. (2011). Quality of life, burnout, educational debt, and medical knowledge among internal medicine residents. *Journal of the American Medical Association*, *306*(9), 952–960. doi:10.1001/jama.2011.1247 PMID:21900135

Wociechowski, M. (2015). *Male Nurses Confronting Stereotypes and Discrimination: Part 1, The Issues*. https://minoritynurse.com/male-nurses-confronting-stereotypes-and-discrimination-part-1-the-issues/

Chapter 11
Lesbian, Gay, Bisexual, Transgender, Queer, Intersex, and Others (LGBTQI+): Providing Comprehensive Care Across the Spectrum

Chasity O'Malley
Wright State University Boonshoft School of Medicine, USA

Samiksha Prasad
Nova Southeastern University Dr. Kiran C. Patel College of Allopathic Medicine, USA

Arkene Levy
Nova Southeastern University Dr. Kiran C. Patel College of Allopathic Medicine, USA

Daniel P. Griffin
Nova Southeastern University Dr. Kiran C. Patel College of Allopathic Medicine, USA

EXECUTIVE SUMMARY

Three scenarios involving LGBTQI+ populations are presented. Case 1 highlights an in-class interaction between a faculty member and two students. A female-to-male transgender student is misgendered by a faculty member in front of the class, resulting in the student leaving the session. A second student acts as an ally when approached by the faculty member about the situation. Case 2 involves a professional development session focused on creating inclusive environments for LGBTQI+ students. One faculty member presents her approach of avoiding knowledge of students' personal lives as an effective tool for protecting students and faculty. Case 3 involves an inclusivity training session that doesn't connect as intended with the audience, resulting in students who are disengaged. Prompt questions promote reflection on what transpired, its impact, and institutional resources to help faculty in building inclusive environments. Readers will consider how to address what transpired both immediately and in the future.

DOI: 10.4018/978-1-6684-5493-0.ch011

BACKGROUND

It is imperative for faculty and staff involved in health professions education to be culturally sensitive in serving an increasingly diverse student population. Cultural humility and sensitivity create a sense of belonging and inclusion for learners while simultaneously modeling behaviors that encourage them to inculcate the same approaches in their professional careers. It is therefore critically important that healthcare professional school personnel acquire the skills necessary to effectively cultivate an inclusive learning environment and train students to appropriately and effectively practice culturally competent health care. Lesbian, Gay, Bisexual, Transgender, Queer, Intersex and other (LGBTQI+) population individuals are an example of such diverse groups that experience disparate outcomes in health care and while there is growing evidence that increasing the representation of gender and sexual minorities in the healthcare workforce could improve the health care experience and outcomes for LGBTQI+ individuals (Phelan et al., 2017; Rowe et al., 2017), health professions students that are a part of this demographic often face many challenges along their educational paths. Health professions students that identify as gender and sexual minorities often face anti-LGBTQI+ discrimination and heterosexism which contributes to a non-inclusive and hence suboptimal learning environment (Lapinski and Sexton, 2014). Gender diverse students are reluctant to disclose their gender in the classroom because of fear of bias, discrimination and marginalization (Dimant et al., 2019). The encounters met by gender diverse students often correlates to increased stress and reduced academic success of LGBTQI+ students (Nama et al., 2017; Ryus et al., 2022).

The challenges faced by LGBTQI+ students may be driven, in part, by explicit and implicit biases of colleagues, faculty, and staff. Explicit biases are attitudes and beliefs that individuals are aware of and can consciously control while implicit biases are attitudes and beliefs that are outside of the conscious awareness of the individual (Phelan et al., 2017). Biases among health professions students toward LGBTQI+ individuals are common and in one large study of heterosexual, first-year medical students greater than 50% exhibited both implicit and biases toward LGBTQI+ individuals (Burke et al., 2015). Similarly attitudes among educators toward LGBTQI+ students are likely a contributor to negative experiences and challenges faced by these individuals.

Several strategies are presented to enhance LGBTQI+ cultural competencies and to create a safe and affirming learning environment. Proficiency training for health care school personnel and students has been shown to mitigate biases, discrimination and microaggressions in learning environments by increasing the knowledge and cultural awareness of the faculty, staff, and students. Such exercises improve cultural awareness and proficiency and translate to improved healthcare outcomes for the LGBTQI+ population.

When discussing LGBTQI+ topics, it is important to consider how microaggressions, especially microinvalidations, may play a role. Microinvalidations are a subtype of microaggressions characterized by communications or environmental cues that exclude, negate, or nullify the thoughts, feelings, or experiential realities of certain groups (Sue, 2010). Creating an inclusive environment and addressing microaggressions against minority groups including gender and sexual minorities is important especially as it relates to preventing burnout (Samuels et al., 2021), preventing attrition, and increasing diversity among healthcare professionals. Non-inclusive environments not only cause undue academic and mental stress to LGBTQI+ students (Ryus et al., 2022) but might negatively impact their academic success. Several strategies have been proposed in health care professions to address microaggressions from the perspective of a bystander or the source or recipient of the microaggression (Poorsattar, Blake, and Manuel, 2021). One such strategy is allyship and advocacy within the learning environment. In this context, an ally is an individual who works to engage with information to improve their understanding of LGBTQI+ experiences and advocates for these individuals. Integrating LGBTQI+ proficiency training longitudinally into health professions curricula for both learners and educators is one avenue that provides an opportunity to understand the lived experiences of gender and sexual minorities. This training also aids in helping individuals to gain the necessary knowledge to amplify the voices of the LGBTQI+ community as an ally when witnessing incidences of discrimination, microaggressions and biases.

This chapter presents cases centered around important LGBTQI+ topics that provide opportunities for self-reflection to different situations, including educator-learner engagement in the classroom, varying faculty philosophies, and navigating reluctance of learner participation in proficiency training. The reader is encouraged to consider the complexities of these cases, challenge their perceptions by considering different possible reasons behind the actions of the characters portrayed, and consider how they would respond if they were the various characters portrayed. The cases provide opportunities to discuss reactions and strategies in these situations and provide guidance for identification of relevant resources.

CASE 1: CLASSROOM CRINGE

Goal

Discuss appropriate responses by faculty, students, and institutions when mistaken gender identity and failure to provide a safe and affirming learning environment occurs in the classroom.

Learning Outcomes

1. Identify effective approaches for creating and maintaining a safe and inclusive learning environment.
2. Elucidate the role of allyship in helping gender and sexual minorities navigate challenges.
3. Recognize the importance of integrating LGBTQI+ proficiency training into healthcare professional program curricula.
4. Reflect on the importance of recognizing personal implicit biases and improving knowledge about gender and sexual minorities.

Case

During a physiology lecture on the female reproductive cycle, Dr. Nguyen asks the class to identify the official start of the ovarian cycle. The class chatters a little amongst themselves, but no one speaks up to answer. Dr. Nguyen calls on Dana to answer and he states (incorrectly) that ovulation is the first day. Dr. Nguyen smirks and says "Dana, I would expect that as a responsible female, you should know that the first day of the cycle is the first day of the menses."

Dana is now quite uncomfortable and doesn't respond but looks down and sinks into his seat. Dr. Nguyen presses the issue, asking Dana "Ok, so if the menses is day 1, what day do you think ovulation might be in a regular cycle?". Dana states, "I'm really not sure" and continues to look down. Dr. Nguyen asks for another student to volunteer to "help Dana out with her question."

At this point, Dana (a female-to-male transgender person) is incredibly frustrated and leaves the room abruptly, leaving his belongings and not returning by the end of the session. Dana thinks to himself, "I experience this every day, but I expected better of the faculty who are trusted to support their students."

After class, Dr. Nguyen asks Charles, the student who was sitting beside Dana, where she went. Charles replies "Dr. Nguyen, I'm not sure how to approach this, but Dana is not a female, he is a male. When you referred to him as a female, he was offended and needed some air." Dr. Nguyen looks perplexed for a second, then states, "Well, he should get a haircut that makes him look like a male if he doesn't want to be confused as a female" and walks away.

QUESTIONS AND ANSWERS

1. Discuss the error, or errors, made by Dr. Nguyen involving Dana. Discuss if this initial mishap could occur innocently, or innately has negative connotation.

Mistaking the gender of another individual can be a rather common occurrence. However, the assumption that a person falls into a specific gender category based on hairstyle brings into question whether personal biases may have played a role. Additionally, the transition of a transgender person from one gender to another is a topic that is not frequently discussed or that has training for faculty. Also, the professor assumes a student should already know topics related to their gender, and publicly challenges the student.

2. Discuss a potential appropriate immediate response from Dr. Nguyen for the mishap.

Dr. Nguyen could have taken the situation as a learning opportunity to learn more about the transition of transgender individuals. They also could have taken the time to recognize that the language used in the classroom was not inclusive. One of the first steps that would be important for them to take would be to meet with Dana and apologize for the way that he was treated and called out in the classroom. To wait to do this in front of the class could create a public spectacle and escalate the situation, making it worse.

3. Discuss a potential appropriate immediate response from Dana and Charles respectively.

Dana's response to the situation was one of frustration. He acted in a way that helped him to remove himself from the situation and avoid potential escalation or further attention being called to him. Charles could be helpful by taking and delivering Dana's belongings, so Dana did not have to worry about how and when to return to class to get them and indicating to Dana that what happened was explained to Dr. Nguyen.

4. Discuss how a bystander may react to the situation. For example, a potential impact onother students in the class.

Dr. Nguyen's behavior has potential to be damaging to other students in the classroom. For example, if another student has been having a tough time due to wanting to transition, seeing the treatment of Dana could negatively impact this student. Additionally, for students who have an unconscious bias against transgender individuals, seeing someone they respect as a professor behave this way may unconsciously reinforce the attitude. Alternatively, a student who is an ally or advocate for the LGBTQI+ community may choose to speak to Dr. Nguyen or his supervisor regarding the behavior to try to prevent it from occurring again. It should be recognized that the power dynamic between faculty and students may present a challenge for an ally or advocate. Processes should be in place at an institution, and well communicated so students can express and/or report their concerns without fear of retribution.

5. Discuss potential escalation of this incident to Dr. Nguyen's supervisor.

In order for remediation of the behavior to occur, Dr. Nguyen's supervisor may need to be involved. When Charles was approached by Dr. Nguyen to discuss the situation, Dr. Nguyen did not appear to recognize how harmful his statements were or that they were inappropriate. Care should be taken to approach the supervisor in a professional manner. Charles, along with any other student in the lecture that day, could report the situation. If not already discussed in Question 4, it should be recognized that the power dynamic between faculty and students may present a challenge for an ally or advocate. Processes should be in place at an institution, and well communicated so students can express and/or report their concerns without fear of retribution.

6. What are some professional development opportunities that Dr. Nguyen can benefit from?
    - Inclusive language training – makes the learner more conscientious about the use of certain expressions/words/ pronouns etc. that might be considered to exclude particular groups of people, especially gender-specific words.
    - LGBTQI+ safe zone training – provides the learner with skills for providing a safe and welcoming environment for those seeking allies.
    - Implicit bias training – to make the learner practice self-awareness and perspective taking to be able to recognize personal biases and ways to mitigate them.
    - LGBTQI+ toolkits – that provide guidance on how to navigate a diverse student body
    - Institutional policies and procedures training – to be updated on expectations and resources available institutionally and encourage active participation in these training.
7. Please take a moment to reflect on the way they imagined the situation, and then share with others as appropriate.

In this scenario, the age, gender, and other identifiers of Dr. Nguyen and Charles were not provided. One should think about how they envisioned this and consider their own biases or assumptions of others and how this may influence their behaviors.

Epilogue

In this scenario, the age, gender, and other identifiers of Dr. Nguyen and Charles were not provided. One should think about how they envisioned this and consider their own biases or assumptions of others and how this may influence their behaviors. LGBTQI+ microaggressions can present subtly and in many ways in the health professions field. In this scenario, Dr. Nguyen has taught the learners for the majority of a semester and has mistaken a transgender male student for a female. This could have been an innocent error; however, Dr. Nguyen assumed that a female would know more about the female reproductive system than a male, which should not have occurred. They then comments that if he doesn't want to be called "she", then his hair should not be so long. This follow-up comment denotes that Dr. Nguyen mistakenly referred to Dana as a female because of external appearances. These comments are often delivered without conscious effort and are expressions of subtle or unconscious biases. However, these statements, though seemingly harmless on the surface, are damaging and can perpetuate LGBTQI+ prejudices. As the situation was explained to Dr. Nguyen by Charles, a student in the classroom, the scenario should be given immediate attention in an appropriate manner to provide remediation. Steps could include Charles discussing the situation with his advisor who could then assist with proper reporting or Charles directly reporting the situation and what he had witnessed to the appropriate college official. There should be processes in place for faculty, staff, and students to anonymously report transgressions. Remediation should include recognition of the harmful statements and a subsequent apology with the intent to modify behavior by Dr. Nguyen.

CASE 2: INTENTIONAL INDIFFERENCE

Goal

Emphasize the importance of validation of students by faculty and the institution to build an inclusive learning environment by affirming and supporting LQBTQI+ life experiences.

Learning Outcomes

1. Recognize the importance of integrating LGBTQI+ proficiency training into healthcare professional program curriculums.
2. Identify effective approaches for creating and being a positive contributor to an inclusive learning environment.
3. Discuss the impact of microinvalidation of gender and sexual minority students on medical education.

Case

During a faculty development session for medical school faculty and staff on diversity and inclusion, the group is discussing effective strategies to interact with students. The group members are Dr. Simmons, Professor and Chair of Anatomy under the Department of Education, who is a self-identifying cis-female faculty member, Dr. James, Assistant Professor of Physiology, who is a self-identifying cis-female faculty member, Dr. Reynolds, Assistant Professor of Anatomy, who is a self-identifying cis-male faculty member and a staff member, are all part of one of the small groups during a breakout activity. Ms. Lynn, senior administrator and self-identifying as cis-female, is serving as the group reporter for this exercise. Following this activity, the groups will come together and discuss their insights as a collective large group. While the topic of creating an inclusive environment for LGBTQI+ students is being discussed, the group members are sharing their experiences with LGBTQI+ students.

The following is part of the small group discussions.

Group Reporter: If anyone would like to start with their experience?

Dr. James: I can start... I try to connect with as many of the students as I can. I feel it's very rewarding to get to know my students, it enhances the whole experience.

Dr. James then goes on to provide examples and personal experiences with some of his students.

Dr. Reynolds: I agree with that. It is very important. I remember when I was a student some of the best faculty, I had were the ones who took the time to get to know us. It created an environment where I felt comfortable approaching them with questions or even concerns, I had about my future in academia.

Dr. Simmons casually explains that she has never been in a situation such as the one mentioned in the scenario and can't relate to what Dr. James and Dr. Reynolds are saying.

Dr. Simmons: My approach is that – students' personal lives are none of my business! I find it best not to know that much about their personal activities or preferences. What they do on their own time is their business and has no bearing on what needs to be taught.

Group Reporter: Can you elaborate more on this?

Dr. Simmons: Well, this is an intentional approach so I can't be seen as treating any of the students differently. I firmly believe that if they aren't hurting anyone, I don't care what they choose to do. They need to learn the material and that's what I am there to help them with.

Dr. James: For me, getting to know my students is important. It helps me to understand better where they are coming from. I want to validate their lived experiences and I learn from them every day. Shouldn't we as faculty members contribute in a positive way to make our learning environment more inclusive? The webinar I attended last week on creating inclusive learning environments really honed in on that. It also mentioned that by faculty modeling this behavior, it encourages our physicians in training to use similar behaviors in getting to know their patients to improve patient care.

Dr. Simmons: What does getting to know your students have to do with inclusiveness? They all have the same opportunity to learn, and we are here to help all of them become great doctors. As far as I am concerned, they should all be seen as medical students. I expect my faculty to focus on covering the learning objectives and not on personal things that would distract from that.

Dr. Reynolds sinks into his chair and focuses on the assignment document without any comment. The facilitator announces that only one minute is remaining before large group reporting and Ms. Lynn asks "what should I report? It seems we haven't come to a consensus and I want to make sure I represent the group accurately".

QUESTIONS AND ANSWERS

1. What is your initial reaction to the comments made by each faculty member?

Reactions may vary depending on learners' past experiences.

The following are the authors' rationale/perceptions of the characters.

Dr. Simmons was written as the senior faculty member with many years of experience, who is also the supervisor of Dr. Reynolds. Dr. Reynolds was written to be brand new to teaching, under the supervision of Dr. Simmons. Dr. Reynolds has an interest in getting to know students, as it was impactful in his past as a student. There is a theme of Dr. Simmons, as a senior faculty member and chair, to have an impact on the behaviors of individuals within her team. This is evident by the way Dr. Reynolds "shuts down" towards the end of the discussion. Dr. James was written to be a faculty member with a few years of experience teaching who has been proactive in professional development. She is in a different department than Dr. Simmons and Dr. Reynolds.

The language we use may invalidate someone else, even if it is not intentional. As members of the health professions, we should be aware that our biases and our language significantly impacts our patients, peers, students, colleagues, etc. Dr. Simmons' comments invalidate and minimize the experiences of students in the classroom, including members of the LGBTQI+ community, and while there were no students in the room during her comments, her beliefs might negatively impact her interactions with all students and hence their learning experience. Other faculty members might also be sensitive to her comments, especially if they identify as members of the LGBTQI+ community. Depending on Dr. Simmons influence and authority she has on others, she may impart a recommendation for how faculty should view students, that might not cultivate a positive environment.

2. Are there any benefits or drawbacks to the approaches by each faculty member?

Dr. Simmons: Someone may think that by avoiding knowing too much about their students, they are protecting their students and themselves. With the driving thought that one cannot discriminate against someone if they don't know about them, this can be seen as a good thing by the individual because they can avoid any type of bias, either based in reality or perceived, because they are intentionally unaware.. There are also concerns by faculty that they need to keep a distance from the students to avoid being seen as inappropriate. However, not knowing about the students does not contribute to an inclusive environment. It does not allow for the faculty member to understand the personal journey travelled by the student and/or keeps the faculty at a distance from students who may benefit from mentorship and guidance by supportive faculty. Being approachable to others and being identified as their ally and an advocate for them creates a safe and welcoming environment. Additionally, it is important to note that "not caring" or avoiding knowing is not equivalent to "not judging or not discriminating against". In fact, a "not knowing" attitude may be detrimental to building a meaningful network.

Dr. James points out the importance of getting to know the students to enrich their learning experience. Dr. James has taken some professional development courses to ensure that the relationships formed with students are appropriate and that she has the proper training to be able to handle situations that may come her way involving the students. It is important to keep in mind that there is a fine line to walk when getting to know your students. There may be situations that are shared that are outside of the scope of what an individual can manage and it is important to know when to ask for additional help, who to go to for assistance, or to seek further training in how to manage delicate situations. Being able to manage and maintain professionalism can become challenging.

Dr. Reynolds appears to want to get to know his students. However, with his supervisor not supporting this, he shuts down and doesn't participate in the conversation any longer. Shutting down as a coping mechanism might seem appropriate at the time for self-preservation, but Dr. Reynolds could possibly benefit from professional development on how to interact with his supervisor when their opinions and values conflict.

3. Do you think Dr. Simmons' approach could impact the perspective of other colleagues?

Depending on the standing of Dr. Simmons, or how influential she is, she may convince/persuade others to follow her lead. This might sound reasonable at face value, but one needs to think of the impact of "not caring" or respecting the distance travelled / life experience of the student. Without proper policies/ procedures and/or training so faculty feel confident in how to approach students, Dr. Simmons approach may be favorable because it avoids risk to the faculty, and it may be seen as protective of the students.

There was an impact on the perspective of Dr. Reynolds based on her direct supervisor, Dr. Simmons's comments.

4. If the excerpts from the case content of the quote was said to a student, how do you think a student would feel about this approach? Quotes include: "all be seen as medical students" and "If they aren't hurting anyone, I don't care what they choose to do."

Students are not seen as individuals ("all be seen as medical students"). The student may question their value and not feel supported by a faculty member who actively avoids engaging with them, thereby diminishing their unique needs and experiences.

The faculty member saying, "If they aren't hurting anyone, I don't care what they choose to do." as a qualifier may beg the question of why the faculty member jumped to considering if someone was being hurt. Even if meant as a positive, the negative connotation may be seen as revealing a bias of disapproval, but not to an extreme where the faculty member would need to become engaged.

5. As a team member in the faculty development session, how would you discuss with Dr. Simmons ways that she may reconsider her approach, and what, if any, potential resources would you suggest would be helpful at your institution?
   - Make sure she realizes that diversity should be embraced and is beneficial to a team. For LGBTQI+, it is a type of diversity that needs to be acknowledged and supported. If knowledgeable, one can refer to disparities faced by this community (mental health, discrimination, health disparity, etc.)
   - The faculty member can be directed to best practices and resources at the institution. If they don't already exist, these can be developed at the institution.
   - An often-overlooked professional development opportunity is that which covers appropriate ways to engage students, colleagues, peers, etc. in an appropriate way. There is a rational fear from faculty that they need to keep distant from students to not be seen as getting too close. Developing a skillset to allow faculty to appropriately get to know and engage students would be beneficial.
6. What are strategies to address microaggressions, especially microinvalidations against LGBTQI+ proficiency training that have potential to cause discrimination.

There could be set institutional policies and standard operating procedures to ensure that faculty attain the correct trainings to limit microaggressions and microinvalidations. Bringing attention to the issues can help to bring awareness to individuals about both implicit and explicit biases they may have that lead to these microaggressions.

Individuals can look for intramural resources at their home institution, such as an office of diversity, equity, and inclusion, office of student affairs or and office of human resources for additional training.

Additionally, they can seek out external resources such as many local, regional and national organizations which offer free training resources for proficiency training. For example, organizations that support medical education such as the American Association of Medical Colleges (AAMC), and the

American Medical Association (AMA) also provide resources to provide cultural competency training that includes LGBTQI+ proficiency. Many local non-profit organizations such also are willing to partner with academic instructions to provide training.

Online Resources:

- The National LGBTQIA+ Health Education Center (https://fenwayhealth.org/the-fenway-institute/education/the-national-lgbtia-health-education-center/)
- Lesbian, Gay, Bisexual, and Transgender Health (https://www.cdc.gov/lgbthealth/health-services.htm)
- The National LGBTQIA+ Health Education Center, Human Rights Campaign (https://www.thehrcfoundation.org/professional-resources/the-national-lgbt-health-education-center)
- Social support agencies such as The Trevor Project Resources for International LGBTQ Youth – The Trevor Project

7. As healthcare professions students, how do you think that microaggressions and microinvalidations portrayed in the case above could translate to provider/patient relationships?

The microaggressions and microinvalidations displayed in the case above may lead to their persistence. As more experienced faculty model the behaviors above, everyone is affected and could "learn" that microaggressions and microinvalidations are acceptable, when in reality they are better to be addressed and mitigated to help foster a more equitable environment. This applies to classroom settings and to future patient care. Microaggressions and microinvalidations have been found to have detrimental effects in the healthcare setting. This could lead to patients not seeking help when needed or encountering misdiagnoses.

Epilogue

Intentional avoidance by faculty of learning "too much" about the personal lives of students may originally be well-meaning. It may be seen as a way of protecting the students from bias and prejudice, and a way to treat them all the same to ensure they have the same opportunities. It may also come from the concerns of faculty that they do not have the necessary training to know how to respond to more personal aspects of and/or challenges faced in students' lives. They may be concerned about crossing a line, putting their career in jeopardy. This case asks the participants to explore the importance of validating students, their distance travelled, and their current state of being as students in the faculty member's classroom. Participants also can either identify policies, procedures, resources and/or training at their institutions that they can utilize and identify where they feel there may be need for faculty to have what they need to support students and their life experiences.

CASE 3: RESISTANT STUDENTS

Goal

Elucidate the importance and effectiveness of outcomes of LGBTQI+ proficiency training for healthcare students.

Learning Outcomes

1. Navigate constructive responses to learner resistance to LGBTQI+ proficiency training
2. Appreciate the need for collaboration with experts for effective training
3. Describe the importance of LGBTQI+ proficiency training as part of health professions curricula
4. Appraise the importance of building an inclusive environment at the institutional-level that supports training

Case

The presenter of an LGBTQI+ proficiency training is a faculty ally/advocate who is not formally trained to sensitively provide training but volunteered to create and provide LGBTQI+ proficiency training for the new cohort of healthcare professional students. This session has been reviewed by faculty peers before implementing to the new cohort of students. The session mixes an informative presentation by the presenter and some small group learning activities where students engage in responding to scenarios regarding providing sensitive, inclusive and appropriate care for LGBTQI+ patients.

One of the scenarios required the students to discuss the parameters of intake process at different healthcare facilities and how they can be more inclusive. One of the student members in the small group asks another student (referred to as Student A) "How have you felt in these situations? Did you say something?". Student A seems a bit taken aback, and replies saying "I don't know, I just fill in the form as much as I can!"

During the rest of the group activity, the presenter recognizes that Student A disengages, as is most evident by them sitting with their arms folded as the rest of the small group members participate in discussion. When the group tries to engage Student A in discussion, they receive at best a short or one-word answer as a response.

After the session, Student A, who self-identifies as a member of the LGBTQI+ community asks to speak to the presenter privately. During the one-on-one meeting, Student A confides in the presenter that they felt isolated and uncomfortable during the discussion of the scenarios provided with cis-gendered students. Student A mentions that the way the cases were provided was not reflective of the experience they have had as an LGBTQI+ individual.

The presenter was taken aback and wanted to further understand the reason(s) behind the discomfort experienced by Student A during the session.

Presenter: "If you are comfortable, can you share why you felt this way?"

Student A: "It would have been nice to have guiding questions or facilitators for the small groups so that it did not fall on me to be the token "gay" kid in the group to lead the discussion and give an inside expert opinion". It was so uncomfortable that I felt I needed to remain quiet to avoid it continuing. With the group dynamic, I was not feeling that I could express how I was feeling, without coming off as combative. I also didn't think it was my place to try to change the group."

Presenter: "I am sorry you had this experience and felt singled out during this session. That was not the intent of this proficiency training session. However, I am glad you shared this with me, and pointed out areas of improvement in the session. The goal was to be as inclusive as possible and provide a safe place where everyone can express themselves and share their questions and experiences so that everyone can learn to address the healthcare needs of the LGBTQI+ community. Although this was always the intention, I can see where we could improve. I am always interested in continuous quality improvements for my sessions, and that is one reason why I provided a session feedback and reflection survey for those interested. I will review these surveys to help find ways to improve the session, and I also hope the future iterations of this training will include an expert to help revise it for achieving its intended goal appropriately."

The next morning, the presenter receives an email from a colleague who was observing the LGBTQI+ proficiency training session. They wanted to bring to the attention of the presenter that a different student (referred to as Student B) who was sitting at the back was quite disruptive to the discussions in their group. This colleague mentions giggling and inappropriate facial expressions displayed by Student B for almost the entirety of the session.

The presenter looks at consent forms provided for a session feedback and reflection survey by participants, and realizes that Student B did not complete one. The presenter then recalls that this was the student who shoved the consent form away a little aggressively when it was first introduced. Even though the feedback and reflection activity portion of the training was voluntary, the reaction of Student B seemed disruptive and unprofessional. However, the presenter was unsure how to approach this situation without taking away the autonomy of the students to decide if they wanted to participate in the feedback and reflection activity. The presenter hoped that any misgivings of Student B would be addressed by engaging in the training session.

QUESTIONS AND ANSWERS

1. Discuss the different reasons why a learner may be disengaged during such a session?

Learning environments are important in fostering student engagement. Students who identify as sexual and gender minorities might not perceive learning environments to be equally as inclusive or supportive when compared to their heterosexual counterparts. This might be for different reasons and these reasons can have minor or major impacts on the level of engagement of students in the classroom and their overall attitudes towards other learners and faculty. For any learner reasons for disengagement may include:

- They are uncomfortable with the unfamiliar
- They have an explicit bias toward the LGBTQI+ community
- They feel that they are targeted in the training
- They feel that they don't need the training because they feel equipped to handle it
- They are struggling with their own sexual orientation and gender identity
- They do not trust the skills and knowledge of the trainer
- There are unrelated outside forces that are distracting the learner

- They struggle to find the value in the training and/or topic
- The timing of the training is not properly placed in the curriculum (for example, placement around their examinations)

2. How could the faculty address the disengagement displayed by the LGBTQI+ identifying student (Student A) in the moment?

Of upmost importance is to not single out the student in front of their peers. Depending on the reasoning, singling out the student may exacerbate the issue that is occurring. If for example, the student feels uncomfortable, calling on them directly could make it much worse. As the trainer walks the room to observe the groups, they can spend some time at the table with the group with the disengaged student. Sometimes the presence of the trainer is effective in promoting communication, or the trainer can hear what the group is saying and ask questions of the group that could provide opportunities for the group members to share,

There are also subtle things that can indirectly give "permission" to the learners to provide commentary. One way is when the presenter is engaging the group, they can eye contact with the disengaged student to include them in the conversation.

A presenter can also provide evidence-based information to address likely questions by the group members. This places the presenter in an objective position since they are not a member of the LGBTQI+ and also helps to avoid placing the sole burden on an LGBTQI+ identifying student to become a representative and authority of the whole community and their experiences.

3. How could the faculty address the disengagement displayed by the disruptive student (Student B) in the moment?

Fortunately, learner engagement is malleable, and can be modified by various interventions to address behavioral, cognitive or emotional aspects of a students' academic experience. Faculty can positively stimulate learner engagement by focusing on the intentions behind the behavior of the students and exploring the thoughts and feelings of the students about the content being delivered. In this case the faculty could also discuss the relevance of the content and importance from the perspective of achieving health equity for LGBTQI+ individuals. Some of the techniques presented in question #2 may also be appropriate to address disengagement by a student who also displays disruptive behavior.

For this student, the intervention may need to have other things added, such as promoting why this type of training is valuable even if it is considered a sensitive topic. Relaying how there are patients that need the best care possible, and there are responsibilities of all healthcare professionals to treat them might help if a student is not happy being in the training.

The presenter can also remind the whole class that the surveys are voluntary, but everyone, even if not taking part in the surveying is expected to contribute equally.

4. What are the roles of other students to cultivate engagement by all team members, and what can the trainer do to promote and reinforce them?

It is the expectation in group settings, that the members of a small group will hold each other accountable for participating. Professionalism is a key component of healthcare training, and it encompasses cultivating an open and safe environment respectful of all opinions, ideas, and values. Students in healthcare professional programs should strive to exemplify professionalism as a competency during the curriculum, healthcare practice, and as part of daily life. These expectations must be clearly delineated by the institution when describing their learning environment, and should be reinforced periodically during program implementation.

While students may decide on roles such as a team reporter, they would each need to also be cognizant of the contributions of others. They can promote contributions of members of the group through a variety of methods, including but not limited to asking questions to promote discussion or agreeing on a method to ensure that everyone has a chance to speak. One caveat will be that they establish an environment that feels welcoming of all contributions of others and is safe to express themselves.

A trainer should not expect team members to naturally have the skillset to establish their roles and expectations of the group, especially when there is limited time to answer a question, as there often is in these training sessions. If team members recognize the content as sensitive topics, they may also not feel that it is appropriate for them to try to "force" engagement of others. The trainer needs to be proactive in establishing a foundation of team function, explaining the intended environment for the training, making expectations for each group member clear, and providing practices they can employ to engage each other. The presenter can also set the stage to let the learners know that some of these topics may be sensitive, and that everyone is expected to be professional, considerate, and empathetic.

5. What are ways that the faculty could address the verbal feedback by the student about representation in the session?
    - Include allies and/or members of the community who share their lived experiences.
    - Invite the student to participate in creating content for the next proficiency training if they are comfortable with sharing their identity in a larger group.
    - Anonymous evaluations to evaluate the level of participation of the student participants
6. What are some avenues to pursue to find resources to improve the training?

Intramural Resources may already be at the home institution, such as an office of diversity, equity, and inclusion, office of student affairs or human resources.

Extramural Resources include many local, regional and national organizations offer free training resources to enhance or develop proficiency training, while others accept fees to create, review, and/or present sessions. For example, organizations that support medical education such as the American Association of Medical Colleges (AAMC), and the American Medical Association (AMA) also provide resources to provide cultural competency training that includes LGBTQI+ proficiency. Many local non-profit organizations such also are willing to partner with academic instructions to provide training.

Online Resources:

- The National LGBTQIA+ Health Education Center (https://fenwayhealth.org/the-fenway-institute/education/the-national-lgbtia-health-education-center/)
- Lesbian, Gay, Bisexual, and Transgender Health (https://www.cdc.gov/lgbthealth/health-services.htm)
- The National LGBTQIA+ Health Education Center, Human Rights Campaign (https://www.thehrcfoundation.org/professional-resources/the-national-lgbt-health-education-center)

Epilogue

This scenario portrays a situation that is more common than one might think. With budget cuts and redirections in universities, there is more opportunity for well-meaning faculty to step in and help to fill a gap and provide training for various topics. While the intentions are good, the faculty may not have the appropriate training to properly be able to handle the situations that may arise. This scenario highlights the importance of ensuring that sessions run to train students are led by properly trained individuals. It would be appropriate for the faculty member in the case to follow up and attend a training seminar to ensure that future iterations of the training are conducted in the most efficient and accurate manner possible.

REFERENCES

Burke, S. E., Dovidio, J. F., Przedworski, J. M., Hardeman, R. R., Perry, S. P., Phelan, S. M., Nelson, D. B., Burgess, D. J., Yeazel, M. W., & van Ryn, M. (2015). Do Contact and Empathy Mitigate Bias Against Gay and Lesbian People Among Heterosexual First-Year Medical Students? A Report from the Medical Student CHANGE Study. *Academic Medicine*, *90*(5), 645–651. doi:10.1097/ACM.0000000000000661 PMID:25674910

Dimant, O. E., Cook, T. E., Greene, R. E., & Radix, A. E. (2019). Experiences of Transgender and Gender Nonbinary Medical Students and Physicians. *Transgender Health*, *4*(1), 209–216. doi:10.1089/trgh.2019.0021 PMID:31552292

Lapinski, J., & Sexton, P. (2014). Still in the closet: The invisible minority in medical education. *BMC Medical Education*, *14*(1), 171. Advance online publication. doi:10.1186/1472-6920-14-171 PMID:25128252

Nama, N., MacPherson, P., Sampson, M., & McMillan, H. J. (2017). Medical students' perception of lesbian, gay, bisexual, and transgender (LGBT) discrimination in their learning environment and their self-reported comfort level for caring for LGBT patients: A survey study. *Medical Education Online*, *22*(1), 1368850. doi:10.1080/10872981.2017.1368850 PMID:28853327

Phelan, S. M., Burke, S. E., Hardeman, R. R., White, R. O., Przedworski, J., Dovidio, J. F., Perry, S. P., Plankey, M. A., Cunningham, B., Finstad, D. W., Yeazel, M., & van Ryn, M. (2017). Medical School Factors Associated with Changes in Implicit and Explicit Bias Against Gay and Lesbian People among 3492 Graduating Medical Students. *Journal of General Internal Medicine*, *32*(11), 1193–1201. doi:10.100711606-017-4127-6 PMID:28766125

Poorsattar, S. P., Blake, C. M., & Manuel, S. P. (2021). Addressing Microaggressions In Academic Medicine. *Academic Medicine*, *96*(6), 927–927. doi:10.1097/ACM.0000000000004029 PMID:33656013

Rowe, D., Ng, Y. C., O'Keefe, L., & Crawford, D. (2017). Providers' Attitudes and Knowledge of Lesbian, Gay, Bisexual, and Transgender Health. *Federal Practitioner: For the Health Care Professionals of the VA, DoD, and PHS*, *34*(11), 28–34. PMID:30766240

Ryus, C. R., Samuels, E. A., Wong, A. H., Hill, K. A., Huot, S., & Boatright, D. (2022). Burnout and Perception of Medical School Learning Environments Among Gay, Lesbian, and Bisexual Medical Students. *JAMA Network Open*, *5*(4), E229596. doi:10.1001/jamanetworkopen.2022.9596 PMID:35486396

Samuels, E. A., Boatright, D. H., Wong, A. H., Cramer, L. D., Desai, M. M., Solotke, M. T., Latimore, D., & Gross, C. P. (2021). Association Between Sexual Orientation, Mistreatment, and Burnout Among US Medical Students. *JAMA Network Open*, *4*(2), e2036136. doi:10.1001/jamanetworkopen.2020.36136 PMID:33528552

Sue, D. W. (2010). *Microaggressions in everyday life: race, gender, and sexual orientation*. John Wiley & Sons Inc. https://www.wiley.com/en-us/Microaggressions+in+Everyday+Life%3A+Race%2C+Gender%2C+and+Sexual+Orientation-p-9780470491409

ADDITIONAL READING

Gaztambide, D. J. (2012). Addressing cultural impasses with rupture resolution strategies: A proposal and recommendations. *Professional Psychology, Research and Practice*, *43*(3), 183–189. doi:10.1037/a0026911

LGBT Health Services. (n.d.). CDC. Retrieved November 15, 2022, from https://www.cdc.gov/lgbthealth/health-services.htm

National LGBTQIA+ Health Education Center - Fenway Health: Health Care Is A Right, Not A Privilege. (n.d.). Retrieved November 15, 2022, from https://fenwayhealth.org/the-fenway-institute/education/the-national-lgbtia-health-education-center/

The National LGBTQIA+ Health Education Center - HRC Foundation. (n.d.). Retrieved November 15, 2022, from https://www.thehrcfoundation.org/professional-resources/the-national-lgbt-health-education-center

ENDNOTE

1 Disclaimer: This chapter took part in the double-blind peer review process and was not compromised due to the authors also being an editor. A non-author editor managed all of the editorial aspects of the chapter.

Chapter 12
Addressing Microaggressions in the Clinical Environment

Nicole Novotny
Ochsner Medical Center, USA

Andreia B. Alexander
Indiana University School of Medicine, USA

EXECUTIVE SUMMARY

Microaggressions are commonly encountered in the clinical learning environment. Although microaggressions may be subtle and/or unintentional, it has been well established that microaggressions can have significant negative impacts on healthcare workers, patients, and patient care, contributing to health inequities. Microaggressions are difficult to address in the clinical learning environment for many reasons. This chapter will provide health professions educators with a framework to effectively teach learners how to recognize and address microaggressions in the clinical learning environment in a non-accusatory way that will build relationships. It will also discuss common barriers to addressing microaggressions in medicine and provide potential solutions.

BACKGROUND

Microaggressions are defined as brief and commonplace daily verbal, behavioral or environmental indignities whether intentional or unintentional, that communicate hostile, derogatory or negative slights and insults toward marginalized groups of people (Sue et al, 2007). While microaggressions are often unintentional and may be subtle, it has been well established that microaggressions can have significant negative impacts on both healthcare workers and patients alike. Microaggressions are associated with lower self-esteem (Nadal et al, 2014). Repeated exposures to microaggressions are associated with increased depression and suicidality (O'Keefe et al, 2015). When patients of marginalized groups experience discrimination, including in the form of microaggressions, it causes them to avoid seeking out healthcare opportunities which further perpetuates health disparities (Casey et al, 2019; Snyder, 2018).

DOI: 10.4018/978-1-6684-5493-0.ch012

To address microaggressions within the clinical learning environment, one must first be able to recognize that a microaggression has occurred and then be able to respond to it. Multiple frameworks have been previously developed to respond to microaggressions directly in a productive and respectful way (Molina et al, 2020; Sagalowsky et al, 2021; Sotto-Santiago et al, 2020; Souza, 2016; Warner et al, 2020). In reviewing these frameworks, the "Open the Front Door" (OTFD) framework is best suited for responding to microaggressions in the clinical environment because it more directly and succinctly asserts the need for behavioral change by ending with a desired outcome (Souza, 2016). The four principles of the "Open The Front Door" framework are observe, think, feel and desire. Many of the other frameworks require longer conversations by asking open-ended questions which may not always be feasible in the healthcare environment. Understanding microaggressions and responding to them by using frameworks such as "Open The Front Door" will facilitate a more inclusive environment for both healthcare workers and patients and will decrease gaps in health disparities among marginalized populations.

CASE 1: HISPANIC PATIENT WITH ACUTE CHOLECYSTITIS

Goal

This case portrays a racial microaggression directed at a Hispanic/Latinx patient. The resident consulting general surgery should recognize the microaggression and respond in a professional manner.

Learning Outcomes

1. Understand the term microaggression and learn how to recognize microaggressions in the clinical environment.
2. Understand the negative impacts that microaggressions can have on patients and healthcare workers.
3. Learn the "Open The Front Door" framework and apply it to the microaggression presented in the case.

Case

The patient is a 35-year-old Hispanic female named Gabriela Lopez Garcia. She is bilingual and speaks both English and Spanish fluently. She initially presented to the Emergency Department for right upper quadrant abdominal pain, fever, nausea and vomiting. She was seen primarily by the resident physician who was being supervised by his attending. After lab studies and ultrasound were obtained, the patient was ultimately diagnosed with acute cholecystitis. The resident physician then consults general surgery for operative management.

Emergency Resident Physician (ERP): Hi, I have a new consult for acute cholecystitis in the Emergency Department (ED) that I would like you to see. Her name is Gabriela Lopez Garcia. She is in room 3.

General Surgeon (GS): Okay. Tell me what is going on.

ERP: She is a 35-year-old female who came into the ED with right upper quadrant abdominal pain, fever, nausea and vomiting. Despite reporting a fever at home, she did not have a fever in the ED. Her heart rate is a little tachycardic at about 105. Her respirations and oxygen saturations have been normal. On exam she is ill appearing and has right upper quadrant tenderness with a positive Murphy's sign. Her labs show a leukocytosis of 15.5K and normal liver function tests and lipase. Her right upper quadrant ultrasound showed a thickened gallbladder wall with pericholecystic fluid and gallstones and was determined to have acute cholecystitis. We have given her IV fluids and medications to control her pain and nausea.

GS: When was the last time she ate something?

ERP: About 6 hours ago.

GS: Okay. Please keep her NPO. What did you say her name was?

ERP: Gabriella Lopez Garcia. And actually, since we've been on the phone, she has become a little more unstable. Her blood pressure is now 89/65 and she is tachycardic to a heart rate of 115.

GS: Okay. Go ahead and start antibiotics and continue with fluid resuscitation. It's close to the end of my shift and we are getting ready to sign out, and I don't have time to get the interpreter and complete this consult, so I will sign it out to my oncoming colleagues, and they will make sure to see her first thing.

ERP: Well, she speaks fluent English. We haven't needed an interpreter.

GS: Yes, that's what they all say, but then I come down there and once I start talking about surgery and going through the consent and everything else, I always end up having to find an interpreter. We'll be down after sign out.

QUESTIONS AND ANSWERS

1. What is a microaggression, what are the different types of microaggressions and what type of microaggression is being exhibited in this case?

A microaggression is defined as brief and commonplace daily verbal, behavior, or environmental indignities, whether intentional or unintentional, that communicate hostile, derogatory, or negative slights and insults towards marginalized groups (Sue et al, 2007). In other words, a microaggression is a brief interaction that can be verbal or non-verbal, intentional or unintentional, hostile or subtle, that attacks someone's identity, particularly someone who identifies with a marginalized group. Microaggressions occur on individual and interpersonal levels.

There are three subtypes of microaggressions: microassaults, microinsults, and microinvalidations. Not all microaggressions necessarily fit into one subcategory, and at times, there can be overlap.

A **microassault** is an explicit derogation characterized primarily by a verbal or nonverbal attack meant to hurt the intended victim through name-calling, avoidant behavior or purposeful discriminatory actions. Microassaults are often intentional. Some examples of a microassault include crossing the street or clutching your purse when passing by certain groups of people, racial profiling, someone stating, "I don't want a black doctor", and name calling. A **microinsult** is a subtle snub or humiliation that conveys rudeness and insensitivity and demeans a person's racial heritage or identity. Microinsults are often unintentional. Some examples of microinsults include statements such as, "You don't sound black" or "You don't seem gay," and questions like, "Where are you from? No, where are you *really* from?" A **microinvalidation** is a statement aimed to exclude, negate, or nullify the personal thoughts, feelings or experiences of an individual. Microinvalidations are often unintentional. Examples of microinvalidations include statements such as, "I don't see color" or "It must have been easy for you to get into this program because you're – black, pretty, etc."

The primary microaggression in the scenario occurs when the general surgeon assumes that the patient is Spanish speaking based on her last name and does not want to come and provide consultation because it will take him longer if he has to use a medical interpreter. Avoiding the consult and delaying patient care is a behavioral indignity, whether intentional or unintentional by the surgeon, directed at Spanish speaking patients. This microaggression would fall under the subtype of microassault.

A second microaggression occurs in this case when the general surgeon did not believe that the patient spoke fluent English, despite the emergency resident physician telling the general surgeon that the patient spoke fluent English. This can be viewed as insensitive to the patient and could be seen as demeaning towards her racial heritage or identity. This microaggression would fall under the subtype of microinsult.

2. The general surgeon is clearly delaying care in a sick patient. Why is this considered a microaggression and not a macroaggression?

Micro and macro-aggressions are similar in concept to micro and macro-economics. Microeconomics deals with the exchange of money and spending on an individual basis, whereas macroeconomics deals with large scale or general economic factors, such as interest rates and national productivity (Encyclopaedia Britannica, n.d.). Along the same lines, microaggressions occur on an individual or group level while macroaggressions occur on an institutional or systemic level and manifest as biased or discriminatory policies, governance, and other practices that disproportionately benefit one group over another (Sue et al, 2019). Macroaggressions refer to when people talk about systemic racism and racist/discriminatory policies.

3. What are the different roles someone can have in a microaggression? What was the role of the emergency resident physician in this case? What was the role of the general surgeon?

The Microaggressions Triangle Model is a framework for understanding microaggressions from a human interaction standpoint (Ackerman-Barger and Jacobs, 2020). The model encourages people to view microaggressions from three different perspectives: recipient, source and bystander.

Recipient – the marginalized individual whom the microaggression is directed towards
Source – the individual whom the microaggression came from
Bystander – an individual who witnesses the microaggression

An "Active" bystander is an individual who chooses to speak out against the microaggression he or she has witnessed. It is also important to note that the source of the microaggression may not always be aware of the impacts of his or her statement or behavior because microaggressions are often unintentional and the product of unconscious bias.

In the above scenario, the source of the microaggression is the general surgeon who was asked to consult on the patient. The microaggression is directed towards the patient who would be the recipient. The resident physician is not the recipient as he is not part of the marginalized group, which in this case, would be Hispanic/Latinx patients. Rather than being the recipient, the resident physician, should he choose to address the microaggression, would be an active bystander.

4. How could the emergency resident physician have responded in this scenario?

In this scenario, it could be implied that the emergency resident physician did not feel comfortable with the general surgeon delaying care for their patient. However, instead of explicitly stating that, the resident let the surgeon know that the patient spoke fluent English. By responding in this way, the resident physician was complicit in the microaggression. There was no indication that the resident felt the surgeon was doing anything wrong. What would the resident's response have been if the patient did need an interpreter? Does it make it okay to delay care then? No, it does not. That is why it is important that we teach our learners to act as an active bystander and address microaggressions, in this case, when speaking with the consultant.

There have been many different frameworks established to address microaggressions (Table 1). Some of these include OTFD (Souza, 2016), XYZ (Molina et al, 2020), ACTION (Souza, 2018), O^3 (Sagalowsky et al, 2021) and GRIT (Warner et al, 2020).

Table 1. Frameworks for responding to microaggressions. Adapted from Molina et al (2020).

Framework	Principles
OTFD "Open the Front Door"	*Observe*: concrete, factual, observable *Think*: thoughts based on observation *Feel*: emotions *Desire*: request or inquire about desired outcome
XYZ	I feel *X* when *Y* because *Z*.
ACTION	*Ask* clarifying questions. *Come* from curiosity not judgement. *Tell* what you observed as problematic in a factual manner. *Impact* exploration: Ask for or state the potential effect of such a statement or action on others. *Own* your own thoughts and feeling around the effect. *Next* steps: Request appropriate action be taken.
O^3	Observation of fact Opinion Open-ended inquiry
GRIT	*Gather* your thoughts. *Restate* the comment or ask the speaker to restate their comment. *Inquire*: Dig deeper and seek clarification *Talk* it out.

Some of these frameworks require lengthier and often probing conversations which may not always be feasible due to time constraints in the clinical environment. For this reason, we recommend the "Open The Front Door" or OTFD framework for the clinical environment (Souza, 2016). The OTFD framework also directly asserts the need for behavior change and provides the microaggressor with a suggested behavior change.

The four principles of the "Open The Front Door" framework include:

Observe: State what you observed. This should be concrete, factual, and observable. For example, if you were to witness a doctor constantly interrupting a nurse, instead of saying, "I heard how you were treating the nurse." You would state, "I heard you repeatedly interrupting the nurse."

Think: State what you think about the situation based on your observation. Some examples include, "I think that is racist (or sexist, homophobic, ageist)." "I think that is inappropriate." "I think that is unsafe for the patient."

Feel: Explicitly name an emotion or feeling. For example, "That makes me feel disappointed (or sad, angry, upset)." In practice, this is the part that is often left out or overlooked. It is important that the "feel" statement is included in your response. First, no one can argue with how you feel. They are your feelings. They may be able to argue with what you observed (e.g., "I didn't say that." Or, "I thought she was done talking.") They may even be able to argue with what you think (e.g., "Well, I don't think it's inappropriate.") However, they cannot argue with how you feel about a situation. Second, it softens the conversation. As we will discuss later in this chapter, one of the biggest barriers to addressing microaggressions in the clinical learning environment is fear of retribution and/or fear of burning bridges. By inserting emotion into your response, your response becomes less confrontational and more inviting for a conversation.

Desire: State your request or inquire about a desired outcome. For example, "I hope we can treat each other with respect moving forward." Or, "I would like you to come see the patient."

Using this framework, an example response from the resident physician could have been:

"I heard you say that you do not want to see this patient because it will take too long to use an interpreter [observe]. I think this would be an unfair and dangerous delay in care for the patient [think]. I am uncomfortable [feel] with this and would like you to come see the patient [desire]."

5. How does the microaggression in this case impact the patient? In the clinical environment, what other effects can microaggressions have on patients and healthcare workers?

Microaggressions in the clinical environment can have many negative impacts on patients. Perceived discrimination has been shown to lead to negative psychological and physical health outcomes (Pascoe and Richman, 2009) and contribute to health disparities among marginalized groups. Patients who experience microaggressions or hear of stories of others experiencing microaggressions may hesitate to obtain or delay health care utilization in the future, further perpetuating health disparities (Casey et al, 2019; Snyder 2018). Furthermore, microaggressions often stem from unfair assumptions (biases) made about patients, which, as in this case, can lead to delayed patient care and poor patient outcomes. This can lead to increased morbidity and mortality.

Microaggressions also have a significant impact on healthcare workers. Microaggressions that occur in the workplace contribute to job dissatisfaction and burnout (Hu et al, 2019). Burnout can lead to suboptimal patient care and medical errors and even increase the risk of suicidality (Ehie et al, 2021).

In this scenario, the microaggression causes a delay in patient care. Delays in patient care can have negative consequences for patients by increasing morbidity and mortality.

Epilogue

This case begins by defining the term microaggression and describing the different types of microaggressions commonly encountered in the clinical environment. Multiple examples of common microaggressions are provided and discussed within this case. The "Open The Front Door" framework is then introduced to teach learners how to address microaggressions in a non-accusatory way that builds relationships. The case concludes by discussing the negative impacts that microaggressions can have on both patients and healthcare workers. By appropriately recognizing and responding to microaggressions, healthcare professionals can facilitate a more inclusive and health equitable environment for both patients and healthcare workers.

CASE 2: INFANT WITH HYPONATREMIC SEIZURE FROM FORMULA DILUTION

Goal

This case portrays a socioeconomic microaggression directed at the parents of an infant patient. The physician in the scenario should recognize the microaggression and respond in a professional manner.

Learning Outcomes

1. Understand the term microaggression and learn how to recognize microaggressions in the clinical environment.
2. Understand the negative impacts that microaggressions can have on patients and healthcare workers.
3. Respond to microaggressions in the clinical environment in a professional manner by applying the "Open the Front Door" framework previously introduced.
4. Identify and discuss potential barriers and challenges to responding to microaggressions in the clinical environment
5. Identify and discuss strategies for overcoming the barriers to responding to microaggressions

Case

The patient is a 3-month-old infant brought in by her mother for seizure-like activity at home. The patient has been having a cough, congestion and decreased appetite over the last three days. The patient's mother has been concerned that she is dehydrated, so she has been trying to hydrate her by adding extra water to her formula. The patient's mother noticed that the patient had an episode of shaking this evening and then was not acting like herself, so she brought her to the Emergency Department. On arrival to the Emergency Department, the patient has another seizure and is treated for status epilepticus. Her labs are significant for hyponatremia which is the result of the formula dilution. The patient is being taken care of by the resident physician who is being supervised by the attending physician. The resident and attending physicians are at bedside re-evaluating the patient and going over the lab work. The patient's mother is also at bedside with her infant daughter. The physicians are unaware that the patient's mother has been diluting the patient's formula at this time, but once they see the labs, it is on their differential diagnosis and needs to be asked about so they can figure out the etiology for the hyponatremia.

Resident physician: Your daughter's sodium level is low. Have you been formula feeding her?

Patient's mother: Yes, I have been mixing her formula.

Resident physician: How have you been mixing her formula?

Patient's mother: I have been giving her one scoop per four ounces.

Resident physician: So you are unable to afford the formula?

The patient's mother becomes visibly upset.

Patient's mother: No, it is because I am trying to prevent her from becoming dehydrated.

Resident physician: Well, you should be giving her one scoop per two ounces instead.

Patient's mother: But I am worried she is dehydrated because she is not eating or drinking much.

Resident physician: I will have our social worker come talk to you so they can help assist you with resources for getting the formula she needs at home.

After the attending and resident finish updating the patient's mother and step out of the room, the resident then turns to the attending and states, "I bet she is buying cigarettes or something else instead of formula."

QUESTIONS AND ANSWERS

1. Review the term microaggression and define the microaggressions in this scenario. Who is the source of the microaggression? Who is the recipient? Was there an active bystander?

As previously discussed, a microaggression is defined as brief and commonplace daily verbal, behavior, or environmental indignities, whether intentional or unintentional, that communicate hostile, derogatory, or negative slights and insults towards marginalized groups.

In the above scenario, the source of the microaggression is the resident physician. The microaggression is directed towards the patient's mother who would be the recipient. The attending physician if he or she would have chosen to address the microaggression, would have been considered an active bystander.

The first microaggression in this scenario occurs when the resident physician makes the assumption that the patient's mother cannot afford the formula as the reason for the formula dilution. This is a microaggression because the resident is making the assumption that the patient's family is of low socioeconomic status without understanding the mother's reasoning for the formula dilution. The mother in this scenario is diluting the formula because she is worried about the patient becoming dehydrated.

There is a second microaggression made by the resident physician privately to the attending physician upon exiting the exam room. The resident physician makes the assumption that patient's mother is spending her money on things other than prioritizing formula for her child by stating, "I bet she is buying cigarettes or something else instead of formula." Both of the microaggressions in this scenario could be categorized as microassaults as they are discriminatory statements that assume the patient's family is of low socioeconomic status. The optimal time for the attending physician to respond to the microaggressions in this scenario should have been after the initial microaggression statement was made to combat this behavior early and prevent additional negative comments.

2. What impact does this microaggression have on the patient and her mother?

As healthcare providers, it is our job to fully understand our patients and their backgrounds so that we can provide the best care possible. In this scenario, the resident physician ignores the patient's mother. The resident physician assumes that the patient's mother cannot afford to buy formula despite her stating that she is worried that her daughter is dehydrated. The patient's mother is not diluting the formula due to lack of resources; instead, she is diluting the formula because she is concerned that her daughter is dehydrated. More history as to why the mother thinks her infant daughter is dehydrated is important to ask here. The resident physician could be missing another diagnosis by focusing on the formula dilution and not addressing the initial cause for dehydration.

The microaggression in this scenario is the assumption that the patient's mother cannot afford to buy formula. While it is still extremely important that the physicians figure out the reasoning behind the formula dilution to prevent poor future outcomes, it should be asked in a non-accusatory, non-judgmental and delicate manner. There are several other causes of formula dilution other than just financial reasons and they should all be considered.

The statements made in this scenario may cause the mother of the patient to distrust physicians and other healthcare workers which in turn could prevent her from seeking appropriate medical care for herself and her child in the future. Whether or not the patient and her mother are of low socioeconomic background, the statements are offensive. Studies show that there is increased morbidity and mortality among minoritized groups as well as in people of low socioeconomic status. These offensive statements may further cause patients not to seek out health care opportunities which can further perpetuate this problem.

3. List and describe the four principles of the "Open the Front Door" framework. How could the attending physician have responded in this scenario using this framework?

The four principles of the "Open the Front Door" framework are observe, think, feel and desire.
Principles:
Observe: concrete, factual, observable
Think: thoughts based on observation
Feel: emotions
Desire: request or inquire about desired outcome
Using this framework, an example response from the attending physician could have been,

"I heard you say that the patient's mother cannot afford to buy formula [Observe]. I think that statement assumes that they are of a low socioeconomic status without knowing their situation and the details that are relevant to the current situation [Think]. I am disappointed [Feel] by this assumption, and I hope that you will listen to and seek to understand your patients' situations before making assumptions in the future [Desire]."

4. What are some potential barriers and challenges to responding to microaggressions in the clinical environment?

There have been many potential barriers identified in the literature when it comes to responding to microaggressions. Responding to microaggressions in the clinical environment also has its own separate challenges. Because healthcare workers and patients come from different backgrounds, it may sometimes be difficult to recognize that a microaggression has occurred. Even when a microaggression has been recognized, there might be a lack of familiarity which what to say or do in that situation. Other barriers include being unsure of the clinical significance of different types of microaggressions, lack of visible allies present to provide support when speaking up, lack of familiarity with institution specific policies and support systems and lastly, fear of retribution.

5. What are some strategies that can be used to overcome the potential barriers to responding microaggressions?

There are many strategies that can be used to help overcome these potential barriers. First and foremost, seeking education to better understand microaggressions and their potential impacts is the most important thing one can do. This education will help provide the knowledge necessary to recognize microaggressions in the clinical learning environment. It is impossible to respond to a microaggression if it goes unrecognized. Becoming familiar with frameworks for responding to microaggression such as the one in this chapter will help turn healthcare workers into active bystanders and facilitate a climate of diversity, equity and inclusivity.

Allies and support systems are institutionally dependent. At minimum, most institutions have mistreatment policies and reporting mechanisms. To overcome fear of retribution, we recommend finding institutional support systems such as human resources, ethics committees, etc. that can spread awareness on policies that protect employees and encourage them to use reporting mechanisms whenever they think a discriminatory or abusive act has occurred.

Epilogue

This case redefines key concepts related to microaggressions and provides an in-depth example on how unconscious bias in the form of microaggressions can negatively impact patient care and lead to health disparities. The principles of the "Open The Front Door" framework are reviewed and applied to the microaggression within the case. Responding to microaggressions is important to foster an inclusive environment for patients and healthcare workers and to decrease the gaps in health disparities. The is not easy and there are many potential barriers and challenges that healthcare professionals face when responding to microaggressions in the clinical environment. This case discusses these barriers and helps to provide potential strategies for overcoming these challenges.

CASE 3: POWER, PRIVILEGE, AND MICROAGGRESSIONS

Goal

This case discusses the role of power and privilege in microaggressions. It addresses the root cause of comments health care workers may receive from their marginalized patients, how these interactions differ from traditional microaggressions, and how to respond to such interactions.

Learning Outcomes

1. Understand the role of power, privilege, and oppression in the definition of microaggression.

2. Describe the role and history of mistrust in the health care system for marginalized populations.
3. Identify how comments/actions from marginalized patients may differ from traditional microaggressions.
4. Discuss how to respond to marginalized patients when they are expressing mistrust in healthcare.
5. Recognize the effects of discriminatory interactions on those observing, but not necessarily involved in, the interactions.
6. Apply the "Open The Front Door" framework.

Case

Cindy, a black female, brings her 15-year-old daughter, Denisha, to the emergency department this evening because Denisha has been having some abdominal pain and feeling tired. Dr. Johnson, a white, male physician, asks the usual history of present illness questions and examines Denisha. Dr. Johnson then turns to Cindy and says, "Based on everything you've said here, and on my exam, I don't think there is anything to worry about with Denisha today. She may be coming down with a stomach bug. As long as she is drinking fluids, I think with some rest over the next couple of days she should start to feel better."

Cindy is not pleased with this and says, "So, you're not going to do anything for her? Or any tests to make sure she's okay?"

Dr. Johnson responds with, "As I said, based on the information you have provided and my exam I do not see any red flags. I think this is a virus, and we do not have a test or treatment for a virus such as this. We can treat her symptoms with Tylenol and ibuprofen, fluids, and rest, and see how she does."

Cindy holds up her cell phone and points to the screen. She then states, "Well, my sister is a nurse and she said that Denisha needs a CBC to check her hemoglobin level and a CT scan of her abdomen."

Dr. Johnson states, "I am a doctor and I have been doing this for a very long time. There is nothing on Denisha's physical exam or history that makes me think any of those tests are indicated."

Cindy, who is clearly getting more frustrated says, "Well, I want those tests done anyway."

Dr. Johnson, who is also getting frustrated at this point says, "I'm sorry, but we will not be doing those tests today."

Cindy stands up and says to Dr. Johnson, "I want to see a Black doctor."

Dr. Johnson then storms out of the room without saying anything more to Cindy. He returns to the physician workroom and starts speaking loudly and in frustration. "I can't believe what this patient just said to me! Just because I won't order a CBC and CT scan like her nurse sister wants, she wants to see a black doctor! Like I can't provide her good care just because I am a white doctor! Who does she think she is?"

In the meantime, there is a Black female physician, Dr. Fleming, who is also sitting in the workroom. Upon hearing these comments, Dr. Fleming pauses, looks around and makes eye contact with one of the Nurse Practitioners in the room. She then quietly goes back to doing her work.

Dr. Johnson continues to complain about the situation. With frustration growing, Dr. Fleming turns to Dr. Johnson and says, "Did you ask her why she felt she needed a Black doctor?"

"Well, no. Why should I have to ask her that? Her comment was inappropriate. I am her doctor, and I am capable of taking care of her," Dr. Johnson responds.

Dr. Fleming says, "Okay, but if you don't want a bad patient experience score, then I would just go back in there and ask her why she feels that way and what you could do better."

Dr. Johnson storms off. Meanwhile, Dr. Fleming looks at her NP co-worker and states, "That was awkward. Does he really think that was okay? I would have said more, but he's scary."

A few minutes later Dr. Johnson goes back into the room to talk with Cindy and Denisha.

Dr. Johnson: "I apologize for leaving the room earlier. I was frustrated by your request for a black doctor. I feel as though I am treating you like I would treat any other patient. What was it about my care that caused you to request a black doctor?"

Cindy: "I am sorry if that made you upset, but I feel like you are not listening to me. This is my daughter. I know her, and she doesn't complain. She plays three sports and is in the band. She is always on the go. She never takes naps and never complains of being tired. So, for her to tell me that she feels so tired that she doesn't feel like playing basketball, I know something is wrong with her! And I don't feel like you believe me, so I'd rather have a doctor that will listen to what I am saying."

Dr. Johnson: "Ok. I can understand what you are saying. I am listening to you. In my opinion, you daughter looks very well, and I don't like to do unnecessary tests on anyone, not just you or my patients of color. Why don't we talk more about the tests you requested?"

Cindy and Dr. Johnson get into a conversation about the utility (or lack thereof) of a CBC and a CT scan. Dr. Johnson takes his time in explaining what information he can gain from each of the tests and how it may change the care Denisha receives. After Cindy has the opportunity to ask more questions, together they decided to obtain a CBC to check Denisha's hemoglobin level but defer the CT scan. The CBC comes back with a mildly low hemoglobin level and Denisha is started on iron supplementation and referred to her primary care physician for further follow-up.

A few weeks later, Dr. Johnson receives a card in his work mailbox. It is from Cindy.

Dear Dr. Johnson,

Thank you for taking care of my daughter, Denisha. I know we didn't start off on the right foot. But thank you for coming back in the room and taking the time to explain things to me and my daughter. This second interaction has helped restore my faith in our medical system. Denisha is doing well and is back participating in all of her activities.

Sincerely,
Cindy

QUESTIONS AND ANSWERS

1. Is Cindy's comment about wanting to see a black doctor a microaggression?

As stated previously, microaggressions are commonplace daily verbal, behavioral or environmental slights, whether intentional or unintentional, that communicate hostile, derogatory, or negative attitudes <u>*toward stigmatized or culturally marginalized groups*</u> (Sue, 2007). Therefore, based on this definition, Cindy's comment toward Dr. Johnson, a white male doctor, is not considered a microaggression because a white male physician is not part of a marginalized group. This is not to say that this physician does not belong to any marginalized groups. For example, he may identify with the LGBTQ+ community, which would be considered a marginalized group. However, because the comment was not targeted at that identity, it would still not be considered a microaggression, even if Dr. Johnson identified as gay.

To unpack this a little more we need to discuss what it means to be marginalized. Marginalized groups are those that are excluded from mainstream social, economic, educational, and/or cultural life. Groups may be marginalized based on race, gender identity, sexual identity, age, physical ability, language, mental ability, and/or immigration status. Marginalization occurs because of unequal power relationships between social groups (Baah, 2019). The diagram below (Figure 1) outlines the various identities and their relationship to power and marginalization (adapted from Duckworth, 2020 and Vanderwoerd, 2016). Identities closest to the center hold the most power/privilege and the identities toward the outer edge (or margins) experience the most oppression, and thus, are marginalized.

When the term was initially coined by Harvard Professor, Dr. Chester M. Pierce, a microaggression was referring to experiences around race and race related interactions (Pierce, 1974). However, the definition of microaggression has since expanded to include people from all marginalized groups. When discussing race, this is racism. When gender is targeted, this is sexism. When sexuality is the focus, we are talking about homophobia and transphobia. And when we are talking about physical ability, this is ableism. Any marginalized identity can have an "ism" attached to it. The "isms" are structured around oppression. In order for something to be a microaggression, it must attack one or more of one's oppressed identities. So, to reiterate, when Cindy asks Dr. Johnson for a Black doctor, this is not a microaggression because Dr. Johnson's white identity is not an oppressed (or marginalized) identity.

2. How is Cindy's remark to Dr. Johnson okay, but it is not okay when a white patient says this to a black doctor?

In short, it's not okay. However, the difference is multidimensional. While Cindy's remark is not a microaggression and is not racist (Racism, 2022) based on definitions, it is still prejudiced (Prejudice, 2022). However, whenever we talk about microaggressions we must talk about impact versus intent. Although most microaggressions are delivered without the intent of harming the recipient, they often do. The black doctor is likely the recipient of microaggressions multiple times per day, while this is possibly the first time the white doctor experienced something like this. When we think about this situation, we should consider equity vs equality. When we look at it from an equality lens (defined as: the state of being equal (Equality, 2022)), yes, both situations are equally wrong and are not okay. However, when we look at it from an equity lens, the difference becomes clearer. Equity considers an individual or group's specific circumstances and allocates the resources and opportunities needed to reach an equal outcome (Murphy, 2021). So, when discussing microaggressions and this specific situation, consider inequity, and the often-cited analogy of mosquito bites. Think of a microaggression as a mosquito bite and apply it to this situation. If you were bitten by one mosquito or received a few mosquito bites over time, it's annoying, but generally it's tolerable. However, if you are bitten by multiple mosquito bites over and over again on a daily basis as you are going throughout your day, that can really affect your quality of life and your ability to live on a daily basis. This is what makes Cindy's comment to Dr. Johnson different from a similar comment made toward a black doctor. In summary, although the two situations are different, neither is okay and both should be addressed. And we will talk more about that below.

Figure 1. The wheel of power and privilege. Identities closer to the center hold the most power/privilege in our United States society, with power/privilege decreasing as we move toward the margins. This is why certain vulnerable populations are considered "marginalized." Many more identities could be added to this wheel, it is not all inclusive. The power structures within certain identities, such as sexuality, are more complicated than a linear relationship between hetero- and homo-sexual. However, they are presented in a linear fashion here to facilitate the understanding of power structures.
Adapted from Vanderwoerd (2016) and sylviaduckworth.com

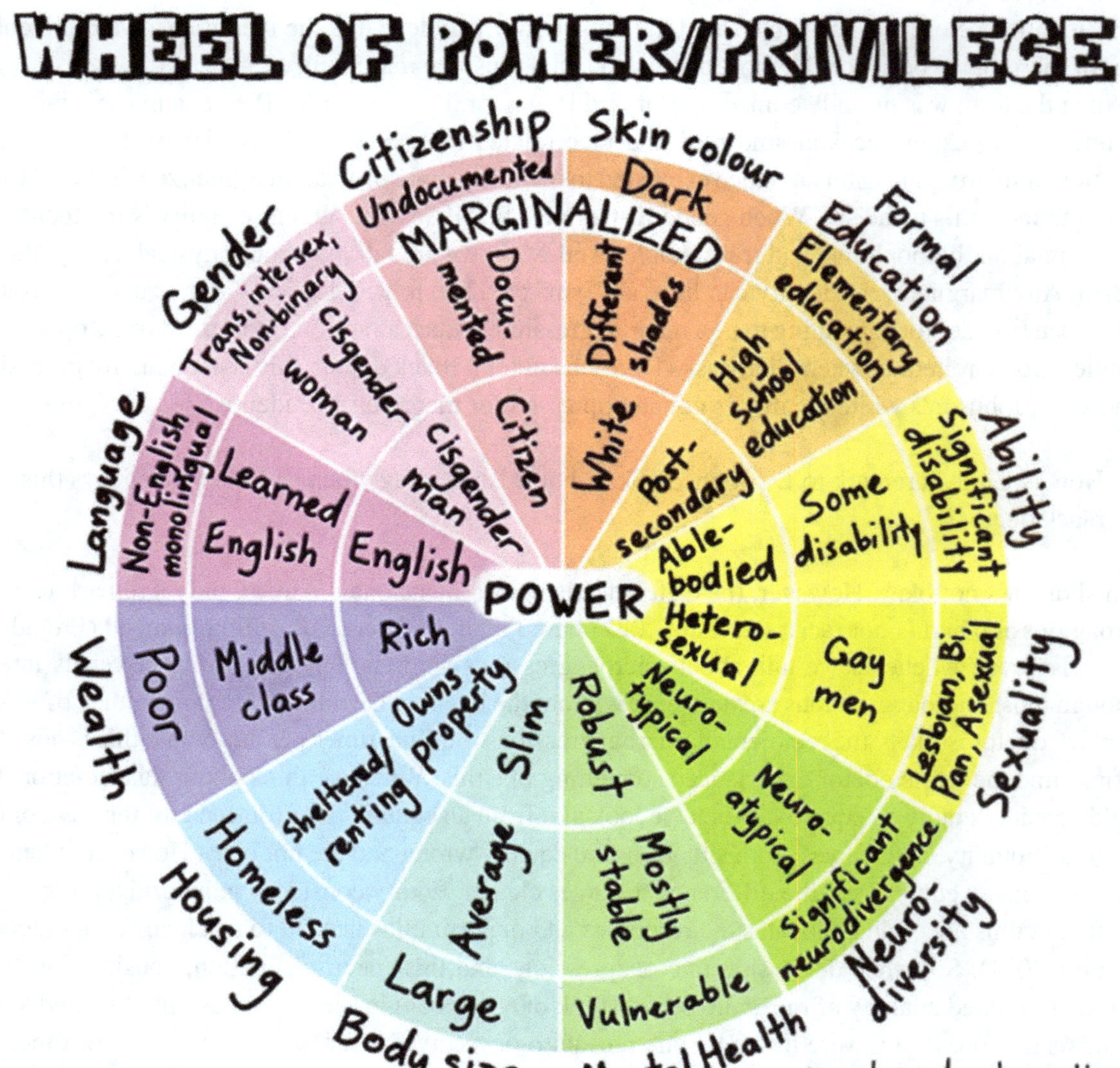

3. As a white health care professional, how do I respond to a black patient asking for a doctor of color?

As a health care professional, we must put our patient's needs before our own, but at the same time we should address these situations so that they do not continue to occur. In this instance, we should recognize the underlying premise of this comment. It is well known that our patients of color have an underlying mistrust of the healthcare system. Although this is often not due to a specific interaction with any one health care professional, it is often manifested as such. Our patients of color often feel that health care professionals, intentional or not, treat minoritized patients differently than White patients. The perception of mistrust from our patients of color is in large part caused by their previous experiences with the health care system or the experiences of others in their community. However, the mistrust is not only in perception but also in reality due to the inherent systemic racism that has permeated our healthcare system for centuries (Kennedy, 2007).

In the book, *So You Wanna Talk About Race,* the author, Ijeoma Oluo, offers readers a way to respond if they've been called a racist in Chapter 16: *I just got called a racist, what do I do now?* While asking for a healthcare professional of color is not explicitly calling someone a racist, the underlying premise is the same. Therefore, a similar approach to the situation would be appropriate. The steps she gives are as follows (Oluo, 2019):

- Listen
- Set your intentions aside
- Try to the hear the impact of what you have done
- Remember that you do not have all the pieces
- Nobody owes you a debate
- Nobody owes you a relationship
- Remember that you are not the only one hurt
- If you can see where you have been racist, or if you can see where your actions have caused harm, apologize, and mean it
- If, after a lot of careful thought, you still do not see your action as racist and feel strongly that this is simply a misunderstanding, do not invalidate that person's hurt

Ultimately, the appropriate thing to do in this situation is to understand why your patient is feeling this way. Remember, many of our marginalized patients do not trust the medical system as is and are already facing tremendous health inequities. The way you react to a statement like this could potentially change the way your patient views healthcare and may even change their life. By taking a moment to understand your patient and why they are asking for a provider of color, you show you care. You have the potential to rebuild trust.

4. How do you think Dr. Johnson's outburst affected Dr. Fleming?

Situations such as these affect not only those directly involved in the interaction, but also those witnessing the interaction and/or response. Dr. Fleming could have stepped in and initiated a conversation with Dr. Johnson, however, she does not have an obligation to do so (Oluo, 2019). Oftentimes, when black health care professionals experience situations such as this in the health care setting their response does not match their internal reaction. While they may experience emotions of anger, embarrassment, and/

or shock, they often use responses that are conflict avoidant to avoid the stereotype of being labeled the "angry black person" or being seen as difficult to work with. This includes ignoring the comments, making jokes about the comment, or even removing themselves from the situation (Alinor, 2022). Although the people witnessing or experiencing the situation may not respond, they are still negatively affected by the interaction and can result in decreased productivity, less effective team interactions (Alinor, 2022), decreased job satisfaction, burnout, suicidality, worse patient care outcomes, and increases in medical errors, as discussed in Case 1 (Molina, 2020). Healthcare professionals should be aware of who is in their surroundings and how their comments may affect those around them.

5. Even though this is not microaggression, can I still apply the "Open the Front Door (OTFD)" framework in this situation?

Yes! There are two places in this case where the OTFD framework could have been applied. First, when Cindy asks for a black doctor. An example response could be:

I heard you say that you would like a black doctor (Observation). I think that comment implies that you feel you would get better care from a black doctor (Think). I am frustrated by this (Feel) because I do feel like I am providing you with the best care possible. I would appreciate if you could explain to me why you would prefer to see a black doctor so I can better understand (Desire).

Additionally, the OTFD framework could have been used by Dr. Fleming to address Dr. Johnson's outburst, but only if she wanted to. An example of this response could be:

I heard you say that you are upset that your patient asked for a black doctor (Observe). I think her comment may be rooted in an underlying mistrust of the healthcare system (Think) and not necessarily aimed at you personally (Think). I feel uncomfortable that you are so upset by this (Feel) and challenge you to seek to understand why your patient feels the need to ask for a black doctor (Desire).

6. What is the difference between Dr. Johnson's first interaction with the Cindy and his second?

Dr. Johnson's first interaction was defensive and volatile. This type of interaction is ineffective and will often escalate the situation. Furthermore, if Dr. Johnson would have left the situation after their initial interaction and sent a different provider into the room, Cindy's mistrust in the health care system would have likely worsened. However, Dr. Johnson's second approach to the situation was much more productive and patient centered. Dr. Johnson sought to understand why Cindy was frustrated with his care. He was able to learn that she felt unheard. He was then able to work with Cindy to (1) understand why Cindy was concerned about her daughter, (2) explain why he does not feel additional testing is necessary, and (3) come up with a plan they both felt comfortable with in caring for Denisha. At the same time, based on the letter Cindy sent to the hospital, Dr. Johnson was able to help Cindy start regaining trust in the healthcare system.

Epilogue

This case helps the learner understand the difference between what is and what is not a microaggression. It reviews key definitions surrounding microaggressions and discrimination and discusses the history behind why our marginalized populations mistrust and distrust the healthcare system. Most importantly, it provides healthcare professionals a framework to respond to patient comments and outward expressions of mistrust and feelings of discrimination in a non-accusatory manner in which the healthcare professional is seeking to understand the patient. Microaggressions, discrimination, and lack of trust are key drivers in health inequities. By appropriately recognizing and addressing these situations in the moment, healthcare professionals have the ability to rebuild trust and begin to eliminate health disparities. However, this is not easy work, and these concepts must be embedded throughout the healthcare professional educational curriculum.

CONCLUSION

Microaggressions are commonly encountered in the clinical learning environment and have negative impacts on patients and health care workers. This chapter provided information on how to recognize and address microaggression in the clinical environment and can be used by health professions educators to teach these concepts. Learning to recognize and address microaggressions in the clinical learning environment is an important step to eliminating health inequities.

REFERENCES

Ackerman-Barger, K., & Jacobs, N. N. (2020). The Microaggressions Triangle Model: A Humanistic Approach to Navigating Microaggressions in Health Professions Schools. *Academic Medicine*, *95*(12S), S28–S32. doi:10.1097/ACM.0000000000003692 PMID:32889926

Alinor, M. (2022). Research: The Real-Time Impact of Microaggressions. *Harvard Business Review*. Retrieved from https://hbr.org/2022/05/research-the-real-time-impact-of-microaggressions

Baah, F. O., Teitelman, A. M., & Riegel, B. (2019). Marginalization: Conceptualizing patient vulnerabilities in the framework of social determinants of health—An integrative review. *Nursing Inquiry*, *26*(1), e12268. doi:10.1111/nin.12268 PMID:30488635

Casey, L. S., Reisner, S. L., Findling, M. G., Blendon, R. J., Benson, J. M., Sayde, J. M., & Miller, C. (2019). Discrimination in the United States: Experiences of lesbian, gay, bisexual, transgender, and queer Americans. *Health Services Research*, *54*(S2), 1454–1466. doi:10.1111/1475-6773.13229 PMID:31659745

Ehie, O., Muse, I., Hill, L., & Bastien, A. (2021). Professionalism: Microaggression in the healthcare setting. *Current Opinion in Anaesthesiology*, *34*(2), 131–136. doi:10.1097/ACO.0000000000000966 PMID:33630771

Encyclopaedia Britannica. (n.d.). Macroeconomics. In *The Britannica Dictionary*. https://www.britannica.com/dictionary/macroeconomics

Equality. (2022). In T. Grant (Ed.), *The Britannica Dictionary*. Retrieved from https://www.britannica.com/dictionary/equality

Hu, Y. Y., Ellis, R. J., Hewitt, D. B., Yang, A. D., Cheung, E. O., Moskowitz, J. T., & Bilimoria, K. Y. (2019). Discrimination, abuse, harassment, and burnout in surgical residency training. *The New England Journal of Medicine*, *381*(18), 1741–1752. doi:10.1056/NEJMsa1903759 PMID:31657887

Kennedy, B. R., Mathis, C. C., & Woods, A. K. (2007). African Americans and their distrust of the health care system: Healthcare for diverse populations. *Journal of Cultural Diversity*, *14*(2), 56–60. PMID:19175244

Molina, M. F., Landry, A. I., Chary, A. N., & Burnett-Bowie, S. M. (2020). Addressing the Elephant in the Room: Microaggressions in Medicine. *Annals of Emergency Medicine*, *76*(4), 387–391. doi:10.1016/j.annemergmed.2020.04.009 PMID:32456801

Murphy, C. (2021). *Equity vs. Equality: Here's the difference*. Health. Retrieved from https://www.health.com/mind-body/health-diversity-inclusion/equity-vs-equality

Nadal, K. L., Wong, Y., Griffin, K. E., Davidoff, K., & Sriken, J. (2014). The Adverse Impact of Racial Microaggressions on College Students' Self-Esteem. *Journal of College Student Development*, *55*(5), 461–474. doi:10.1353/csd.2014.0051

O'Keefe, V. M., Wingate, L. R., Cole, A. B., Hollingsworth, D. W., & Tucker, R. P. (2015). Seemingly Harmless Racial Communications Are Not So Harmless: Racial Microaggressions Lead to Suicidal Ideation by Way of Depression Symptoms. *Suicide & Life-Threatening Behavior*, *45*(5), 567–576. doi:10.1111ltb.12150 PMID:25556819

Oluo, I. (2019). So you want to talk about race. Academic Press.

Pascoe, E. A., & Smart Richman, L. (2009). Perceived discrimination and health: A meta-analytic review. *Psychological Bulletin*, *135*(4), 531–554. doi:10.1037/a0016059 PMID:19586161

Pierce, C. (1974). *Psychiatric problems of the black minority. Vol. American Handbook of Psychiatry*. Basic Books.

Prejudice. (2022). In T. Grant (Ed.), *The Britannica Dictionary*. Retrieved from https://www.britannica.com/dictionary/prejudice

Racism. (2022). In T. Grant (Ed.), *The Britannica Dictionary*. Retrieved from https://www.britannica.com/dictionary/racism

Sagalowsky, S. T., Woodward, H., Evins, J., & Kessler, D. O. (2021). Responding to Microaggressions: Further Frameworks From Simulation Debriefing. *Annals of Emergency Medicine*, *77*(3), 381–382. doi:10.1016/j.annemergmed.2020.10.006 PMID:33618815

Snyder, C. R., Wang, P. Z., & Truitt, A. R. (2018). Multiracial Patient Experiences With Racial Microaggressions in Health Care Settings. *Journal of Patient-Centered Research and Reviews*, *5*(3), 229–238. doi:10.17294/2330-0698.1626 PMID:31414007

Sotto-Santiago, S., Mac, J., Duncan, F., & Smith, J. (2020). "I Didn't Know What to Say": Responding to Racism, Discrimination, and Microaggressions With the OWTFD Approach. *MedEdPORTAL: the Journal of Teaching and Learning Resources*, *16*, 10971. doi:10.15766/mep_2374-8265.10971 PMID:32754635

Souza, T. J. (2016). *Managing Hot Moments in the Classroom: Concrete Strategies for Cooling Down Tension. Faculty Focus Special Report: Diversity and Inclusion in the College Classroom*. Magna Publication.

Souza, T. J. (2018). *Responding to Microaggressions in the Classroom: Taking Action*. Magna Publication. https://www.facultyfocus.com/articles/effective-classroom-management/responding-to-microaggressions-in-the-classroom/

Sue, D. W., Alsaidi, S., Awad, M. N., Glaeser, E., Calle, C. Z., & Mendez, N. (2019). Disarming racial microaggressions: Microintervention strategies for targets, White allies, and bystanders. *The American Psychologist*, *74*(1), 128–142. doi:10.1037/amp0000296 PMID:30652905

Sue, D. W., Capodilupo, C. M., Torino, G. C., Bucceri, J. M., Holder, A. M., Nadal, K. L., & Esquilin, M. (2007). Racial microaggressions in everyday life: Implications for clinical practice. *The American Psychologist*, *62*(4), 271–286. doi:10.1037/0003-066X.62.4.271 PMID:17516773

Vanderwoerd, J. R. (2016). The promise and perils of anti-oppressive practice for Christians in social work education. *Social Work & Christianity*, *43*(2), 153–188.

Warner, N. S., Njathi-Ori, C. W., & O'Brien, E. K. (2020). The GRIT (Gather, Restate, Inquire, Talk It Out) Framework for Addressing Microaggressions. *JAMA Surgery*, *155*(2), 178–179. doi:10.1001/jamasurg.2019.4427 PMID:31774484

Chapter 13
Making Room for Religion in Health Education:
Institutional Discrimination and Dismantling the Framework

Sherrica Taylor
Nova Southeastern University Dr. Kiran C. Patel College of Osteopathic Medicine, USA

Christina Brown-Wujick
Nova Southeastern University Dr. Kiran C. Patel College of Osteopathic Medicine, USA

EXECUTIVE SUMMARY

A light review of historical practices can provide what some may consider a superficial evolution of higher education and its practices. Specifically, in the field of health professions, a shift that is easily identifiable is the move from black and white photos of white male physicians in coats and nurses in starched white dresses to a more diversified student body adorned with white coats. However, are the current systems in place supportive of the individual needs and beliefs of these students or are students inadvertently being required to alter who they are to fit into systems not supportive of their individuality, especially as it relates to their religious beliefs? How do we undo the practices of a one-size-fits-all approach to educating students and move towards a goal of inclusivity for all faiths by providing students educational environments and curriculums purposefully designed to support students of different religions?

BACKGROUND

Approximately seventy percent of those with postgraduate degrees identify religion as being at least somewhat important in their lives (Religious Landscape Study, 2022). In this same population, only twenty percent of them can attest to participating in religious practices such as prayer and religious studies recently (Religious Landscape Study, 2022). With statistics such as these, it leads one to question if a lack of participation in religious activities by health professionals can be a direct result of learned behaviors obtained during intense periods of educational attainment and if potentially the percentage

DOI: 10.4018/978-1-6684-5493-0.ch013

of importance decreased due to an inability to merge one's beliefs into their educational process. In one study, a medical student reported "*I feel like we lose that sort of internal "This is who I am*." A sentiment that medical students and faculty both experience as it relates to religion, spirituality, and its intersection with the medical school curriculum (Balboni, et al., 2015). Balboni et al. (2015) note that the spiritual principles upheld by many religions are consistent with the values that are ideal in many professions. Yet the spaces and opportunities to operate within one's religious beliefs are not made evident as recommended by Patel et al. (2015). In fact, policies and practices that reinforce institutional discrimination and create barriers to those from specific faith backgrounds to practice their beliefs often take the form of recommendations related to professionalism, curricular requirements, and patient safety (Ruzycki et al, 2022). In health professions education, much of what is taught directly or indirectly, is eventually applied in clinical practice. As such, the knowledge, skills and ability acquired in the classroom often influence the quality of the skills and care afforded to patients in the long-term. Allowing students the opportunity to infuse their faith backgrounds with proper patient care in the learning environment can lead to higher quality, and more holistic patient care in the future.

It has been demonstrated that spirituality and religion are important coping mechanisms in patients experiences with illness and death, and national standards related to hospice and palliative care explicitly require training for medical professionals in this area (National Consensus Project, 2009). However, there are often times formal and informal barriers that inhibit students in the health professions from learning how to integrate their religious beliefs into their professional identities. In clinical practice, most patients report that many healthcare professionals fail to discuss their religious beliefs with them even when there is acknowledgment that it might be helpful for the patient and/or their families. It has been found that inadequate training in the formal curriculum, and lack of thorough cultural competence education provided by clinical sites and/or as part of continuing education requirements, is the most common reason for this (Balboni et al, 2014). If it is understood that students entering into health professional programs come from diverse backgrounds and have unique expectations as it relates to the incorporation of their religious beliefs into their clinical identities and patient care (Devi et. al, 2016), then it is imperative that we create spaces that support these populations and their religious beliefs on a personal and academic level through curricular integration and policies supportive of students from diverse faiths.

Religious beliefs can have a positive impact on academics and professional acclimation throughout a students career. A greater sense of responsibility and empathy felt towards patients was reported from students who had strong religious beliefs (Sarcahmi et al, 2020). This means that students who have experienced the rigors of a health professions program and were able to maintain their beliefs, are more equipped to speak firsthand on the ability to use one's beliefs to get them through challenging periods. This can transition to the provider/patient relationship by making the provider more relatable and, in some instances, more trustworthy. Even learners who do not exercise personal beliefs, can benefit from exposure to others who do and environments who welcome them to do so. These learners, by experience and exposure, are more equipped to offer holistic care moving forward. A worthy goal is to implement a curriculum that creates an awareness of all belief systems and how to properly interact with them in healthcare environments. As noted by Puchalski and Larson (1998), a learner taught in their education to address and respect the spiritual and physical concerns of patients will be better equipped to offer compassionate care and foster healthy rapport with future patients.

The goals of this chapter are to explore how and where students' religious identities can be better recognized and included in the formal and informal curriculum; and how cultural competence training related to religion can positively influence student success and patient health outcomes. The first case-study focuses on barriers that influence proper patient care and student instruction. The second explores ways in which the systems created to educate our health professional students can make room for religious identities from the time that students are accepted until they graduate. These cases are used to outline best practices to dismantle the framework of systems that uphold narrow-minded or oppressive practices that disadvantage those from minority religious backgrounds, and encourage discussions that promote more inclusive learning environments for future and practicing health professionals.

CASE 1: FAITH MANDATED PROVIDER GENDER REQUIREMENT

Goal

This case portrays barriers to culturally competent care, as well as microaggressions, experienced by a student during a clinical training experience.

Learning Outcomes

1. Identify religion-related barriers to health care experienced by the patient.
2. Identify microaggressions experienced by the Muslim medical student during clinical rotation.
3. Describe best practices for religious inclusivity in healthcare education.
4. Discuss best practices for cultural competence education that allows room within the curricula to adequately review topics such as religion for faculty and students.

Case

Mrs. A is a 55-year-old female Muslim patient who was recently diagnosed with diabetes. She presents to the clinic due to intermittent tingling and numbness in her left foot over the last two months, and the formation of an ulcer over the last two weeks that started to emit a discharge. She is greeted at the clinic by an administrative assistant who informs her that the wait should be very short today. Within five minutes she is then escorted to an examination room by a female medical assistant, Ms. C, and is asked to wait for the physician who will be in shortly.

After 10 minutes, Mrs. A is greeted by a male physician who walks in without knocking and states, "My name is Dr. I and I am here with my medical student who is shadowing me today. He will introduce himself, take your vital signs and history for me."

Male Student Doctor S immediately realizes that his patient, Mrs. A is a Muslim and that this might introduce some challenges to the provision of her care. He greets Mrs. A by saying, "Hello, I am Student Doctor S, I apologize for not knocking before we entered. As Dr. I stated, I am a student doctor who is here to learn and hope to do that by assisting Dr. I with your care today if you are comfortable with that?"

Mrs. A thinks for a minute and then says, "I have no problem with you introducing yourself, but as you can see, I am a Muslim woman and do have a gender preference for my providers. I would prefer to be seen by females for my care if possible."

Dr. I then lets out a big sigh and says to Mrs. A, "Student Doctor S is obviously a Muslim as well. You can see that, right? Can he assist me since he is Muslim and should understand your religious customs?"

Mrs. A then interjects "Actually he is male, so I am not allowed to have him touch my foot. My provider should really be a female."

Dr. I sighs again, and says, "Okay. I will have our medical assistant Ms. C come in and take your history while we see if we have anyone else on staff to assist you." He then leaves the room with Student Doctor S and asks, seemingly annoyed, "You guys cannot provide care to each other? You are both Muslim for goodness sake. I thought that is why we recruited for diversity in admissions, so we do not have to deal with this all of the time! How many of you do we need to let in!" Then he calls Ms. C and asks her to go take Mrs. A's history and vitals. Dr. I walks to the nurse's station to see if there are any female physicians or medical students on shift. The desk assistant stated that a female physician would not be in for another thirty minutes, but that there was another female medical student just finishing with another doctor. Dr. I requests that she come with him once Ms. C is finished with the patient. Student Doctor S looks down at his iPad with the patient's chart on it, obviously uncomfortable with the exchange.

Ms. C knocks on the exam room door and Mrs. A asks her to enter and is very friendly and grateful for the knock. Ms. C introduces herself and asks the patient to explain her history and what brought her in. Mrs. A shares that "she was diagnosed with non-insulin-dependent diabetes (NIDDM) about 5 years ago. She had previously been on insulin but had stopped about 6 months ago. She noticed the progression of symptoms from her foot had been escalating and she shared that she recently had not been monitoring her blood sugar very well. She also mentions that she just concluded her participation in Ramadan fasting, so she suspected that might be a contributing factor with her foot. She noted that she does not drink or smoke, but that she does not always eat well. Ms. C thanks Mrs. A for sharing this information with her and tells her that the doctor will be back shortly and excuses herself from the examination room.

Ms. C then waives at Dr. I, male Student Doctor S, and female Student Doctor T who had recently joined them and walks over to briefly present the patient's history and chief complaints. After this, Dr. I thank Ms. C. for the information and asks her to stay for a moment. He then motions for everyone to head towards the examination room. On the way, Dr. I informs Student Doctor T, "this patient is a Muslim so you'll be doing the physical exam since we can't touch her." Student Doctor T asks, "why is that again?" Student Doctor S then takes it upon himself to inform her that, "it is a customary practice in the Muslim religion for patients to ask for providers of the same gender due to beliefs related to modesty and physical touch." Then, Student Doctor T takes it upon himself to also explain that "it is considered polite to knock and introduce yourself before entering an exam room, and it is also very normal for patients to request that you maintain their modesty when examining them."

As they walk towards the room, Student Doctor S takes the lead and knocks before entering the examination room. He explains the purpose of the visit and introduces the team from the door before entering to follow-up on Mrs. A's care. Mrs. A says, "please come in."

Dr. I begins by telling Mrs. A that there are no female physicians currently available for the next 30 minutes. However, Student Doctor T is happy to perform the physical exam. Mrs. A agrees saying, "as long as it is done as modestly as possible. Also, I would very much like for the female physician to see me once she becomes available." Dr. I says that this will not be a problem and then excuses himself and Student Doctor S from the examination room. Student Doctor T and Ms. C remain. Student Doctor T introduces herself and proceeds with the physical exam, carefully explaining what she would be examining and for what purpose as she went along. After she concludes, she informs Mrs. A that she would return to discuss the physical exam with Dr. I as she is only a Student Doctor and cannot provide her with the next steps in her care based on her current training level. Mrs. A indicates that she understands and very much appreciates both Student Doctor T and Ms. C for accommodating her requests.

Student Doctor T then leaves the room with the medical assistant, Ms. C. As they are exiting, they approach Doctor I and Student Doctor T. Dr. I is hurriedly addressing a female physician, Dr. E, who has arrived early for her shift. As they approach, they hear Dr. I inform Dr. E that "the patient in examination room 12 has requested a female physician. It's a diabetic foot issue. Student Doctor T just concluded the physical exam with Ms. C and will present the case to you to catch you up. I will let Student Doctor T stay with you as well as he is also Muslim, as you can see. Might be helpful."

Dr. I then walks away and Dr. E processes what has just been told to her and sees the questioning looks from her Student Doctors. She then asks them, "so, I assume that did not go so well with Dr. I based upon your looks and what I just heard?" Student Doctor S responds, "the whole thing made me feel extremely uncomfortable. I would prefer not to work with Dr. I again as well, to be honest."

QUESTIONS AND ANSWERS

1. How did Dr. I fail to provide an inclusive learning environment for students of non-dominant religious backgrounds?

In the learning environment that Dr. I facilitated, he failed to foster a clinical learning experience that showed inclusivity to patients and students of diverse faiths. By failing to do so, he demonstrated that he was either unfamiliar with, or had forgotten, any formal training on cultural competence related to world religions and how the customs of some might impact potential interactions within the healthcare environment. Cultural competence here is defined as "a set of consistent behaviors, attitudes and policies that enable a system, agency or individual to work within a cross-cultural context or situation effectively" (Watt et.al, 2016). If Dr. I had been better trained; he would likely have been able to anticipate customary requirements of religious patients such as a preference for female providers and maintenance of modesty during the physical exam as shown in the example case. It is unclear if Dr. I was trained to consider religious differences in medical school, or from the site where he was employed. However, by failing to model inclusive care to a religious minority, he failed to serve as a role model and educator on the importance of this for those students under his direction, and in doing so failed to uphold common professionalism standards related to cultural competence education required by many accrediting agencies such as the Liaison Committee on Medical Education and the Commission on Osteopathic College Accreditation.

Although an extreme example, it is not necessarily uncommon for preceptors. This is problematic because across health professions there is a focus on reducing the pervasiveness of health disparities that patients from diverse backgrounds encounter, and this has become a focal point in the curricula that faculty and students are aware of and engaged in improving nationally. Furthermore, accrediting bodies for health professional schools such as the Liaison Committee on Medical Education (2003) and the Commission on Osteopathic College Accreditation (2019), amongst others, have made cultural competence in the formal curriculum and in faculty training a requirement that must be met as a part of accreditation standards. As such, colleges and schools must be actively engaged in finding novel and innovative methods to help ensure that faculty and students are well-trained in cultural competence, including the provision of inclusive care for patients of diverse religious backgrounds.

2. How could the student trainees' home institution better ensure a more culturally competent clinical learning experience that models inclusivity to patients of diverse faiths?

A recommendation that would address this issue would be to have colleges ensure that all faculty that teach students clinical skills are required to undergo annual comprehensive cultural competence training. This training should be provided by the students' home institution. It is not uncommon for clinical supervisors to report that they do not feel equipped to evaluate and train on this topic, and as such there is a need for more training of clinical faculty so that they can better approach these issues in their patient care and teaching (Berger et al, 2014). When this training is provided by the college, it allows for more purposeful design to ensure that topics that are commonly lightly reviewed, such as religion, receive adequate attention. This also ensures that what is taught is aligned with institutions' policies, procedures and instructions. These trainings should be annually evaluated to ensure that the four major tenets of cultural competence education: awareness, attitudes, knowledge, and skills (LCME, 2003) are adequately covered and related to how race, ethnicity, religion, gender identity, sexual preference, socioeconomic status, political and geographic factors, and others are interrelated and impact patient populations and interprofessional interactions within the healthcare environment.

To help ensure that these topics are comprehensively addressed, and ensure that the teaching methods used are engaging, it is important to incorporate clinically relevant case studies and regularly required assessments to ensure faculty are actively learning the topics being covered. Ideally, this training will also model what is being taught to the students in their preclinical years so that those serving as clinical educators can better identify gaps in knowledge in the clinical environment and find opportunities for expanding upon them when opportunities arise. Puchalski and Larson (1998) note that many patients want to be able to engage in spiritual conversations with their physicians, which means that a level of cultural competence and awareness related to the world's religions must be present. To do this successfully, it is imperative that students receive adequate training from these faculty during their clinical years.

Anderson & Vanderbilt (2018) recommended that adopting a train-the-trainer model of cultural competence education in which the same pre-clinical faculty that teach student physicians these skills also be employed to train the faculty teaching them in their clinical years. This would help to better ensure that there are fewer gaps between students' cultural competence training and behaviors in clinical practice.

3. In this case, how did Dr. I's comments create a hostile learning environment for the Muslim student shadowing him for his clinical rotation?

Dr. I's comments showed a lack of understanding of Islamic culture and how it influences patients' expectations related to healthcare delivery. In doing so and by commenting on it, he also created an uncomfortable learning environment for his Muslim student on his rotation. Specifically, his multiple audible sighs and comments such as "Student Doctor S is obviously a Muslim as well. You can see that, right?" when speaking to the patient could be interpreted as a belief by Dr. I that the students' manner of dress and/or facial hair implies a specific religious denomination that stands out from the norms within the field. This could make the student question whether his religion and its customs are truly accepted in the occupation he is studying. Similarly, when Dr. I leaves the room and says, "You guys cannot provide care to each other? You are both Muslim for goodness sake. I thought that is why we recruited for diversity in admissions...How many of you do we need to let in!" his comments can be interpreted by students to show both frustration with the rules of a non-dominant religion practiced by Student Doctor

S, as well as frustration related to the acceptance of students from non-dominant religious backgrounds into the occupation as a whole. Dr. I's comments about the incorporation of diversity in the admissions process made the learning environment extremely uncomfortable for the Muslim student under his tutelage. By not being familiar with basic customs he forced Student Doctor S to serve as a cultural bridge between the dominant religious culture of his faculty instructor and fellow student to the Muslim patient. In so doing, it did not only interfere with Student Doctor S's ability to focus on his clinical learning, but it also was insulting when he was forced to endure comments that could be viewed as disrespectful of his religious customs, and which would have been better left unsaid. These types of actions and the institutional ineffectiveness of whatever cultural competence training related to religion that Dr. I and Student Doctor T had been exposed to, demonstrates a disregard for the positive role that religion, and religious customs, can play in both patient and student trainees' personal wellness and ability to cope with the mental strain of illness and death (Posner, Ali, and Douglas, 2019).

Dr. I's comments about religious diversity in the admissions process were a blatant microaggression. First coined in the 1970's by Dr. Chester Pierce, microaggressions are meant to give a name to the "commonplace behavioral indignities, whether intentional or unintentional, communicating hostile, derogatory or negative attitudes towards marginalized groups," which can be found historically throughout man's existence (Ehie et al, 2021; Pierce, 1974). This microaggression is one that Student Doctor S could reasonably interpret to mean that Dr. I believed that religious diversity was encouraged in the admissions process only to facilitate the ease of dealing with patients from diverse faith backgrounds for those from mainstream belief systems, like himself. This assumption could further be interpreted to mean that Dr. I believed that students from these faiths might not otherwise be qualified for admission if that assistance was not needed, which creates a hostile environment. As many students already struggle with imposter syndrome, defined as the inability of one to view their position and accomplishments as having been earned based upon effort, skills or merit, and finding a way to integrate their faith backgrounds into their new professional identities as professional students, this type of comment could have long-term detrimental effects on the professional identity formation of Student Doctor S (Balboni et al., 2015). Better and regular training on how and why diverse student populations are important for faculty will continue to be a need as it is vital in combatting the potential for such negative experiences occurring with future students. These faculty should be made aware that the Institute of Medicine (2020), amongst others, has endorsed the importance of recruiting more physicians from underrepresented communities in order to help reduce disparities patients face within medicine.

4. How could Dr. I's behaviors have influenced his Muslim patient?

Dr. I's comments do not just constitute a microaggression to the student on his service, but it also was a microaggression that could have both immediate and long-term impacts upon the patient for whom he was responsible. Ethie et al. (2021) note that microaggressions cannot just "influence one's access to power, resources, and opportunity, but...also contribute to the persistent disparities faced by marginalized groups among healthcare professionals as well as patients (p. 131)." In the case above, Dr. I's comments have the ability to potentially lead to negative effects related to clinical diagnosis and the provision of care for Mrs. A. When studying the effects of microaggressions in healthcare, Pascoe and Richman (2009) found that perceived discrimination is a significant predictor of disparities in hypertension, cardiovascular diseases, diabetes, and respiratory conditions. This could be because in the short-term, when patients like Mrs. A. face discrimination in healthcare settings, they are unlikely to be as candid about physical symptoms that could be relevant, as well as about mental, behavioral, and environmental factors that can be important in the diagnostic process. Long-term, when patients encounter providers who are discriminatory, they are less likely to follow-treatment plans and attend follow-up appointments. As such, Dr. I's behaviors could have both short and long-term negative impacts on Mrs. A's overall health and perceptions of what one should expect when interacting in the healthcare environment, due to the potential for prolonged issues related to provider mistrust.

5. In what ways could the students have been better supported by their home institution and clinical rotation site in their cultural competence training as it relates to religion?

One way in which greater support could have been provided to the student trainees is by offering training on the provision of culturally competent healthcare prior to entering a clinic setting with real patients. This training could have been offered by their home school, or clinical rotation site. In this case, Student Doctor T was unfamiliar with the common expectations of patients from different faith backgrounds. Student Doctor S felt that he had to explain these cultural practices to her as both she and the attending physician were unfamiliar with common requests from patients within the Muslim community given their responses. Placing students in a position where they feel compelled to serve as a spokesperson for their culture or religion places a potential barrier on the quality of training and education they receive, due to it splitting their attention between this task and their clinical learning, and as such it can create a level of mistrust between the clinical faculty member and trainee. This is especially true if the actions and attitudes as displayed by Dr. I demonstrate purposeful ignorance and/or an unwillingness to learn.

Many healthcare educational institutions have short, required lessons on cultural sensitivity in the provision of care as part of their standard curricula as it is an accreditation requirement. However, when overlapped with more rigorous coursework, students who are stressed and overwhelmed are at risk of not retaining these lessons. Especially if they are not recurring throughout the curriculum. A quick resolution to this would be a cultural competence thread implemented from day one until graduation. In so doing, programs can expand upon the original training in various components of cultural competence across the curriculum by integrating these lessons into evaluatory exercises assessing clinical acumen and foundational science knowledge. Programs can utilize their standardized patients by ensuring they represent patients of diverse faith backgrounds when students are initially trained on how to interact in the clinical environment. Another method for integrating this knowledge into practical applications would be to purposefully design clinical vignettes used for testing that incorporate variables related to different religious customs that can impact what tests are recommended or treatment options are available in the provision of care. By putting students' training and knowledge about patients of diverse faith backgrounds into practice, students' ability to retain and apply it in future clinical scenarios will be greatly enhanced. This will allow these future providers to better serve diverse patient populations as well as allow students of diverse faith traditions the opportunity to not feel forced to serve as a cultural bridge for those from the religious majority by providing higher quality training to all.

These types of educational approaches should then undergo regular evaluation, as longitudinal studies of these interventions will be crucial in the establishment of more rigorous best practices over time (Brottman, et al., 2020). There is also debate about the role of integrating a religion and spirituality class into either the formal or informal curriculum as it would be a way to address religious competency more purposefully in clinical settings (Mitchell et al., 2016).

Epilogue

In the "Gender Preference" case noted above, the negative impacts of healthcare professionals not receiving adequate cultural competence and inclusivity training as it relates to religion in healthcare are demonstrated when both the Muslim patient and medical student trainee must explain religious norms to those from the dominant culture. Experiences like these can lead to patients from religious minorities delaying initial and follow-up care. Also, during these encounters, students from religious minorities might not feel accepted within their professional environments and might find that successful integration of religious beliefs and customs into their new professional identities is a challenging part of their professional acculturation process. This can be detrimental to the student trainee as spirituality has been linked to a better ability to handle the stress inherent in the health professions. Health professions educators must be willing to look at the formal and informal curriculum of their programs and identify areas in which students from religious backgrounds might encounter barriers to both their education, and feelings of inclusion within their professional communities, in order to purposefully and meaningfully target areas in which improvement is needed. Furthermore, integration of such new programming must be added into the annual curricular review process. It is imperative that schools engage in this continuous review in order to keep up with necessary improvements that will be needed over time as students' needs related to their faith backgrounds change in step with cultural evolution and how that influences individuals' religious beliefs and experiences in their training.

CASE 2: ADMITTED & EXCLUDED

Goal

This case depicts the unintended institutional challenges that limit a student's ability to acclimate into a health professions program without losing their spiritual identity on the road to becoming who they want to be.

Learning Outcomes

1. Outline ways in which the onboarding process can be enhanced for those from diverse religious backgrounds prior to beginning a health professions program.
2. Identify challenges that are faced by students from various religious backgrounds.
3. Identify means for providing religious accommodations to students.
4. Determine types of policies that should be implemented to support students of various religious backgrounds.
5. Outline ways in which common barriers to inclusivity can be dismantled within one's organization.

Case

Q is a 24-year-old first-generation health professions student. Upon being accepted to her professional program, she joined various web-based groups to prepare her for what to expect. While these groups did provide some insight as to what to expect from her institution, she was curious as to how this institution would specifically address her religious needs. Although she believed that many of her questions would be addressed during orientation, Q decided to be proactive and did research focused on concerns that directly impact her. Q comes from a very religious family and believes that her beliefs are the cornerstone of who she is. She has faced many challenging periods in her life, both personally and academically, and can attest that it is her faith that has brought her to this point. Outside of her amazing work ethic and dedication to her community, she believes that it was always a higher being that provided her with the tools to succeed.

Q began to look for evidence in the student handbook and on the school website for policies focused on religious support and accommodations offered by the institution. When her research fell short, she decided to reach out to the institution. Not finding much guidance online as to who to contact at the school, she reaches out to Student Affairs. Immediately upon realizing that the student has yet to matriculate, the Student Affairs office forwards her to the admissions department to address her concerns. Ms. L in admissions congratulates Q on her acceptance and confirms that she has satisfied all of the requirements to begin school. Identifying no issues preventing Q from beginning her program she asks the reason for the call. "Thank you for taking my call, Ms. L, I have been reviewing the student handbook and the school website and I am curious about accommodations offered to students of various religious backgrounds."

A bit stumped, "What kind of accommodations are you looking for sweetie," responds Ms. L.

"In my religion, there are observances that I would like to take part in that might require me to miss class or exams at various times throughout the year. In the past, I have been able to work with my instructors so that I do not miss any work assigned to me."

Ms. L. responds, "Well I imagine here would be the same. You would need to work with your professors to figure out the specifics. I know we offer accommodations… but the specifics would be handled in Student Affairs."

Q begins to ask a number of other questions related to orientation, faculty support, and student organizations. Each time she was met with the same response, "I am not sure" or "Student Affairs." Realizing that her questions would not likely be addressed until orientation, Q leaves the call underwhelmed and slightly questioning her fit within the profession.

A month later Q decides to move forward, relocates to begin college, and participates in orientation. While everyone is pleasant, she realizes that the outline of orientation is set to welcome students, orient them to the college, and set the tone of what to expect in the program. After days of orienting, Q is still left with many questions and finally heads to Student Affairs for a one-on-one meeting. As a result of her meeting, she finds that there is a strict adherence to uniform requirements, students are limited in the number of days they are allowed to be absent, and the support offered to students were the same across the board promoting equality but not necessarily equity. A little defeated, yet still determined, Q begins her program.

During the course of her program, Q becomes acquainted with other students of various religious backgrounds. Many students share the same concerns regarding their inability to observe their religious holidays, adhere to cultural/religious attire requirements, and a lack of spaces dedicated for prayer throughout the day. During a town hall meeting, several students begin to speak out regarding the issues they believe are impacting their academic and personal success. Q decides to speak up for herself and her colleagues citing the benefits of not only supporting the religious practices of the students, but the need to implement them within the curriculum. Immediately after her statements, leadership within the college mentions the need to maintain policy in an effort to graduate professionals able to excel in their fields, thereby continuing to support the policies and procedures currently in place.

A bit distraught, Q begins to formulate a petition and virtually distributes it to her peers. Inside this petition, Q mentions that she believes that the school is bringing in individuals from diverse backgrounds but is not allowing them to learn in an accommodating environment and is thus producing conformed beings lacking in cultural competence and empathy. She concludes her letter by stating, "How can I learn to respect my patients and interprofessional colleagues' religious beliefs and needs in the clinical environment, and how they might be similar or different than my own, if I am not provided an educational environment that respects the religious diversity of its students enough to incorporate their needs into the systems built to educate us?

QUESTIONS AND ANSWERS

1. What steps can be done to enhance the onboarding process of students from various religions?

It is noted that a properly structured onboarding program can provide networking opportunities for students and is effective in enhancing the learning and retention within one's program (Pajarillo & Korn, 2021). Ellaway et al. (2014) points out that many orientations held for medical students are similar in that they offer ceremonies marking the development of students' professional identities as physicians. In this case, Q found it challenging to obtain direct answers to her religious concerns. Prior to entering the institution, her questions were answered haphazardly, and they were still not addressed during her orientation. During onboarding, Q may have received tips and "best practices" meant to help students in her program. However, this session may have missed a crucial opportunity to show or explain how the school was willing to make room for her faith. Even if what Q was looking for did not exist, acknowledging that the current offerings are not extensive and explaining the willingness of the administration to support new initiatives can aid in creating a welcoming and safe environment. A statement with inclusive language is invaluable as it shows a willingness to acclimate to the needs of students and can take less than a minute to vocalize. Onboarding processes are ripe with the opportunity to facilitate a greater understanding and awareness of religious differences and in some instances a greater understanding or appreciation of one's own beliefs. While there are many topics of necessity that should be covered during these sessions, and time constraints are always a concern, there is always an opportunity to be proactive and broach spirituality and religion in order to create a more inclusive setting.

It is important to create an onboarding process that identifies and understands that a student entering a health professions program is more than an incoming student and future professional, but one who has an identity that precedes admissions into an institution. A few things that could be done to enhance the onboarding process are 1) the administration of a matriculating student questionnaire similar to that offered through AAMC (AAMC, 2022). Outside of identifying experience and career interests, these questionnaires can be designed to identify the demographics of the incoming class. Information garnered from such a questionnaire can then be used to tailor onboarding practices to make sure that the needs and concerns related to the religion of incoming students are being met and can be used to begin the process of preparing for concerns that may arise based upon the religious identities identified. 2) While many orientations/onboarding processes have a focus on providing knowledge of the professional campus, policies, and curriculum, the opportunity to provide social engagement within one's religious community through providing lists of on-campus clubs and local religious organizations, could be another avenue to better enhance the onboarding process (Ellaway et al.,2014). It is during these opportunities that students can get to know each other and potentially connect with others of similar backgrounds.

2. What can be done to provide religious accommodations for students of various religious backgrounds?

Patel et al. (2015) notes the importance of institutions creating policies that identify how to address issues or concerns relating to religion and procedures that properly address requests or concerns that may arise. In some instances, students who are not allowed to observe their religious holidays and afforded reasonable accommodations could view this as a form of discrimination. This could be a Title IV violation prohibiting equal educational opportunities regardless of religious belief or affiliation (The United States Department of Justice, 2022). One way to accommodate and support students of various religious backgrounds is by allowing them to observe their religious holidays. To mitigate any claims of discrimination a process should be formalized which allows students to identify early in the curriculum, ideally during the onboarding process, dates that conflict with their religious observances. Many institutions have adopted a policy that allows students to provide this notification but limit it to work-restricted required religious holidays in order to mitigate the disruptive effects of requested observances in large student populations with great success. When notification is provided within a set time frame, accommodations such as alternative exams and/or exam dates can be provided to allow the student an opportunity to meet the requirements of the course. Creating easy-to-access formalized policies to support these types of processes allows students the opportunity to honor commitments to both their religious beliefs and their future profession without feeling like both identities can't coexist in harmony with each other.

Creating interfaith spaces on campus close to where students study is another way that institutions can accommodate students and eliminate any perceived barrier to their religious belief and professional identity not being able to coexist. Providing spaces in close proximity to where students spend the majority of their time, eliminates the challenge of having to trek across campus and make it back to classes on time for those who wish to practice their beliefs during the school day. Proactively offering these spaces near where students frequent based on their program of study limits the barrier of access. Various religions observe prayer, meditation or quiet moments throughout the day and having designated spaces can help to eliminate the added stress that students from these religious groups would experience if they were required to do more by asking them to go on long journeys across campus to practice their faith versus those students whose religious beliefs do not require such accommodations.

Lastly, offering student support for those with specific religious needs will require the adoption of novel advising methods. Many campuses currently offer counselors for students on campus. Academic counselors, mental health counselors and wellness coaches are just some examples. Perhaps the adoption of interfaith advisors/counselors within these subspecialties would allow for additional support based on students' faith backgrounds. This would allow students the opportunity to reach out to faculty and staff with similar religious backgrounds to identify opportunities for religious engagement, and to offer guidance for students looking to advocate for change that will support their educational experiences and the experiences of others. A few schools that offer interfaith advisors include Swarthmore College, who offers Religious Advisors; and NYU who offers Spiritual Life Advisors (Religious Advisors,2022; Spiritual Life Advisors, 2022). Another college to note is DePauw University, which offers Spiritual Life staff and advisors and outlines for students' spiritual affiliates and instructors in their organization (Staff and Advisors, 2022). This can help build community for students based on their beliefs and show them professionals and organizations within their institution who are willing to let them share their beliefs.

While an interfaith support structure can be unique to each institution, in many cases, knowing that it exists can be impactful for many.

3. What types of policies should be created to ensure proper support for students from various religious backgrounds?

The creation of policies can help a student fulfill obligations that they deem important in both their spiritual and academic journeys. In a study conducted by Haghnegahdar et al.(2021), it was reported that on average, participants of the study spent 1.88 hours a week participating in religious activities and attended on average 21.8 religious services per year. The study went on to note that students who took part in services on religious holidays had significantly lower burnout scores than others tested. With wellness being a focal point, it's important to create policies that are supportive of the mental, physical, and academic health of our students.

As noted in the answer above, policies regarding exam accommodations can limit a student's stress and need to prioritize their belief versus their education. It is equally important that all representatives of the college are familiar with this policy. Awareness of such policies and training on how to execute these policies appropriately, are important (Patel et al., 2015). Faculty, staff, and students should all receive formalized training in order to understand the purpose and importance of these policies and the positive benefits it has on student success.

Policies regarding dress code are important as well. In a study conducted by Ruzycki et al. (2022), various types of discrimination were identified in a number of dress code policies. This article described dress code policies that allude to 'proper dress' and 'professionalism standards' that focused on norms and standards found in mainly White or affluent communities. It is suggested that students who seek accommodations for attire be accommodated. The failure to support religious or culturally mandated attire is more than the failure to support a student, it is also a failure to support a culture. It has been noted that failure to support certain garments as required by beliefs can be viewed as a lack of respect for one's religion and can ultimately impact students' decisions regarding what fields they decide to practice in (Malik, et al., 2019). Malik et al. (2019) documented the impact that religious attire of Muslim women had on their ability to practice as surgeons. It was noted that 51.5% of the participants in this study experienced issues when attempting to wear their hijabs. 14.3% of these participants noted that these experiences impacted their choice to go into surgical specialties. We thus suggest that healthcare educational institutions go further than just offering accommodations. We suggest that schools expect to enroll students with diverse cultural and religious attire requirements and build into the onboarding process policies that outline how these beliefs are accommodated It will be equally important that institutions partner with clinical training sites that share the same values or are willing to support these students in a similar fashion. We further suggest that schools and clinical training partners publish these accommodations in a manner that is easy for students and potential students to access. This will allow students, and those still considering careers in the healthcare field, to feel supported and know that their beliefs do not have to be in conflict with their desired professional identities.

Policies that focus on support of religious and cultural practices that might impact students' training are also important. Alvord (2013) presents the challenges of addressing the needs of a Navajo student who is unable to work with cadavers. In this work, she notes an instructor's refusal to accommodate or work with students in similar situations, and how that can create a barrier to the completion of their program and ultimately impact the diversity of the overall profession. Creating policies and procedures to address known obstacles where various religious requirements might impact career choice and training, and how students can receive alternative forms of instruction, can serve as a form of institutional support.

One common course in many health professional programs that requires special consideration for students of various religious backgrounds, is the gross anatomy cadaver lab. An example of institutional support is how many schools have started to incorporate ceremonies that are part of the formal curriculum that acknowledges the human value of the body to be dissected in the anatomy cadaver lab course. Ceremonies such as the Thai ajan yai ceremony involve inviting students, families, and Buddhist monks to read aloud the names of the cadavers, give them ritual flower bouquets, and bestow upon them the title of "great teacher" (Winkelmann and Guldner, 2004). Ceremonies such as these are an example of a best practice of blending the need for education with an acknowledgment of how some faiths require acknowledgment of the human body as sacred.

Another example of how some health professional programs are accommodating students with religious customs that can impact their education in the cadaver lab, is the labeling of the dissection room as a cemetery. This accommodates the Jewish requirement that mandates bodies must be physically buried immediately, and that those who come into contact with them, if they have not been, will become unclean. These spaces are required to be physically separated from the rest of the teaching classrooms in order to foster a feeling within students of being in a different mental space when working with the bodies. Programs that follow this also usually will require that all bodily tissues, blood, and organs of cadavers be kept together in order to emphasize that all of these parts belong to an individual whose life should be honored in the educational space (Notzer, 2006). Actions such as the purposeful design of educational spaces and the incorporation of ceremonies acknowledging religious beliefs about the body, are great examples of steps educational institutions can take to further the work of dismantling structural barriers student encounter to merging their religious faiths with the requirements of their professional identities and education.

4. What are some ways that the institution could have addressed the expectations of Q and supported her prior to the start of her program?

One way in which the institution could have addressed Q's desire to know about what's to come, is by establishing an admitted student's page. This page can provide a checklist to help students identify what should be done prior to starting classes as well as an outline of what will be covered in the orientation program. This page can also include a contact list and important deadlines, allowing students to plan and prepare ahead of time. A list as such could have helped Q identify specifically who she needed to contact to address questions about religious accommodations.

Another way that Q could have been better supported by her home institution would be if the Student Affairs and Admissions staff had received better training on how to handle student inquiries. This training should emphasize the concept, if you don't know the answer to something, the best course of action is to tell the student you will ask and get back to them. Had this been exercised, student Q would have had a vastly different experience. Instead of guessing at the answers, Ms. L. could have shown better support by identifying answers to her questions. Entering into a new program can be daunting, so ensuring that all college personnel know that if they cannot directly provide aid to students, they should take it upon themselves to lead them in the proper direction is a best practice related to onboarding. This ensures that students feel supported and can alleviate stress even when easy answers to questions are not readily identifiable.

5. What are some steps to dismantling the framework for religious students?

The concept of dismantling processes and policies that limit inclusivity in various environments is not new. Yet specific steps to outline practical ways to remove the barriers that would allow our future healthcare professionals to thrive in their academic and professional environments without compromising their religious beliefs are limited. The authors of this chapter have compiled a few steps that can be considered in order to start the process of removing religious barriers. Below are steps one can use to identify and address discriminatory practices and begin the process of dismantling the policies, procedures, and institutional norms keeping them in place.

- **Be Aware**-The first step is for health education programs to recognize that the health professionals that are being groomed today are different in appearance, beliefs, and understanding from those that came before them. Then they can begin to purposefully plan out curricula and support structures that can benefit not only these students but the surrounding communities in which they will live and serve.
- **Listen**- While many that educate our students are professionals in their respective fields, they can be biased toward the needs of their students by assuming that the current generation of students is fundamentally the same as those that came before them. This bias can be remedied by listening to what is needed by our current student population, especially as it relates to their religious beliefs, and then actively working to provide it. In doing so we are teaching our future health professionals two lessons. First, paying attention to the customs and needs of those you serve is important. Second, the power of collaboration. By collaborating with our students and creating safer spaces that they can thrive and grow in, we are modeling how we hope that they will also treat their future patient populations.
- **Partner**- Many schools partner with their students by offering them the opportunity to serve on student leadership boards. While this may provide an opportunity for students to be vocal regarding their concerns, many in college leadership positions miss the opportunity to help students understand why policies and procedures are in place in the interactions on these committees. With greater understanding comes increased opportunities. If students are oriented to the challenges that prevent change, collectively with leadership, a synergy of ideas can be developed to dismantle barriers for students
- **Act**- Long gone are the days when educators can ignore the changing faces present in our health professions programs. Ignorance is no longer an excuse when, from the point of interest to the application process, students are requested to provide information that clues us into their differences and potential needs based upon their multiple identities. However, a note of caution, before we move to action based on our assumptions of what students need, partnerships with them as noted before will allow educators to act with intention and not just from the prism of our own beliefs and experiences with students who have come before. There are many ways in which institutions of higher education can foster religious and culturally inclusive environments. While the solutions represented in this section are not exhaustive, it is imperative that we keep in mind all solutions are not a one size fits all remedy. In order to best support our students, we must create solutions that are tailor-made for them.

Many of the concepts above are generic in terms of who can benefit from these steps. Yet they are universal enough to support the desire to change how things are currently done and promote acceptance and understanding of our students. Especially those whose religious beliefs often come into conflict with their desired professional goals. While many try to separate ideas of religion and education, one cannot do so without separating the student who believes from their beliefs, and as such the adoption of policies and procedures that allow better integration remains the goal for fostering progressively more inclusive educational environments.

Epilogue

Merriam-Webster defines dismantle as, "to disconnect the pieces of" (Dismantle, 2022). If we are looking to disconnect the pieces of systems that make it challenging for students of diverse religious backgrounds to thrive in our health professions programs, we must first review the Mission and Vision of our programs and that of external partners brought on to educate our students. We must make sure that our values and purpose strive to be impartial and promote fairness. It is equally important that those whom we partner with mirror our impartiality. We first dismantle the framework by making it clear what we will and will not stand for through our mission and vision. We then break down policies that might be limiting, offensive or inconsiderate for any minority group. Finally, we must be willing to pivot. Our world is ever-evolving and so are the people that live in it. We must be willing to always stop, listen and improve our practices to meet the needs of our students. This means the work of dismantling is a continuous process. However, its successful implementation provides us with a workforce of future healthcare professionals that are culturally competent and able to serve patients from diverse faith backgrounds. Of equal importance, it also creates healthcare professionals who did not have to sacrifice a part of who they were to become who they want to be.

REFERENCES

AAMC. (2022). Retrieved from Matriculating Student Questionnaire (MSQ): https://www.aamc.org/data-reports/students-residents/report/matriculating-student-questionnaire-msq

Alvord, L. A. (2013). Medical School Accommodations for Religious and Cultural Practices. *The Virtual Mentor*, *15*(3), 198–201. doi:10.1001/virtualmentor.2013.15.3.ecas3-1303 PMID:23472807

American Osteopathic Association. (2019). *Accreditation of Colleges of Osteopathic Medicine: COM Continuing Accreditation Standards*. Commission on Osteopathic College Accreditation. Microsoft Word - 2019 COM Continuing Accreditation Standards Rev 2-20.

Anderson, P. M., & Vanderbilt, A. A. (2018). Bridging the gap between physician and medical student education: Using the Train the Trainer model to improve cultural competence training in the clerkship years of medical school. *Advances in Medical Education and Practice*, *9*, 495–498. doi:10.2147/AMEP.S163485 PMID:29983602

Association of American Medical Colleges & Liaison Committee on Medical Education. (2003). *Functions and structure of a medical school: standards for accreditation of medical education programs leading to the MD degree*. Liaison Committee on Medical Education.

Balboni, M. J., Bandini, J., Mitchell, C., Epstein-Peterson, Z. D., Amobi, A., Cahill, J., Enzinger, A. C., Peteet, J., & Balboni, T. (2015). Religion, Spirituality, and the Hidden Curriculum: Medical Student and Faculty Reflections. *Journal of Pain and Symptom Management*, *50*(4), 507–515. doi:10.1016/j.jpainsymman.2015.04.020 PMID:26025271

Balboni, M. J., Sullivan, A., Enzinger, A., Epstein-Peterson, Z. D., Tseng, Y. D., Mitchell, C., Niska, J., Zollfrank, A., VanderWeele, T. J., & Balboni, T. A. (2014). Nurse and physician barriers to spiritual care provision of the end of life. *Journal of Pain and Symptom Management*, *48*(3), 400–410. doi:10.1016/j.jpainsymman.2013.09.020 PMID:24480531

Berger, G., Conroy, S., Peerson, A., & Brazil, V. (2014). Clinical supervisors and cultural competence. *The Clinical Teacher*, *11*(5), 370–374. doi:10.1111/tct.12170 PMID:25041671

Brottman, M. R., Char, D. M., Hattori, R. A., Heeb, R., & Taff, S. D. (2020). Toward Cultural Competency in Health Care: A Scoping Review of the Diversity and Inclusion Education Literature. *Academic Medicine*, *95*(5), 803–813. doi:10.1097/ACM.0000000000002995 PMID:31567169

Devi, N. J., Kumari, A., & Murty, D. (2016). The impact of orientation program for first M.B.B.S students in the transformation of perceptual learning into experiential learning-An insight. *IOSR Journal of Dental and Medical Sciences*, *15*(6), 40–45. doi:10.9790/0853-1506084045

Dismantle. (2022). Retrieved from Merriam-Webster: https://www.merriam-webster.com/dictionary/dismantle

Ellaway, R. H., Cooper, G., Al-Idrissi, T., Dubé, T., & Graves, L. (2014). Discourses of student orientation to medical education programs. *Medical Education Online*, *19*(1), 23714. doi:10.3402/meo.v19.23714 PMID:24646440

Haghnegahdar, M., Sharma, P., Hubbard, K. P., & White, W. A. (2021). The Influence of Religious Belief on Burnout in Medical Students. *Missouri Medicine*, *118*(1), 63–67. PMID:33551488

Institute of Medicine (US) Committee on Institutional and Policy-Level Strategies for Increasing the Diversity of the U.S. Healthcare Workforce. (2004). *In the Nation's Compelling Interest: Ensuring Diversity in the Health-Care Workforce.* National Academies Press (US). Available at https://www.ncbi.nlm.nih.gov/books/NBK216009/

Malik, A., Qureshi, H., Abdul-Razakq, H., Yaqoob, Z., Zahra Javaid, F., Esmail, F., ... Latif, A. (2019). 'I decided not to go into surgery due to dress code': A cross-sectional study within the UK investigating experiences of female Muslim medical health professionals on bare below the elbows (BBE) policy and wearing headscarves (hijabs) in theatre. *BMJ Open*, *9*(3), e019954. Advance online publication. doi:10.1136/bmjopen-2017-019954 PMID:30898792

Mitchell, D. L., Bennett, M. J., & Manfrin-Ledet, L. (2006). Spiritual development of nursing students: Developing competence to provide spiritual care to patients at the end of life. *The Journal of Nursing Education*, *45*, 365–370.

NCP Clinical Practice Guidelines for Quality Palliative Care. (2009). National Consensus Project. Available at: http://ww.nationalconsensusproject.org/guideline.pdf

Notzer, N., Zisenwine, D., Oz, L., & Rak, Y. (2006, July). Overcoming the Tension between Scientific and Religious Views in Teaching Anatomical Dissection: The Israeli Experience. *Clinical Anatomy (New York, N.Y.)*, *19*(5), 442–447. doi:10.1002/ca.20312 PMID:16683239

Pajarillo, E. J., & Korn, K. H. (2021). Equitable academic preparation: A structured onboarding program for incoming graduate nursing students. *Journal of Nursing Education and Practice*, *11*(7), 1. Advance online publication. doi:10.5430/jnep.v11n7p1

Pascoe, E. A., & Smart Richman, L. (2009). Perceived discrimination and health: A meta-analytic review. *Psychological Bulletin*, *135*(4), 531–554. doi:10.1037/a0016059 PMID:19586161

Patel, E., Baxter, K. B., & Silverman, N. (2015). Leadership Practices for Interfaith Excellence in Higher Education. *Liberal Education*, *101*, 48–53.

Pierce, C. (1974). *Psychiatric problems of the black minority. Vol. American Handbook of Psychiatry*. Basic Books.

Posner, P., Ali, M., & Douglas, S. (2019). Religion and Spirituality Among Medical Students. In D. Zappetti & J. Avery (Eds.), *Medical Student Well-Being*. Springer. doi:10.1007/978-3-030-16558-1_6

Puchalski, C., & Larson, D. (1998). Developing curricula in spirituality and medicine. *Academic Medicine*, *73*(9), 970–974. doi:10.1097/00001888-199809000-00015 PMID:9759099

Religious Advisors. (2022). Retrieved from Swarthmore: https://www.swarthmore.edu/interfaith-center/religious-advisors

Religious Landscape Study. (2022). Retrieved from Pew Research Center: https://www.pewresearch.org/religion/religious-landscape-study/educational-distribution/

Ruzycki, S. M., Daodu, O., Hernandez, S., & Lithgow, K. C. (2022). The contribution of undergraduate medical education dresscodes to systemic discrimination: A critical policy analysis. *Medical Education*, *56*(9), 949–957. doi:10.1111/medu.14854 PMID:35688162

Sarcahmi, R., Rajael, S., & Aalaei, S. (2020). Evaluation of the relationship between religious beliefs and academic achievements of dental students. *Journal of Education and Health Promotion*, *9*(305), 305. Advance online publication. doi:10.4103/jehp.jehp_576_19 PMID:33426109

Spiritual Life Advisors. (2022). Retrieved from NYU: https://www.nyu.edu/students/communities-and-groups/student-diversity/spiritual-life/religious-and-spiritual-life-on-campus/chaplains-circle.html

Staff and Advisors. (2022). Retrieved from DePauw University: https://www.depauw.edu/campus-life/spiritual-life/center/staff-and-advisors/

The Joint Commission. PC.02.02.13. 3.7.0.0 ed. (2011). Available at: https://www.jointcommission.org/assets/1/6/LTC_Core_PC.pdf

The United States Department of Justice. (2022). Retrieved from Types of educational opportunities discrimination: https://www.justice.gov/crt/types-educational-opportunities-discrimination

Watt, K., Abbott, P., & Reath, J. (2016). Developing cultural competence in general practitioners: An integrative review of the literature. *BMC Family Practice*, *17*(1), 158. doi:10.118612875-016-0560-6 PMID:27846805

Winkelmann, A., & Güldner, F. H. (2004). Cadavers as teachers: The dissecting room experience in Thailand. *BMJ (Clinical Research Ed.)*, *329*(7480), 1455–1457. doi:10.1136/bmj.329.7480.1455 PMID:15604182

Chapter 14
Inclusion for Wellness:
Fostering Wellness Through Inclusive Dialogue, Environments, and Practices

Delores Amorelli
Kaiser Permanente School of Medicine, USA

Nicole Lawson
Kaiser Permanente School of Medicine, USA

EXECUTIVE SUMMARY

It is well-established that medical students and practicing physicians alike continue to suffer from extreme burnout, despite growing efforts to attend more closely to wellness. This often takes the form of mindfulness practices, community activities, transparency around work expectations, mentor and support groups, and the like. However, less attention is paid to how efforts towards inclusive learning experiences can themselves support wellness. This chapter will explore how to build a truly inclusive and justice-oriented environment in the service of student wellness by looking at three key moments of the medical education journey, exploring where things often go awry, and offering possible solutions to enhance them. Specifically, the cases will leverage the didactic experience as a student, clinical encounters as a resident, and physician educator encounters with colleagues to illustrate how enhancing inclusive dialogue, environments, and practices in these spaces can also support practitioner wellness.

BACKGROUND

From the beginning of their medical education all the way through residency to becoming a practicing physician, many medical providers struggle with issues related to health and well-being. Research suggests that over fifty percent of providers experience symptoms related to burnout including exhaustion, detachment, and self-doubt (Rotenstein et al., 2018). A similar trend regarding rates of exhaustion has been seen in medical students as well as residents and fellows (Dyrbye et al., 2014). It is clear that the stressful demands of practicing medicine predispose physicians to burnout, and that the entirety of the

DOI: 10.4018/978-1-6684-5493-0.ch014

medical profession has a wellness problem. However, the factors at the root of this wellness issue and the strategies we might use to enhance health and well-being for healthcare workers are less evident.

This chapter suggests that one measure of wellness that is often overlooked is individual provider feelings of inclusion and belonging, and specifically, belonging and inclusion through a Diversity, Equity, and Inclusion (DEI) lens. Inclusion has been described as "a sense of belonging; feeling respected, valued for who you are; feeling a level of supportive energy and commitment from others so that you can do your best work" (Miller & Katz, 2002). Research shows that enhancing wellbeing at any level has positive benefits on retention, satisfaction, and ultimately improved outcomes for patients (Ripp et al., 2017). We also know that factors such as lack of representation, microaggressions, unconscious bias, and other stressors negatively impact mental health, a key indicator of wellness (Tsai & Muindi, 2016). Here, through the use of case studies we illustrate how successfully promoting and engaging in inclusion efforts at the individual, practitioner, group, and institutional level is critical to enhance wellbeing across the spectrum of learning and practice.

CASE 1: ON BEING SEEN

Goal

This case illustrates how medical student classroom learning experiences afford opportunities to not only teach basic science and doctoring skills, but also to cultivate space where neuro-diverse students can feel seen and integrated into the learning community.

Learning Outcomes

1. Identify how a learning disability may affect student academic and social experiences
2. Describe appropriate ways for students to attend to their own well-being
3. Articulate ways for faculty educators to enhance inclusion in course content, facilitation, and student relationships
4. Identify actions and structures at an institutional level to enhance inclusion and support well-being for neurodiverse students

Case

Jess Walters is a first-year medical student. They were accepted to many schools, even by one offering free tuition, but decided to attend this school because they were so impressed by the diversity of the faculty and staff they met during the interview process. There were folks of different races, country of origin, gender, ability status, etc.; they were hopeful this was the right learning environment for them. Jess had been diagnosed with dyslexia as a child, and always had challenges keeping up, but was certain they wanted to become a pediatrician. During the interview process, one staff member mentioned the resources the school had available to students, including accommodations and counseling, not to mention a health training partnership with a local daycare, and a hiking club that is intentional about choosing activities in which wheelchair-bound folks could also participate (Jess thought to themselves, my friend Pedro would love this!). With that range of activities and opportunities, Jess was certain the school would be a good fit. They started medical school optimistic that maybe they had found a place where all aspects of Jess' identity, from their outdoorsy interests to their passion for caring for kids, and even their dyslexia was welcome and represented in both the curriculum and the community.

As the first weeks went by, things were going pretty well. Jess had made a few close friends in one of the physiology classes, and even managed to go hiking with the outdoors club once. However, academically things proved challenging. It was hard to keep up and most of the material was not built for non-typical learning needs – lots of text, fast pace, not all lectures were recorded, etc. Not to mention the standardized multiple-choice exams were particularly taxing for Jess. Jess began to struggle and started noticing that maybe other students were too. One incident was really sticking with them, and they weren't sure what to do about it. In lecture one day, Jess was trying to focus on the material – they had gotten used to the other students fidgeting and had found a spot near the front so those distractions would be less obvious, but this instructor was making it hard. Dr. Lee was speaking softly, and wearing a mask, making it hard to follow along but Jess told themselves they would just rely on the textbook and review the lecture video after class to understand everything. But another student, Anthony, raised their hand looking confused - "I guess I'm not the only one having a hard time" Jess thought. Dr. Lee finished his slide and called on Anthony, who shared that it was really hard to follow, given how quiet the teacher was and how fast he was going. Dr. Lee replied, saying "Sorry about that, I'll try to speak louder, but we've got a lot of material to get through so we're going to go pretty quick. Good thing there is a recording to watch after class!" Dr. Lee then picked back up with his lecture; he was a bit louder at first, but it quickly tapered off. Between the sound, the speed, and the amount of text on the slides, Jess was feeling increasingly lost. They glanced at Anthony who was also looking frustrated and disappointed.

The more Jess thought about that incident that day, the more it bothered them. Someone had spoken up, but it didn't really change anything. Jess questioned too why they didn't also speak up? Maybe if more than one student said something it would have had more of an impact. But Jess didn't want to be "that student." Medical school was hard enough without everyone thinking that Jess couldn't keep up. Increasingly, Jess was feeling dissociated from the school community, and questioning whether their decision to attend was the right one. Despite the initially apparent diversity and welcoming environment, and the new friends and awesome hiking club, Jess wished the school did more to make learning more accessible for students like them. Jess started to feel like at best they might be the only one with a disability, except maybe Anthony; at worst, maybe the school just didn't really care? Jess was heading to lunch and happened to see Dr. Amina, their Health Systems instructor, eating alone. As Dr. Amina was one of the faculty members with whom Jess felt a connection, they gathered their courage and sat down to talk.

Jess greets their instructor, saying, "Hi, Dr. Amina, do you have a minute?"

Dr. Amina replies, "Of course Jess, how can I help?"

Thoughtfully, Jess replies, "Well I'm just having a hard time with classes, and I'm really struggling to keep up. I spend so much extra time reviewing material which means less time prepping for the next day of class. But I want to stay on top of things, so I end up staying up really late, not getting enough sleep. I'm just worn out and it's only the first semester! I don't know how I'm going to make it once things get really tough. I feel like my needs aren't really being met, and people like me are just completely invisible. It feels like the curriculum was made for your typical learner, not me."

Somewhat concerned, Dr. Amina asks, "Do you mind sharing more about what you mean when you say 'like you'?"

Trying to open up, Jess replies, "Well, I've always struggled with dyslexia. But I've had it so long I've come up with my own coping mechanisms and never really needed to report it to the Office of Disability. In undergrad I studied environmental studies, which was a lot of experiential learning and it worked great for me, so I didn't have too much of an issue. But here, the way some of the faculty teach makes it really hard to learn and feel like I'm actually doing a good job. They go too fast, they use these text-heavy slides in tiny font, not to mention all the students in the room fidgeting and making noise making it hard to concentrate. Like it's already hard to learn this stuff, and this just makes it that much harder."

"Hmm, I'm sorry to hear that, Jess. I know we do a good job with integrating race and gender and stuff into our curriculum, I guess folks aren't thinking much about disabilities. I admit I don't even know much to be honest and haven't really had any experience with it. Have you talked to the office of disability?" asks Dr. Amina.

A little put off, Jess replies, "No, like I said I don't want to stand out, and I don't really see it as a disability. And I've learned to mostly manage it so it's more that the extra effort I put in is wearing on me. I'm so tired all the time, and always behind. And honestly, it leaves a bad taste in my mouth in a school that emphasizes the diversity of students and staff and faculty but doesn't seem to do much to support different learning needs, not to mention other disabilities. I'm increasingly anxious about the upcoming exam – if I'm this tired now and this far behind, how will I catch up in time to study successfully? My anxiety which had been pretty well managed till now is really showing up, and I feel tense and irritable more often than I would like."

Dr. Amina tries to be supportive, saying "I don't know Jess, it's a tough problem. I would still recommend reaching out to the office of disabilities, they can help you find appropriate resources, and then knowing you, and since you said you have your own coping mechanisms, I know you'll get through this! After all, medical school is notoriously tough for everyone. But you've got this! I think I heard yoga might be a good practice for folks with dyslexia and other learning conditions, but I'll have to dig up the article where I saw that. I'd be happy to share it with you. Listen, I have to run to class, but definitely reach out again if you want to talk more, ok?"

Tersely, Jess replies, "Sure. Thanks, Dr. Amina."

Jess left that conversation feeling worse than before, and even more anxious. If medical school is notoriously tough, how are they going to get through it? Dr. Amina was nice and all, but seemed clueless about what to do, and worse, resigned that this is just how it is. Jess headed toward the parking structure to leave school, maybe being at home would help. As they approached their car, they passed a couple of students from Dr. Lee's class who were talking about school. Jess overheard them say "Man, Dr. Lee doesn't stop mumbling and speed-talking! Trying to hear and keep up with him might be harder than the exam!" The other student replied, "For real! And those slides are a nightmare... At least we only have one more year of classes with him."

That conversation reinforced Jess's fears that this environment was not made with people like them in mind. It seemed like when people talked about diversity and inclusion, they really were thinking about race and gender. Jess agreed these were important, the school actually was doing a pretty good job providing formal and informal support structures for those areas, and the curriculum seemed pretty inclusive. As a non-binary person Jess definitely felt like that identity was at least somewhat visible. But this other piece of themselves, the invisible piece, was completely absent beyond the standard disability accommodations which Jess wasn't comfortable pursuing. The more Jess thought about it, and about how isolated they were and how difficult the work would be, the higher their anxiety. They went home that day thinking that they may have made the wrong decision with medical school, or at least with this school.

QUESTIONS AND ANSWERS

1. How do we know Jess' well-being is impacted by not feeling included?

In this case, there are many moments where Jess is trying to articulate how this situation is making them feel unwell. It is easy to brush off the workload of medical school as a given, however, a more evidence-based approach highlights the extent to which the resulting fatigue and stress can result in burnout, which itself is a sign of poor well-being (Frajerman et al., 2019; Dunn et al., 2008). The biggest indicator of an impact on Jess's well-being is their increased anxiety levels. Anxiety in dyslexic students is a common issue in higher education, particularly in the sciences (Elgendi et al., 2021). Importantly, Jess specifically identifies experiencing fatigue which takes a toll on physical and mental wellness, but also mentions falling behind in the work, which can negatively impact students' feelings of self-efficacy. Finally, pointing to the impacts on their wellbeing, Jess remarks feeling "invisible," a powerful indicator of a lack of belonging and inclusion, and one which affects the self and a sense of community and safety and has been described as a form of neglect (Romanski et al., 2020).

2. Why should neurodiversity be a part of inclusion efforts?

Neurodiversity is generally invisible, and therefore unrecognized and highly stigmatized. Often misinterpreted as such, neurodiversity is in fact not a deviation from normal, but rather, represents natural variation in the human genome (Robinson, 2013). Just like race and gender and many other identities that are often the subject of exclusion and discrimination, neurodiverse traits like Asperger's, ADHD, dyslexia, and many others are simply variations on normal. Making neurodiverse traits and experiences explicit rather than invisible, and considered part of the normal spectrum, aligns with the broader DEI movement (Myers et al., 2014). Unfortunately, too often businesses and universities neglect including disability or accessibility in their DEI initiatives – one report from the Return on Disability Group found that although 90% of companies claim to prioritize diversity, only 4% consider disability in those initiatives. This is a significant gap in DEI work, and one that is slowly beginning to be rectified. If DEI work is about representing and valuing difference and creating space where everyone feels heard and like they belong, this should also include neurodiverse and differently abled people.

3. What can Jess do to support their own wellness?

Medical school is notoriously difficult and pushes the limits of student wellbeing (Dyrbye et al., 2019). While institutions are increasingly providing resources for students with disabilities, many of these students develop their own techniques and coping mechanisms to combat the fatigue, stress, and anxiety that results from these conditions, especially in unsupported environments. Some best practices Jess could use include implementing time management strategies, leveraging simple tools and tech, asking for help, and embracing the power of dyslexia. Jess already seems to have a good handle on their dyslexia and not letting themselves be defined by it. Time management, such as breaking up big projects, trying to stay ahead, making outlines, working in a quiet place, making flashcards, etc. are all good techniques that it sounds like Jess is engaging in. Jess also maintains self-care activities like the hiking club, critical to create an outlet from the stressors of medical school. Jess also asked for help, but unfortunately, the person they spoke to did not have the training or resources to adequately support them. Basic supports exist, such as extended time for exams; however, if this doesn't support their needs, Jess can work on articulating for themselves what might help and advocating for that support.

4. How could faculty support Jess better? What about their peers?

This scenario is intended to guide educators to provide support resources for differently abled students resources, normalize diversity of learning in curricular design, and create spaces for open discussion. In that vein, there are many tools and best practices for faculty to cultivate an inclusive learning environment. Universal Design for Learning (UDL) is one core frameworks to create that kind of environment. UDL recommends providing multiple means of representation (how material is presented), multiple means of engagement (allowing for autonomy and co-creation), and multiple means of action & expression (varied activities and assessments) such that all learners have an equitable opportunity to succeed (Luke, 2021; Rose, 2000). These principles also align with best practices for accommodating learning differences such as dyslexia (Wright, 2000). For example, instead of large lectures with text-heavy slides and unreliable recording which creates a learning burden specifically for students like Jess, faculty can consider breaking students into small groups, employ problem-based learning, or incorporate independent projects. Additionally, the faculty member in this scenario was somewhat dismissive of Jess' concerns, repeatedly suggesting they talk to the Office of Disability even though they had explicitly stated they didn't want to, and unfortunately reaffirming the narrative that medical school is just hard and that they would figure it out. Instead, in keeping with tips provided by students at the Yale Center for Dyslexia and Creativity, some best practices this faculty member could have employed include empathizing with the student, actively listening to their concerns, and admitting their own limitations and work to find other resources (dyslexia.yale.edu, 2022). Finally, peers can play an important role in serving as a support network and building community for each other, especially if the environment creates space for inclusion and normalization of differences.

5. What can the institution do?

Ultimately, student coping or adaptation mechanisms and the ability of individual faculty to respond to concerns are only small elements of success. To cultivate an inclusive learning environment for all students, initiatives and resources at the institutional level are critical (Williams et al., 2005). Faculty development on Universal Design for Learning as described above should be required, so students like Jess do not need to struggle through endless lectures and text-heavy slides without support. Instructionally, using pass/fail for grading or creating learning communities to provide informal support can offer structural and community supports to students (Dyrbye, 2019). Integrating neurodiversity and differing abilities into ongoing well-being and DEI initiatives such as well-being curricula, informal activities like mindfulness and physical activities, and making wellness a graduation competency are a few structural modifications to support students like Jess. Importantly, many schools have also created dedicated roles responsible for student well-being such as a director of student well-being or dean of students, and also having a student well-being committee with funding to support student-led activities (Dyrbye, 2019). Again, much of the literature focuses on well-being writ large, or on culture-specific or gender-oriented groups and activities. It is just as important to consider how to include diverse abilities in these approaches to ensure the institution reaches all students, including those whose differences may be invisible.

Epilogue

World Bank estimates show that about 15% of the global population lives with a disability; in the United States, around 5-10% of Americans have dyslexia (worldbank.org 2022). Chances are, there will be at least 1 student in each medical school classroom with an invisible disability or who is neurodiverse. Because of this invisibility, students like Jess are left to struggle on their own, or with minimal accommodations such as extended test time, without acknowledging the many other ways institutions, faculty, and peers can support neurodiverse students. Additionally, without these structures and supports, students like Jess risk ending up more and more behind in their studies, fatigued from trying to keep up, and anxious from the struggle and common concerns like timed standardized test taking. All of these in turn profoundly affect student well-being. Solutions to counter these effects include institutional imperatives to offer formal and informal supports destigmatizing neurodiversity, faculty development and efforts to implement pedagogy best practices such as Universal Design for Learning, and student socialization and awareness to better support their peers. In doing so, students like Jess will feel included, and their well-being will benefit.

CASE 2: BURNOUT & GENDER BIAS

Goal

This case illustrates how gender bias and discrimination can take a significant mental and emotional toll on residents and highlights key opportunities for achieving gender equity and supporting health and well-being in the academic medicine community.

Learning Outcomes

1. Discuss factors that contribute to resident burnout, including issues of equity, inclusion, and diversity
2. Discuss symptoms of resident burnout in the health professions
3. Identify strategies for communicating with health professions students experiencing burnout due to equity, inclusion, and diversity issues
4. Develop strategies for using equity, inclusion, and diversity principles to support the health and well-being of residents

Case

Marion Harmons is an emergency medicine resident nearing the midpoint of her PGY2 year. She has just finished the first week of a 4-week rotation in the medical ICU, where she is caring for several patients with critical pulmonary disorders. Being around patients with these disorders has been difficult for Marion, who is the primary caregiver for her 65-year-old mother who suffers from advanced COPD. Marion has no time for socializing as she spends most of her time at work or caring for her mother. She knew it would be hard to balance her responsibilities when she began her residency, but she assumed that being so closely involved in her mother's care would actually give her an advantage when working with patients who are suffering from pulmonary diseases. Instead, Marion finds herself distracted thinking about her mother throughout the day, and she finds that she needs to study late into the night to prepare for her patient care rounds. If she puts in the extra hours, she is able to skillfully present pertinent patient history, physical exam findings, as well as information from consultation services, but it is at the expense of feeling exhausted the entire next day. When she doesn't put in the extra hours, Marion struggles to organize her presentations and often leaves out pertinent information. Her attendings have noticed and have given her some feedback about being adequately prepared.

While Marion was excited to begin this stage of her training, she has been feeling less excitement and more pressure than ever before. She finds herself exhausted all the time and dreads going in for her shifts most days. While she has done well with the technical requirements of this rotation, such as setting up and adjusting ventilators, she now finds herself struggling when it comes to doing such tasks. One of the attending physicians on her service, Dr. Adams, recently told her, "You need to get this down yesterday. It's something you should be able to do in your sleep." He made this comment in front of several others, including a nurse, a respiratory therapist, and another resident. Marion didn't have a chance to respond, as Dr. Adams left the room immediately after making the comment, but the other resident in the room sighed and said, "Well, that was really harsh." Marion was not initially upset because she knows she can do better and believes that if she just had more rest everything would be fine. She knows that working in the emergency medicine department is going to require her to engage with high-risk patients who require urgent, complex care, and her attending is just reminding her of this fact with his comment.

The more Marion thinks about this exchange with Dr. Adams, though, the more it bothers her. Many of her colleagues are men, and they are almost never given any kind of negative feedback in front of others. Marion remembers a recent encounter she observed where one of her male colleagues, Brian, was unable to answer several questions during rounds, and Dr. Adams simply moved on and asked someone else for the answer. Another male resident on the team, Darren, made a pretty significant medication error with a patient, and was even patted on the back by Dr. Adams who said, "Don't worry yourself too much. These things happen in this kind of environment." Over the next few days, she finds herself thinking about these incidents and how it only ever seems to be men who get away with not knowing the answers or making mistakes. When interacting with patients, she is constantly worried that she will make a mistake and that she will be called out for it. During rounds, Marion stops raising her hand first when her attendings pose questions, even when she is sure she knows the answer. After a few days of this, Brian says to her: "What gives? You always have something to say during rounds." Marion doesn't know what to say. She just gives Brian a look and walks away. At home, she continues to feel the exhaustion she has been experiencing over the last few weeks. She finds that she is less patient when caring for her mother and feels bad about this. She begins to have trouble sleeping, even when she gets to bed at a reasonable time.

Now Marion's MICU rotation is halfway over, and she finds that she can't fully concentrate on her studies. It's taking her twice as long to review charts because she has to reread everything multiple times. As hard as she tries, she can't stop letting thoughts about how unfair things are creep into her mind, and she's still worried that she is going to mess up and hurt someone else. She isn't getting enough rest and she knows this can't continue. She tries to talk her colleague, Angela, who is one of the two other women in her ED residency program. Marion begins, "Hey Angela, have you ever noticed how some of the guys around here seem to get away with not knowing things?"

Angela laughs and says, "Oh, all the time. This is a boy's club if I have ever seen one."

Marion replies, "Doesn't that kind of tick you off, though? I mean we work so hard and give up so much to be here, and there is so much at stake. I think we all need feedback to get better, but I don't see why we're all not treated the same. It's just really upsetting."

Angela says, "It used to make me upset, but I know what the reality of this field is. I've come to accept it for what it is. I just keep my head down and make sure to study as hard as I can."

Marion wants to say more, but she isn't sure what else she can. It sounds like Angela has become accustomed to dealing with this kind of treatment, and Marion isn't sure she'll find any sympathy about the matter.

Feeling dissatisfied after this exchange with her colleague, Marion decides to talk with one of her attending physicians, Dr. Pierce, who has also just stepped into the role of career advisor in her program, about how she is feeling and the challenges she is facing. She's never had a personal conversation with Dr. Pierce before, so she's a little nervous to start the conversation with him about something so sensitive. She finds herself wishing that her program had at least one career advisor who was a woman. Marion begins by saying, "Well, umm…I've been feeling a little unsure of my skills lately, and part of this has to do with how exhausted I've been, but also it has to do with how I've been given feedback by some of the attendings here. I feel like it's starting to affect some of my work and…"

Dr. Pierce cuts in and says, "I know a lot of residents feel like we don't give enough feedback, or any at all, but honestly I feel like that's all we do."

Marion replies, "No, it's not that. It just feels like some of us are being given feedback and others aren't, even when we make the same mistakes, and the tone of the feedback sometimes is just kind of unprofessional."

Dr Pierce shakes his head and sighs, and then he says, "You residents are all so competitive with each other. You're constantly worried about what everyone else is doing when you should just be worried about your own skills."

Marion is taken aback and responds, "This doesn't have to do with being competitive. It's just that I wanted to be treated the same as everyone else here, and it seems like that's not happening."

Dr. Pierce replies, "What exactly are you suggesting is the problem, Marion?"

"I see a lot of my male colleagues making the same mistakes as I am, and instead of being given constructive feedback they're being given pats on the back. When I am told to improve, it's in such a demeaning way—like I should be able to do this job in my sleep," Marion says.

Dr Pierce says, "I haven't noticed anything like this here, and I've been here for quite a while. It is true that there are more men in emergency medicine. That's just a fact, but I don't think it means we get any sort of privilege, especially when we're still training. This is just a tough specialty. Everyone here has to prove themselves, and sometimes the feedback can be a little harsh but there are lives at stake."

Dr. Pierce gets a page and has to excuse himself before Marion can respond to his comments. She is disheartened by this conversation and begins to question whether she has chosen the right specialty. She knew this would be difficult, but she feels alone and that she has no good role models to help her navigate the complexities of residency. She continues to worry that she might make a mistake that could endanger one of her patients.

QUESTIONS AND ANSWERS

1. In this case, what factors are contributing to Marion's feelings of burnout?

Burnout is a work-related stress syndrome that results from chronic exposure to stressors on the job (De Hert, 2020). In this case, Marion is experiencing burnout due to both external and internal factors. The external factors include the high demands of her residency, such as the time pressure of dealing with patients in critical conditions and her experience of a negative work environment that stems from unequal treatment of residents. The internal factors contributing to Marion's burnout include high expectations of herself and using work as a substitute for a social life. Of all these factors that contribute to burnout, the unequal treatment of residents in her program is perhaps the most problematic, and it is likely compounding the other job-related stress she is dealing with. Marion notes a pattern of behavior in her department, where women are oftentimes receiving unprofessional feedback about their mistakes while men receive constructive feedback or are given a "pass." This lack of equity in her residency program has increased the stress in an already stressful working environment and is impacting Marion's performance. Gender bias and discrimination such as this can have far-reaching effects, even beyond burnout, on the physician workforce and ultimately on patient care (Spector et al., 2019).

2. Which symptoms of burnout is Marion experiencing?

Quantifying burnout can be difficulty can be difficult, as it is an internal experience that is on a continuum. The Maslach Burnout Inventory (MBI) is one of the most commonly used measures of physician burnout, which considers the following components: emotional exhaustion, depersonalization, and reduced personal accomplishment (Maslach, Jackson, & Leiter, 1997). In this case, Marion is experiencing some of the classic symptoms of burnout, including exhaustion and depersonalization, and she is also experiencing a lack of efficacy (Drummond, 2015). Exhaustion is her most prevalent symptom of burnout at the beginning of the case. Because she is worried about her performance, she's sleeping less and spending more time trying to prepare for her rounds. As the situation at her residency program continues, she begins to experience depersonalization, evidenced by how quickly she begins to lose patience with her ailing mother while caring for her. Finally, Marion begins to doubt the choice she made to enter emergency medicine, and she even worries that she will make a mistake if she continues down this path. While both men and women in medicine suffer from exhaustion and depersonalization equally, there is evidence to suggest that women in medicine are much more likely to experience lack of efficacy, where they doubt the meaning and quality of their work (Houkes et al., 2011).

3. What mistakes did Dr. Pierce make when discussing Marion's experiences with her? How should he have responded in this conversation?

Marion demonstrated vulnerability by approaching her attending Dr. Pierce with the concerns about how the residents in her program are being treated differently. Dr. Pierce wrongly assumed Marion was going to complain about not getting enough feedback and did not give her the space to share her feelings without jumping in first. When she shared why she was upset, he refused to acknowledge or validate Marion's feelings. Instead, he reminded her of the reality of the gender imbalance in the profession and denies that men in their emergency medicine program benefit from any privilege. He notes that all of the residents have to work hard to succeed in the program. None of these responses address the issues that Marion is facing. In fact, his responses are dismissive of something that is having a profound impact on Marion's day-to-day life. Dr. Pierce should have listened actively to Marion's concerns and approached her with empathy. He should have asked follow-up questions to try and understand more about Marion's experiences and her feelings of uncertainty about her skills. Furthermore, he should have acknowledged the potential for gender bias or discrimination in the workplace and planned to talk with or further train other physicians and staff in the program about the importance of equity and inclusion in the learning environment.

4. How might equity, inclusion, and diversity initiatives help to decrease Marion's feelings of burnout?

Equity, inclusion, and diversity (EID) have a huge role to play in supporting wellness in the for physicians and physicians in training. Spaces where physicians feel that they belong, regardless of identity, and are treated equally to their peers can help to foster the best performance and help individuals grow their skills (Ayyala et al., 2022). The workplace environment in this case is not one in which Marion feels that she belongs. Her gender identity makes her one of the least represented persons in this specific residency program, which has heightened her feelings of inherent biases and made her feel like she is somehow being held to higher and different standards than others. Leaders in Marion's residency program need to work towards building an inclusive environment, where all learners, regardless of identity, feel treated fairly and that their opinions and perspectives are valued. Part of this effort might include more training around EID issues; however, the failure to recognize gender bias and discrimination calls for more than just a simple, one-and-done approach to training. Instead, it calls for long-term, sustained work in this space, which should also include more opportunities for mentorship, especially mentorship by women in specialties like emergency medicine where women are in the minority (Agrawal, 2020). Additionally, efforts to promote more women into leadership positions in academic medicine, such as career advisors, could have provided Marion an opportunity to talk with a potential role model about her experiences.

Epilogue

This case focuses on how gender bias and discrimination can impact resident well-being, ultimately leading to burnout, which has the potential to impact patient care. More specifically, it illuminates how unequal treatment of women in health professions can lead to depersonalization and doubt about career trajectory and purpose. The failure of organizations to even acknowledge the existence of gender bias in medical education is highlighted in Marion's conversation with her attending physician/career advisor. Refusing to acknowledge these disparities has created a non-inclusive environment that is detrimental to her health and well-being. To thrive, Marion needs to be in an inclusive environment where there is a culture of support and professional development around equity, inclusion, and diversity. Such efforts in residency programs can positively impact students' health and well-being and make it less likely for them to experience burnout.

CASE 3: CREATING ANTI-RACIST SPACES

Goal

In this case, we explore the persistent and pervasive ways in which subtle racism has ramifications both on clinical practice, but also on the relationships in the clinical space, and the impacts to well-being that result when racism goes unchecked and people feel excluded.

Learning Outcomes

1. Identify where racism may persist in the clinical space
2. Explore the relationship between belonging and well-being
3. Discuss how encounters with racism may affect individual well-being
4. Identify strategies to respond to and prevent microaggressions

Case

Alex was thrilled to start his first day as the Family Nurse Practitioner in a small primary care practice. He had just moved to Phoenix and didn't know too many people but was excited about exploring a new place and putting down some roots after all the bouncing around from undergrad, nursing school, and residency. He might even find someone to settle down with! He planned to arrive early – he knew from prior meetings with the senior physician there that Dr. Paulson was very particular about timeliness, and he wanted to make a good impression. He had heard great things about this physician, and how he treated the other members of the care team as equal partners, so wanted to make sure they had a good working relationship.

When he arrived, Dr. Paulson was there in the waiting room to greet him. "I'm so glad you're joining us Alex! You're going to love it here. And given how much our patient population is changing, you're going to be a real asset," said Dr. Paulson. Alex thought that was kind of an odd thing to say, but he dismissed it. Maybe she was just referring to his age and the new ideas and practices he might bring, after all his paper published in the American Journal of Nursing was starting to get some buzz. "I wonder if she's implying something about me being Black…? Nah I'm just overthinking it," he thought to himself. When he glanced up at the receptionist, a woman named Rosa who seemed like she might be Latine, she gave him a look that seemed to say "no, you didn't imagine that." He shook it off and followed Dr. Paulson into the back.

Since he hadn't been able to visit in person due to the pandemic, he got the grand tour. Dr. Paulson was friendly, if perhaps a little too enthusiastic, and showed him to his workspace. He was so excited he finally got his own space, he decided not to address the fact that his space was in a dark corner of the floor, like it used to be a storage room. "That's nothing some good lighting can't fix," he thought to himself. They continued without any further incident, and Alex decided it was probably just nerves and he was just overreacting. By the end of the day, he was more than ready to head home to his new apartment and try to do some unpacking. Dr. Paulson enthusiastically wished him well and said she looked forward to seeing him tomorrow.

The next morning, Alex was up early, the concerning comments from the day before mostly forgotten. He got to the clinic and started his day, intaking new patients and taking his time to get to know them.

Many seemed glad to see him, a few even commented explicitly that it was nice to see a Black male provider for a change. He tried to correct them that he wasn't a doctor, but they said either way they were glad to have more folks that look like them helping with their care. Alex was feeling like he had found his niche. As the days passed, he was feeling pretty comfortable, and was so busy he didn't often have time to talk with Dr. Paulson, though he noticed a couple of her patients had switched over to him. He didn't think too hard about why. A couple weeks into the job, Dr. Paulson stopped by his office to chat and see how things were going. Alex was glad she came by, she was after all the reason he got the job, and it would be nice to get some feedback and get to know her a little better.

Dr. Paulson stops by Alex's desk, asking, "Hey Alex, how are you settling in?"

Enthusiastically, Alex replies, "I'm good! I love it here. The staff is great, and I really love the community, it feels like a bit like where I went to nursing school, in a good way."

Dr. Paulson casually remarks, "That's great, you were at Howard right?"

With a smile on his face, Alex replies, "That's right!"

In a matter of fact way, Dr. Paulson says "That makes sense then."

Slightly confused, Alex stammers "Uhhh, yeah. So anyway, is there anything I should know about our patients as I'm getting to know them and want to make sure I can give them the best care."

Dr. Paulson replies, "Hmm, I mean I don't think so, they pretty much speak for themselves in their visits. Truth be told we see so many patients, I don't have time to talk about much beyond their chief complaint, you know how it is! Oh, there is one thing, I'm sure you've heard about the GFR change recently? I did some CME recently and figured I'd sign up to hear the latest on GFR, not realizing it was really all about anti-racism. I mean I'm all for diversity – that's one reason why you joined after all! – but sometimes I think we take it too far. I don't put much stock in it, changing all of the calculators in clinical practice. I mean between you and me, based on my decades of practice I can tell you I have seen a difference between my Black patients and my Caucasian or Hispanic patients, not to mention all of the studies that have used these for decades! So, to me the race corrections have been actually beneficial to my own patient outcomes."

Trying to be tactful, Alex comments, "Well, actually there is a lot of good data to back removing race corrections from GFR calculations, so many people got under or over diagnosed when it was in place…"

Dismissively, Dr. Paulson says, "Maybe elsewhere, but not here. I have never had a problem and my patients haven't complained."

Alex offers, "I'd be happy to walk you through the rationale for the change if you'd like?"

Quickly Dr. Paulson replies, "Oh no no, no need. I won't be changing it anyway, but you go ahead and do what you like. Oh, and one other thing, some of these Hispanic patients, especially the older ones, put too much stock in, what do you call them? coo-ran-dare-eeyahs?"

Alex delicately says, "Curanderos?"

Dr. Paulson shrugs and says, "Yeah that. They say they help them feel better and sometimes even go to them instead of us! I usually just smile and nod and continue with our usual approach, since it usually works just fine. Just watch out for that, though you probably know more about that anyway. Oh, is that the time? Sorry gotta run. It was great chatting with you! Let's definitely do this more often, and for longer. I'll have Rosa set us up some time. See you later!"

Alex left that conversation completely overwhelmed by what he had heard. It was obvious Dr. Paulson had some deep-seated beliefs about providing care, and about Latine people and racial differences, and it didn't look like she was interested in changing anytime soon. He decided to talk to the office clerk, Rosa, about his concerns. As he suspected based on the look she gave him that first day, this was no surprise to her. Rosa told him she had tried and tried to teach Dr. Paulson some basics around being inclusive of her patients' beliefs, and seeing beyond race, but it just didn't work. She said the more she tried, the more unhappy and isolated she felt. These were significant concerns and there was no way to address them, and moreover being Latine, Rosa felt attacked by some of Dr. Paulson's beliefs despite how kind Dr. Paulson was to her personally. Having Alex around was actually a huge boost to her well-being and feeling like she might not be alone. But she warned him, if he didn't want this place to get to him and start eating away at him, it was best to just come in, do the job, and go home. Eventually, Dr. Paulson would retire, and they could all breathe a little easier. That just made Alex more concerned – if the office clerk was that resigned given she had been there for nearly 10 years, what could he do?

As the weeks and months went by, the lack of recognition and valuing of his identity, and the constant microaggressions he experienced or overheard chipped away at Alex. He had a hard time meeting other providers of color locally just because he worked so much and was still settling in, so that didn't help either. He spent so much time at work because he cared so deeply about his patients, the constant belittlement began to make him anxious to go in every day, and increasingly made him feel like this wasn't the right place for him after all. Finding something new would be hard, and he wasn't sure he could invest in that effort right now. Alex became worried about his future and started showing signs of depression.

QUESTIONS AND ANSWERS

1. How would you characterize the work environment in this case?

The work environment in this case can be characterized as unhealthy or toxic. A toxic work environment is one in which there is a repetitious pattern of abuse, harassment, or discrimination over time that is ignored, allowed to exist and/or supported by the employer and no adequate steps are taken to correct the situation (Shain, 2009). Both Alex and Rosa have experienced repetitious harassment or discrimination at the hands of Dr. Paulson, although sometimes it is subtle in nature. In Alex's case, most of this abuse takes the form of microaggressions; these microaggressions in turn stem from implicit and in some cases explicit biases and assumptions Dr. Paulson holds both about Alex's identity, and also of race as a determinant of disease (Feaster et al. 2021). These include comments about the changing patient population and how Alex is going to be an asset, about how Alex feels so at home with a patient population that is similar to his community at Morehouse, about how Alex was hired because of a belief in diversity, and even disparaging comments about some of the personal beliefs of Hispanic patients. Even more egregious than this is Dr. Paulson's strongly held beliefs about race-based medicine and her refusal to engage with Alex and the data behind removing race corrections from GFR calculations. While we do not have very specific information about Rosa's interactions with Dr. Paulson, we do know that she feels attacked by some of Dr. Paulson's beliefs about Hispanic people and racial differences and has tried to speak with her about being more inclusive, but nothing is done to correct the situation.

2. What impact is the work environment having on Alex and Rosa?

An unhealthy work environment can act as a driving force for physician burnout and overall decreased well-being (Morgantini, 2020). In this case, both Alex and Rosa are feeling isolated in their workplace and that their identities are not being valued. Being constantly devalued and subjected to microaggressions has caused Alex to experience anxiety, and he is also showing signs of depression. While Alex has only been in the practice for a few months, he is already starting to feel that he made the wrong choice and needs to start looking for a new practice. Rosa has been in this environment for a much longer time, nearly 10 years, and she acknowledges that she has become less engaged in the workplace over the years. The more she tried to engage Dr. Paulson in conversations about race and diversity, the more isolated and unhappy she felt, and this caused her to disengage from those conversations. She delivers a warning to Alex about how the toxic environment would eat away at him if he tried to be more engaged. For both Alex and Rosa, the lack of belonging or inclusion they feel in their workplace is negatively impacting their well-being.

3. What strategies could be used to respond to or prevent microaggressions in this case?

Alex is the primary target of the microaggressions in this case, and he uses several different upstander strategies (defined as actively intervening in or standing up to microaggressions and unsafe environments, see Ehie et al. 2021) for dealing with them. Initially, Alex simply ignores some of the microaggressions aimed at him, such as when Dr. Paulson suggests that he will be a real asset to the practice now that the patient population is changing. Alex isn't certain about what this comment implies and actually thinks about whether or not he may be overthinking things, but it does make him question whether Dr. Paulson is making a reference to him being Black. When Dr. Paulson makes another race-based comment, Alex takes a different approach of trying to refocus the conversation on patient care. This can be seen as an attempt to distract the perpetrator. Another approach that could be taken in this case would be to directly confront Dr. Paulson about the microaggressions and how they are impacting the work environment. Alex could tell Dr. Paulson that her comments are making him uncomfortable and ask her to stop. Another direct approach Alex could take would be to ask Dr. Paulson to clarify what she means by some of these comments, such as when Dr. Paulson notes that she is all about diversity and that is why she hired Alex. This would allow for a dialogue about the issue, which would force Dr. Paulson to interrogate her own thinking. One of these more direct approaches to dealing with those who commit microaggressions may prevent them from occurring in the future, as they can surface the feelings and impact that microaggressions have on individuals who experience them.

4. How can professional structures like mentoring programs or CME programs prevent this situation?

Alex and Rosa are working in an unhealthy environment where a senior physician is contributing to their feelings of lack of inclusion and belonging. This, in turn, is having an impact on their health and well-being. Many of the missteps by Dr. Paulson could have been prevented with the help of professional structures likes mentoring programs and CME programming. While the traditional mentoring approach in medicine pairs senior physicians with junior physicians, there are many skills that even senior physicians need to develop. Equity, inclusion, and diversity is one such area, and a mentorship program focused on these skills could have enhanced Dr. Paulson's skills in this area. A mentoring program also would have benefited Alex in this situation. If he could easily have connected with other providers of color in his area, he would have had a sounding board to discuss his experiences. This may also have helped him take a more direct approach to dealing with microaggressions in his clinic. Ongoing participation in CME focused on anti-racist practices and foundational implicit bias training in the clinical environment could also have helped Dr. Paulson. Importantly, though, this would need to be a sustained effort, as Dr. Paulson attended one CME session, deemed it contrary to her own experience and beliefs, and then continued to practice race-based medicine.

Epilogue

This case catalogues the persistent and pervasive ways in which subtle racism can impact well-being and lead to a lack of inclusion. Ultimately, leaders in medicine have a moral obligation to promote healthy work environments and personal well-being for providers at all stages of training and practice (Ripp et al., 2017). When medical professionals are subject to microinvalidations and microaggressions, this has a direct impact on their sense of self, belonging, and ultimately well-being, often resulting in significant mental health concerns like depression and anxiety (Berk, 2017). Additionally, these impacts are amplified when there is a perceived power differential as Alex is a FNP while Dr Paulson is a physician, potentially amplifying her dismissiveness of Alex's needs (Manderino and Berkey, 1997). This case also seeks to offer best practice recommendations on how to transform these environments from unsafe and exclusionary to brave and inclusive. Here we illustrate upstander best practices at an individual level, recommend mentoring and other social supports at the community level, and promote creating ongoing opportunities for learning at the institutional level. In concert, working across multiple spheres of influence and practice is critical to transforming the workplace environment and enhancing well-being and inclusion for all involved.

REFERENCES

Agrawal, P., Madsen, T. E., Lall, M., & Zeidan, A. (2020). Gender disparities in academic emergency medicine: Strategies for the recruitment, retention, and promotion of women. *AEM Education and Training*, *4*(S1), S67–S74. doi:10.1002/aet2.10414 PMID:32072109

Ayyala, R. S., Artunduaga, M., Morin, C. E., & Coley, B. D. (2022). Leveraging diversity, equity and inclusion for promoting wellness in the radiology workplace. *Pediatric Radiology*, *52*(9), 1–6. doi:10.100700247-022-05292-z PMID:35088132

Berk, R. A. (2017). Microaggressions trilogy: Part 1. Why do microaggressions matter? *Journal of Faculty Development*, *31*(1), 63.

De Hert, S. (2020). Burnout in healthcare workers: Prevalence, impact and preventative strategies. *Local and Regional Anesthesia*, *13*, 171–183. doi:10.2147/LRA.S240564 PMID:33149664

Disability Inclusion Overview. (2022, April 14). World Bank. Retrieved December 8, 2022, from https://www.worldbank.org/en/topic/disability

Dunn, L. B., Iglewicz, A., & Moutier, C. (2008). A conceptual model of medical student well-being: Promoting resilience and preventing burnout. *Academic Psychiatry*, *32*(1), 44–53. doi:10.1176/appi.ap.32.1.44 PMID:18270280

Dyrbye, L. N., Shanafelt, T. D., Johnson, P. O., Johnson, L. A., Satele, D., & West, C. P. (2019). A cross-sectional study exploring the relationship between burnout, absenteeism, and job performance among American nurses. *BMC Nursing*, *18*(1), 1–8. doi:10.118612912-019-0382-7 PMID:31768129

Dyrbye, L. N., West, C. P., Satele, D., Boone, S., Tan, L., Sloan, J., & Shanafelt, T. D. (2014). Burnout among US medical students, residents, and early career physicians relative to the general US population. *Academic Medicine*, *89*(3), 443–451. doi:10.1097/ACM.0000000000000134 PMID:24448053

Ehie, O., Muse, I., Hill, L., & Bastien, A. (2021). Professionalism: Microaggression in the healthcare setting. *Current Opinion in Anaesthesiology*, *34*(2), 131–136. doi:10.1097/ACO.0000000000000966 PMID:33630771

Elgendi, M. M., Stewart, S. H., MacKay, E. J., & Deacon, S. H. (2021). Two aspects of psychological functioning in undergraduates with a history of reading difficulties: Anxiety and self-efficacy. *Annals of Dyslexia*, *71*(1), 84–102. doi:10.100711881-021-00223-3 PMID:33786751

Feaster, B., McKinley-Grant, L., & McMichael, A. J. (2021). Microaggressions in medicine. *Cutis*, *107*(5), 235–237. doi:10.12788/cutis.0249 PMID:34288848

Frajerman, A., Morvan, Y., Krebs, M. O., Gorwood, P., & Chaumette, B. (2019). Burnout in medical students before residency: A systematic review and meta-analysis. *European Psychiatry*, *55*, 36–42. doi:10.1016/j.eurpsy.2018.08.006 PMID:30384110

Houkes, I., Winants, Y., Twellaar, M., & Verdonk, P. (2011). Development of burnout over time and the causal order of the three dimensions of burnout among male and female GPs. A three-wave panel study. *BMC Public Health*, *11*(1), 1–13. doi:10.1186/1471-2458-11-240 PMID:21501467

Langness, S., Rajapuram, N., Marshall, M., Rahman, A. S., & Sammann, A. (2022). Risk factors associated with student distress in medical school: Associations with faculty support and availability of wellbeing resources. *Public Library of Science ONE*, *17*(4), e0265869. doi:10.1371/journal.pone.0265869 PMID:35395007

Manderino, M. A., & Berkey, N. (1997). Verbal abuse of staff nurses by physicians. *Journal of Professional Nursing, 13*(1), 48–55.

Maslach, C., Jackson, S. E., & Leiter, M. P. (1997). *Maslach burnout inventory*. Scarecrow Education.

Meeks, L. M., Herzer, K., & Jain, N. R. (2018). Removing barriers and facilitating access: Increasing the number of physicians with disabilities. *Academic Medicine*, *93*(4), 540–543. doi:10.1097/ACM.0000000000002112 PMID:30248081

Morgantini, L. A., Naha, U., Wang, H., Francavilla, S., Acar, Ö., Flores, J. M., Crivellaro, S., Moreira, D., Abern, M., Eklund, M., Vigneswaran, H. T., & Weine, S. M. (2020). Factors contributing to healthcare professional burnout during the COVID-19 pandemic: A rapid turnaround global survey. *PLoS One*, *15*(9), e0238217. doi:10.1371/journal.pone.0238217 PMID:32881887

Myers, K. A., Lindburg, J. J., & Nied, D. M. (2014). Allies for Inclusion: Disability and Equity in Higher Education: ASHE Volume 39, Number 5. John Wiley & Sons.

Ripp, J. A., Privitera, M. R., West, C. P., Leiter, R., Logio, L., Shapiro, J., & Bazari, H. (2017). Well-being in graduate medical education: A call for action. *Academic Medicine*, *92*(7), 914–917. doi:10.1097/ACM.0000000000001735 PMID:28471780

Robinson, D. (2022). Neurodiversity in medical education: How can we improve postgraduate learning for neurodiverse doctors? *Medical Teacher*, *44*(5), 564–566. doi:10.1080/0142159X.2022.2039383 PMID:35236237

Romanski, P. A., Bartz, D., Pelletier, A., & Johnson, N. R. (2020). The "invisible student": Neglect as a form of medical student mistreatment, a call to action. *Journal of Surgical Education*, *77*(6), 1327–1330. doi:10.1016/j.jsurg.2020.05.013 PMID:32507361

Rose, D. (2000). Universal design for learning. *Journal of Special Education Technology*, *15*(3), 45–49. doi:10.1177/016264340001500307

Rotenstein, L. S., Torre, M., Ramos, M. A., Rosales, R. C., Guille, C., Sen, S., & Mata, D. A. (2018). Prevalence of burnout among physicians: A systematic review. *Journal of the American Medical Association*, *320*(11), 1131–1150. doi:10.1001/jama.2018.12777 PMID:30326495

Shain, M. (2009). Psychological safety at work: Emergence of a corporate and social agenda in Canada. *International Journal of Mental Health Promotion*, *11*(3), 42–48. doi:10.1080/14623730.2009.9721791

Spector, N. D., Asante, P. A., Marcelin, J. R., Poorman, J. A., Larson, A. R., Salles, A., Oxentenko, A. S., & Silver, J. K. (2019). Women in pediatrics: Progress, barriers, and opportunities for equity, diversity, and inclusion. *Pediatrics*, *144*(5), e20192149. doi:10.1542/peds.2019-2149 PMID:31548337

Ten ways to support learners with dyslexia. (n.d.). Cambridge English. Retrieved September 30, 2022, from https://www.cambridgeenglish.org/blog/ten-ways-to-support-learners-with-dyslexia/

The UDL guidelines. (2022, September 2). UDL. Retrieved September 30, 2022, from https://udlguidelines.cast.org/

Tips from students. (n.d.). Yale Dyslexia. Retrieved September 30, 2022, from https://dyslexia.yale.edu/resources/dyslexic-kids-adults/tips-from-students/

Tsai, J. W., & Muindi, F. (2016). Towards sustaining a culture of mental health and wellness for trainees in the biosciences. *Nature Biotechnology*, *34*(3), 353–355. doi:10.1038/nbt.3490 PMID:26963557

Williams, D. A., Berger, J. B., & McClendon, S. A. (2005). Toward a model of inclusive excellence and change in postsecondary institutions. Washington, DC: Association of American Colleges and Universities.

Wright, D. (2000). Educational support for nursing and midwifery students with dyslexia. *Nursing Standard, 14*(41), 35.

Chapter 15
Work-Life Integration in Medicine:
Unlearning Medical Culture and Establishing Boundaries

Elimarys Perez-Colon
University of South Florida, USA

EXECUTIVE SUMMARY

As defined by the International Classification of Diseases 11th revision, burnout is a syndrome conceptualized as resulting from chronic workplace stress that has not been successfully managed. It is characterized by three dimensions: feelings of energy depletion or exhaustion, feelings of negativism or cynicism related to one's job, and reduced professional efficacy. Multiple studies using the most widely accepted standard for burnout assessment—the Maslach Burnout Inventory—reported an increased incidence of burnout amongst all healthcare workers, particularly physicians. The most reported factor leading to burnout is the lack of appropriate work-life integration (WLI). WLI is a complex issue that requires prioritization, value alignment, boundary setting, and lifelong work. This chapter highlights a few of the many barriers to WLI in medicine, the impact of burnout on the delivery of quality care, and strategies to achieve a goal-based WLI for healthcare workers offering direct patient care during and after training.

BACKGROUND

Healthcare delivery can bring intellectual challenges, meaningful relationships with patients, and personal fulfillment, yet more than 50% of healthcare workers in the United States report burnout at some point in their careers. Data from other countries are less extensively available, but the existing literature suggests that similar issues are present worldwide (West et al., 2018). The COVID-19 pandemic exacerbated the rate of burnout among healthcare workers owing to increased workload, unsustainable emotional demands, and lack of public and systemic support leading to moral injury (Murthy, 2022).

DOI: 10.4018/978-1-6684-5493-0.ch015

Healthcare worker burnout carries substantial consequences. Burnout has been associated with patient safety concerns, poor quality of care, and increased healthcare costs. Burnout also impacts the physical and mental health of healthcare workers (Patel et al., 2021). Contributing factors include long working hours, high and oftentimes unsustainable productivity goals, lack of support from leadership, administrative work, chronic underinvestment in public health infrastructure, increased screen time, and greater overall difficulty with work-life integration (WLI) (Singh et al., 2022).

Satisfaction with WLI has been reported as lower for physicians than for the average U.S. worker (Shanafelt et al., 2012). Similar findings have been documented for other healthcare workers with direct patient care. Current literature indicates that both individual and organization-focused interventions are complementary and effective (Shanafelt et al., 2019). Individual strategies include mindfulness, stress management training, communication skills training, exercise programs, and self-care efforts. Adequate WLI is key in the treatment of burnout. Studies suggest that satisfaction with WLI inversely correlates with healthcare worker burnout. However, WLI is a complex problem requiring complex solutions. Healthcare culture teaches healthcare professionals to quell personal needs for their patients and these sacrifices can make maintaining adequate WLI challenging. Research shows that physicians report the poorest WLI among healthcare workers (Sexton et al., 2017). Although typically regarded as an individual intervention, WLI requires culture changes and systemic/organization-focused interventions (Schwartz et al., 2019). Adequate WLI offers great benefits to both the individual and the organization (Marques and Berry, 2021).

The cases outlined in this chapter discuss some of the barriers to adequate WLI and delineate potential individual and organizational strategies to improve WLI for healthcare workers.

CASE 1: MY NAME IS YES

Goal

This case portrays barriers to work-life integration due to unsustainable productivity expectations leading to over-commitment.

Learning Outcomes

1. Discuss setting and respecting boundaries.
2. Discuss strategies to choose tasks that will help achieve your goals.
3. Discuss the concept of "minority tax".
4. Describe how over-productivity can lead to burnout.
5. Discuss impostor syndrome and how it affects work-life integration.
6. Discuss potential organizational/system solutions to burnout.

Case

Dr. R is a 31-year-old female physician who recently completed her Internal Medicine residency. She identifies as Black. She was regarded as one of the most talented residents and was elected as chief resident for her last year of residency. Dr. R subsequently landed a job as an assistant professor and academic hospitalist at a renowned academic center. Her new job consisted of a total of nine months of ward service with a resident team and three months of administrative time, all split into 2 week-blocks. She also committed to working a weekend every six weeks. As soon as she started her dream job, she followed the advice of her residency mentor to say yes to every project, committee, and opportunity that was presented to her. Without fully finding her footing as a new attending physician, she was asked to be a part of the medical school admissions committee, the physician lead for the hospital's sickle-cell anemia quality improvement project to reduce readmissions and cover two extra weekend calls that weren't assigned by mistake.

After two years at her job, she was named the associate program director for their internal medicine residency program where she was in charge of recruitment efforts. She was also the chair of the hospital's diversity, equity, and inclusion (DEI) committee, and a member of multiple hospital committees, including peer review, pharmacotherapy, and readmission prevention. She is consistently assigned to mentor any resident from underrepresented backgrounds and was recently tasked to create a DEI curriculum for the residency program. She is also a faculty mentor for a student-run clinic serving uninsured patients. She often precepts the residency's daily case conference and is the to-go person to cover other attending physicians when they need coverage. Her hard work has been recognized with multiple teaching awards and induction to multiple honor societies.

On a personal level, Dr. R is single and not dating as she is "too busy building her career to date". In her off time, she volunteers with multiple non-profit organizations locally and frequently leads community outreach programs. She enjoys running by the nearby lake although she has not been able to run for the past couple of months due to lack of time. During residency, she used to have brunch most Sundays with her brother and parents but lately, she has been canceling often due to extra coverage or project deadlines. She often finds herself catching up on emails, evaluations, or patients' notes late at night after her workday. Recently, she had tickets for her favorite Broadway musical but could not make it as she had to stay late at the hospital while covering two resident ward teams at a time. She often makes plans with her friends only to cancel last minute as she needs to "catch up with work".

Dr. R's yearly review with the chairman of Internal Medicine Dr. X is coming up and she is excited to update her Curriculum Vitae (CV). She stayed late preparing herself for the meeting, dressed for success, and was at Dr. X's office 15 minutes before their meeting time. Right on time, Dr. X called her in and ask her, "How are you doing?". Dr. R said she was well and that she loved her job and is thankful for every opportunity. After Dr. X took some time to quickly review her CV, he said, "I see that you have been very productive from the educational and leadership standpoint, but you have only published a couple of case reports and haven't landed any research grants." Dr. R's demeanor changed completely as she listened attentively. Dr. X continued by saying, "You must find a way to publish the work that you are already doing and participate in clinical trials. I recommend that you look at active projects and see how you can incorporate yourself into them." He finished the meeting by saying, "You are doing very well. Residents and faculty respect you, but you have not reached your full potential! You just need to work harder." Dr. R got up shook Dr. X's hand and said, almost in a whisper, "Thank you." As Dr. R was walking out, shoulders down, Dr. X said, "We are recruiting a new division director for Infectious Diseases, and I think you would add diversity and perspective to the recruitment committee. Are you interested?" Dr. R responded, "Would be happy to help," with a half-smile on her face.

The next day she scheduled a meeting with her mentor, Dr. E who is a well-respected, nationally recognized internal medicine-pediatrics professor and program director for the Internal Medicine-pediatrics residency program. Dr. E is also a mother and a wife and holds multiple leadership positions in the university, for which she has worked for 17 years. After Dr. R explained that the yearly review with the chairman did not go as well as she predicted, Dr. E said, "It is hard to balance it all, but publications are important for promotion and as a junior faculty you cannot afford to say no. Remember what we talked about? If you say no, they will not offer you an opportunity the next time." Dr. R sat there holding tears back and said, "I don't think I can do all of this. I feel like an impostor at times. Maybe I am not good enough for academic medicine." Dr. E replied almost instantly, "Nonsense, it happens to everyone. You do belong. Just need to try and find a way to balance your time better." Dr. R nodded and thanked Dr. E for her time.

As per recommendations, Dr. R joined an active clinical trial and vowed to work on publishing at least five case reports every academic year. She even joined one of her colleagues in applying for a grant to start a mobile clinic for underserved patients. Six months later, while rounding with her team, Dr. R was having a difficult time remembering details of patient care that were just discussed. Furthermore, after her team explained to her that Mr. A, a patient that has been admitted for over two weeks, is finally medically stable for discharge but he just lost his lease and has no place to go; she responded, "Talk to the social worker to give him a list of shelters. We cannot solve the homeless crisis." Her response was so out of character that her senior resident asked her after rounds, "Dr. R, are you ok?" Shortly after, she received multiple complaints from nursing staff as she would dismiss their requests or concerns in a "condescending way". Before this, she was recognized as the provider of the month for her "patience and compassion while educating patients and families". After these events, she met with Dr. E again. As soon as she stepped inside Dr. E's office, she blurted, "I am not sure that I want to continue in academic medicine. I think I may be going through burnout. I constantly feel over-committed yet underproductive."

QUESTIONS AND ANSWERS

1. How can Dr. R prioritize tasks that will help her achieve her goals?

Goal setting, value alignment, and boundaries. Many physicians chose a career in medicine as a calling to serve while still being intellectually challenged. The journey to becoming a physician, however, is long and paved with obstacles and expectations. Furthermore, the general culture in medicine does not support self-care as a priority. Physicians are taught in medical school that patients always come first, even at the expense of their own health. During the post-graduate years, training hours are long and there is very little time for medical appointments, exercise, and self-care. In fact, the term "resident physician" originates from early physicians in training spending most of their time "residing" in the hospital. Later in their career, long hours, administrative duties, teaching engagements, maintenance of certification, committees, continuing medical education, and many other responsibilities quickly fill up physicians' time. With all the demands that come with being a physician, it is important to prioritize tasks, responsibilities, and projects that will help you reach your own goals.

First, she must delineate her goals as they are different for every individual. It is imperative to set goals that are strong, detailed, and carry a plan. S.M.A.R.T. (Specific, Measurable, Attainable, Relevant and Timely) goal-setting framework was initially introduced by Doran in 1981. S.M.A.R.T goals create a clear plan towards success. Once she figures out what her goals are, it's time to write them down. Write them down somewhere accessible so she may go back to them, make herself accountable for them, and have clarity on what things, people, or activities would help her achieve them (Marku, 2019).

Once she has clarity on what her goals are, it is important to evaluate value alignment. Value alignment is very important since burnout is not only about long hours but also about the fundamental disconnect between health workers' mission to serve and the organization's mission. Working for an organization whose values do not align with hers will not allow Dr. R to reach her goals.

The next step is to set her boundaries. Boundaries are like an imaginary fence around your well-being, and one cannot exist without the other. Boundaries are there to protect your time, energy, and goals. Especially at the beginning of our careers, we tend to say yes to every opportunity owing to the fear of not being offered opportunities in the future. Saying yes to everything can lead one to feel over-committed, over-functioning, and undervalued. In Dr. R's situation, she must determine what opportunities will allow her to achieve her goals. Now is the time to revise the goals that she wrote and decide which opportunities will take her closer to those goals- while avoiding those which take time away from her goals. This is where boundary setting comes in. Maybe she will determine that chairing the DEI committee and overseeing residency recruitment are aligned with her goal of improving the house-staff diversity yet being part of other recruitment committees does not.

Once she determines what her boundaries are, she needs to enforce and protect them. Boundary enforcement does not come without backlash. Healthcare workers are service-oriented; therefore, they tend to say "yes" because they want to help -- when the answer is "no", people are taken aback (Shillcutt, 2022). One cannot control another's response but if someone resents us for setting boundaries around our well-being, they probably do not have one's best interests in mind. What if there is an opportunity that may not help one's goals but would result in immense joy? Well, that is the beauty of boundaries they are set up by oneself and they can be flexible.

2. What is the "minority tax" and how does it manifest itself? How does Dr. R's case support this concept?

The Association of American Medical Colleges (AAMC) defines underrepresented in medicine (URMM) as "those racial and ethnic populations that are underrepresented in the medical profession relative to their numbers in the general population". URMMs generally include Blacks or African Americans, Latinos/Hispanics, Native Americans, and Pacific Islanders. Minority tax is generally defined as "the burden of time and resources placed on minority persons to represent and advocate for their communities". It is characterized by the synergistic effects of cultural isolation, lack of mentorship, disparities in clinical assignments, and additional responsibilities that hinder career advancement for those who are URMM (Campbell et al., 2019).

In academic medicine, this manifests as an expectation of gratitude to the academic institution, and to future generations of URMMs, for being awarded the opportunity to be a physician. URMM faculty are often asked and expected to lead DEI efforts for the institution, mentor URMM students, residents, or junior faculty, and be a part of recruitment committees solely based on a shared experience and not considering their skill sets or personal goals. This sense of indebtedness to the academic institution can at times diminish one's sense of accomplishment and stimulate a continuous desire to pay back the perceived debt at the expense of one's academic promotion and personal goals. Although such a service is very meaningful and undoubtedly important, it is not always compatible with traditional metrics of academic success. In other words, the overtime spent in some of these activities comes at a cost, a charge known as minority tax.

As a Black female physician, Dr. R falls under the URMM category. She was asked to mentor all URMM residents, oversee the DEI curriculum and committee and participate in diversity-focus recruitment efforts, leaving very little time for career-advancing activities such as research. Her mentor, Dr. E, failed to recognize the impact of minority tax and recommend prioritization of goal-directed activities. Mentoring is particularly important for URMM faculty to help them navigate the complex process of academic promotion and foster inclusion (Rodriguez et al., 2015).

3. What are some signs of burnout that Dr. R presented with?

As defined by the International Classification of Diseases 11th revision, burnout is a syndrome conceptualized as resulting from chronic workplace stress that has not been successfully managed. It is characterized by three dimensions: feelings of energy depletion or exhaustion, feelings of negativism or cynicism related to one's job, and reduced professional efficacy. The most widely accepted standard for burnout assessment, the Maslach Burnout Inventory report (MBI), evaluates three major categories: emotional exhaustion, depersonalization, and personal accomplishment (Maslach et al., 2017).

Burnout incidence has consistently been increasing in the United States across different disciplines in healthcare. Frontline physicians including emergency medicine, family medicine, internal medicine, and obstetrics/gynecology are at particularly high risk for burnout, and female physicians are more likely to experience burnout than their male colleagues (Reith, 2018). The higher risk for burnout for female physicians may be explained by the societal expectations on women to sustain a full-time job while maintaining a full load of household tasks (Shillcutt, 2022).

Dr. R shows signs of exhaustion as not remembering patient details, depersonalization, or decreased compassion as per her response toward their homeless patient situation, negativism, or cynicism as per interactions with nursing staff, and decreased professional efficacy. Dr. R should be evaluated for burnout using MBI.

4. How does impostor phenomenon present? How can it impact work-life integration?

Impostor phenomenon or syndrome (IP), first described by Psychologists Clance and Imes in 1978, is not a diagnosable psychiatric disorder but rather a constellation of feelings of inadequacy despite objective success and competence. IP is defined as a psychological construct characterized by the persistent belief that one's success is undeserved rather than due to personal effort, skill, and ability (Clance et al., 1978). Several tools have been developed to assess impostor syndrome, yet the cutoff and interpretation varies amongst published literature (Bravata et al., 2020).

Although impostor syndrome was first described in high-achieving women, newer data found no difference in the rates of men and women suffering from IP. There have been other factors that seemingly increase the prevalence of IP including being a member of ethnic minorities (Bravata et al., 2020). Recent literature showed that experiences of IP were more prevalent among physicians than workers in other fields. Furthermore, IP correlated with burnout and inversely correlated with professional fulfillment (Shanafelt et al., 2022). In Dr. R's case, her feelings of "not belonging in academic medicine" could represent IP and may lead to professional dissatisfaction and issues with work-life integration.

5. What can organizations/systems do to prevent physician burnout?

Burnout is a systems issue, not an individual one. Studies show that physicians demonstrated higher levels of resilience than the general working population in the US yet higher burnout rates (West et al., 2020). Organizations can help reduce burnout by instituting initiatives that increase healthcare worker efficiency and decrease their burden. Effective leadership is imperative, leaders must be invested in the well-being of healthcare workers. Value alignment is very important to ensure that healthcare workers and organizations are committed to similar goals (West et al., 2016).

Equally important are strategies that can decrease duty hours, such as optimizing workflow and electronic medical records to work efficiently for the healthcare worker, nonphysician staff support to offload clerical burdens, and fair productivity targets. Allowing flexibility in the work schedule can significantly improve work-life integration. Acquisition of knowledge and skill sets via workshops to facilitate work-life integration can promote positive drivers of career satisfaction for early career physicians (Pirte et al., 2017).

Organizations should also provide easy access to mental health resources for healthcare workers. Lastly, and most importantly, supporting a culture of well-being. In recent years, there has been increased awareness of physician depression and suicide. However, only about 1% of medical students with major depressive disorder disclose it as a disability (Haque, Stein, and Marvit, 2021). This illustrates a culture of suffering in silence and a lack of appropriate accommodations. Thus, a culture of well-being that encourages disclosure, treatment, and accommodations of mental health disorders is of the utmost importance.

6. What can Dr. R do to improve her work-life integration?

Dissatisfaction with work-life integration usually referred to as work-life balance, has been shown to directly correlate with burnout (Karash et al., 2019). Balance is defined by Oxford's English dictionary as an even distribution of weight enabling someone or something to remain upright and steady. The term work-life balance suggests that one should spend equal time, energy, and effort at work and in their personal/family life. This ideology is not realistic for healthcare workers as many factors may interfere with the day-to-day duties of healthcare workers, patient-related emergencies, administrative duties, notes, pandemics, natural disasters, emotional trauma, and others. Additionally, the COVID-19 pandemic has put extreme stress on healthcare workers in the United States, leading to workforce shortages as well as increased healthcare worker burnout. Studies suggest that three in ten healthcare workers report wanting to quit their profession (Wan, 2021).

Work-life integration refers to coordinating or blending elements of your life by allocating enough time and energy to each of them. As previously discussed, WLI is a complex issue that requires both organizational and individual action. What can Dr. R do? To start, she should grab a calendar and write everything that she is responsible for in there— her work duties, calls, personal time, self-care, brunch with family, time with friends, time to read, etcetera. Everything that gives her joy helps her to achieve her goals, makes her who she is, or is mandatory and inevitable, should be written down. Once her calendar is completed, that is her bandwidth. Those are the things that she identified as priorities and has time for. It is important to recognize that journaling with a calendar can be time-consuming, therefore adding to her individual workload and stress. However, this will allow her to have a clear visualization of her available time. Journaling with a calendar and adhering to the schedule is crucial to maximizing productivity (Gade and Yeo, 2019).

Next, comes the hardest part— she needs to make sure to say no to anything that doesn't fit into said calendar. This stage is when boundaries are important; she must protect her time and energy to avoid feeling overwhelmed with endless tasks. The truth is that in our service-oriented careers, we are expected to say yes— hence when we say no, it is deeply uncomfortable (Shillcutt, 2022). Saying no may cause backslash, maybe they will say that she is not a team player or maybe she just cannot say no as she owes that person some coverage; it is not simple. Holding strong boundaries is of the utmost importance as a weak boundary can result in spillage from one domain to another happening frequently and easily, while a strong boundary is less permeable, and spillage rarely happens (Marques and Berry, 2021). As uncomfortable and complex as protecting one's boundaries may be, not doing so leads to over-commitment and absolute exhaustion, and a stressed-out, run-down physician cannot be an effective caregiver.

Epilogue

This case illustrates how over-commitment and a lack of boundaries can lead to burnout, job dissatisfaction, impostor phenomenon, and poor work-life integration. It also illustrates the potential cost and burden of "the minority tax". Dr. R took on more tasks/projects than she was able to effectively manage, leaving her overwhelmed and having impostor feelings. Following her mentor's advice, she said yes to every opportunity without stopping to think if it would help her accomplish her goals. Appropriate work-life integration (WLI) is complex for healthcare workers and entails prioritization, value alignment, and setting boundaries. WLI requires coordinating work, family, friends, and self-care by allocating enough energy and time to each of them. Medical culture carries the unspoken expectation of living a work-dominated life, which creates extra barriers for healthcare workers. This mindset brings significant consequences including a much higher rate of burnout than the general population, physical and mental illness, poor work performance, and/or career change (Gade and Yeo, 2019).

To attain adequate WLI, one must undergo a process of self-evaluation to establish S.M.A.R.T goals and priorities, both work-related and personal. Once goals are established, it is important to create a calendar/schedule that is attainable and realistic. Calendar journaling should include activities and commitments from all areas of your life, to determine your availability. Most importantly, one needs to establish boundaries around your calendar to prevent over-commitment, and potentially, burnout. One's boundaries need to be shared with those around you for two reasons, to help them know where your limits are and to help you with accountability. Achieving one's goals is easier by choosing an environment that contains resources and people who will provide support. Mentors, for example, are there to help guide oneself in achieving short- and long-term goals. One's boundaries must be protected to prevent spillage from the work domain to the personal domain and vice-versa. Being a YES person without boundaries may leave you over-committed and an exhausted healthcare worker cannot provide effective and high-quality care. Lastly, WLI is a life-long journey that requires flexibility and frequent re-evaluation of one's goals.

CASE 2: COMPETING DEMANDS

Goal

This case portrays barriers to work-life integration owing to competing demands at work and personal life.

Learning Outcomes

1. Discuss prioritization of family time.
2. Describe strategies to include all required work tasks within expected work hours.
3. Explain how extenuating circumstances, such as the COVID-19 pandemic, affect the work-life balance for healthcare workers.
4. Outline the significance of setting and respecting boundaries.
5. Discuss the importance of attention to self-care.

Case

Nurse E is a 30-year-old male who has been working as a bedside critical care nurse at a large county hospital. He identifies as White. He has been working at the medical intensive care unit (ICU) for seven years and has received multiple awards for his excellence in nursing care. On a personal level, he is married to a nurse anesthetist who works at the same hospital, and they have a five-year-old daughter and a three-year-old son. He enjoys working out at the CrossFit gym, hiking, swimming, reading, and spending time with his family. He finds himself being outdoors often. Nurse E gets along with most people at work, has a close friend group, and participates in work events and team spirit activities. Nurse E has always enjoyed his job because of the complexity of bedside medical care, the multidisciplinary and collaborative approach to ICU care, and the never-ending learning. Most of his patients were on mechanical ventilation and/or sedated, hence, he couldn't converse with them. However, he enjoyed updating, educating, and supporting families when they visited. His wife asked him often if it wasn't sad that most of his patients were very ill and a substantial amount ended up passing away, but he still enjoyed caring for them and supporting patients and families through the end-of-life process. He proudly described his job as "an honor to serve patients at their most vulnerable moments". Even if patients are unable to communicate verbally, he would check on them often and calm them down with stories and reassurance.

At home, Nurse E shares parental and household responsibilities with his wife. He is regarded as a great father and is very involved in his children's lives. He generally works three 12-hour shifts per week, and he is the primary parent during his days off. Twice a month, he works as the ICU charge nurse, an opportunity he earned through his leadership and helping colleagues. His wife works four 8-hour shifts Monday–Thursday every week. When both are off service, they take road trips to visit family or check out national parks with their kids. They enjoy seeing their kids play outdoors and connect with nature so they traveled as often as they could. In February 2020, Nurse E and his wife found out that they are expecting their third child. They were happy and immediately started planning and adjusting to their new life.

In March 2020, the SARS-CoV-2 virus that caused the coronavirus disease (COVID-19) global pandemic was announced and as front-line providers, they were both needed for the hospital response. With all the uncertainty around this novel virus and the lockdown orders, their lives became more complicated. To reduce potential infection risk and cover childcare, they decided that his pregnant wife should stay home. Nurse E was happy to serve as a front-line nurse but quickly the extra hours and shifts, the shortage of ventilators and personal protection equipment, and the isolation from family and friends made it very hard. Instead of his usual schedule, he was obligated to work four to five days a week and shifts often lasted up to sixteen hours due to staff shortages. Despite his busy schedule, the constant support from his wife, family, and the public, made him proud to be part of this historic moment. The walkway into the hospital was filled with signs such as "heroes work here" and "we are thankful for you", which motivated and inspired Nurse E before every shift. As an ICU nurse, he was taking care of critically ill patients with COVID-19, many of whom unfortunately passed away. Visitors were not allowed; thus, he felt a bigger need to offer support and compassionate care to these patients, often holding their hands as they died. His routine of coming home, changing his clothes in the garage, and then debriefing and often crying with his wife became all too familiar. Family time was significantly reduced for obvious reasons and traveling to decompress was not an option.

In December of 2020, the long-awaited COVID-19 vaccine was released and shortly after, Nurse E's third child arrived. The couple and the family were elated to welcome their youngest son. Nurse E and his wife were amongst the first healthcare workers to get vaccinated, and he was able to enjoy some time off. They were able to take a family road trip and decompress. In mid-January of 2021, another COVID surge arrived.

This surge was different, Nurse E was asked to take extra shifts and his wife was to return to the hospital after maternity leave soon after. With the protection from vaccination and enough personal protection equipment, they were excited to be able to spend more time with patients, yet they now had three kids to care for. To complicate things further, as misinformation spread the relationship between healthcare workers and the public became contentious. As the surge progressed, Nurse E experienced increasingly difficult encounters with patients' family members accusing the healthcare team of not caring for patients appropriately, owing to their decision to not get vaccinated. It became increasingly hard to continue to offer compassionate care as this emotional abuse became more common. He had to work longer hours due to the virus spread affecting staffing. The job that he loved felt less fulfilling and his hours felt longer.

Nurse E's routine when he got home began to feel different. He was not just sad but also angry; particularly at those spreading misinformation and felt guilt for not feeling compassion for them. He also felt exhausted, physically, and emotionally, and had very little energy to help with childcare and household work. At work, he was tired and unmotivated. At home, he felt guilty for being away and overwhelmed with family responsibilities. Nurse E and his wife started fighting over mundane things and she suggested that he should seek therapy. He agreed to see the hospital's clinical psychologist. At his first appointment, he sat down after initial greetings and immediately started sharing, "It was just horrible. These patients were parents, grandparents, sons, daughters, and friends, all fighting this horrible disease alone in an isolated room and many of them didn't make it."

QUESTIONS AND ANSWERS

1. How can Nurse E prioritize his family time?

At the family level, work-life integration promotes greater marital stability, family cohesion, and perceived happiness (Rao et al., 2010). As a healthcare provider, there are many factors that determine how much of your time you spend at work. Most healthcare workers choose their careers to serve others. Hence, it is not surprising that most jumped into action amid the pandemic. Apart from the unprecedented demands associated with the COVID-19 pandemic, there are many factors that may contribute to imbalances in time spent at work and personal time, including national shortages in healthcare workers. To prioritize family time, Nurse E must be intentional in his actions. As previously discussed, scheduling family time/responsibilities into your daily schedule assists with time management. It is of the utmost importance to be present during that designated time, especially when the time is reduced by extenuating circumstances. When Nurse E is with his family, he should attempt to disconnect from work, put away his computer, not check emails on his phone and/or find non-work-related topics to discuss with his wife. Part of being present is to remind yourself of your priorities. If Nurse E had to miss bedtime during some of his shifts, it might be important for him to be in charge of bedtime on the days that he is not working. Another important strategy is not to be afraid to get help. Maybe they would have to pay for childcare from time to time to spend some time as a couple. Most importantly, Nurse E should be flexible and realistic with his goals and give himself grace; no one gets it right all the time.

2. What are some strategies that he can use to improve his work-life integration?

Work-life integration (WLI) can be challenging when there are so many competing demands that require your time and energy. Improving WLI has been tied to decrease burnout rates and improved job satisfaction (Karash et al., 2019). There are many strategies to better your WLI, but first, Nurse E must determine what are his immediate goals or priorities. One way to do this is using the 5/25 rule, assumed to be attributed to Warren Buffet, where you write down 25 life goals and then circle your top five, those will be your priorities. These priorities may change as you progress through life. But right this moment, those are all you have time for. Once his priorities are identified, it is important to schedule his time around those. It may seem silly to schedule bedtime, reading time, or date night. But when you do, you keep yourself accountable and make sure to have time for the activity. When preparing your schedule/calendar, it is important to be realistic and flexible.

Other strategies to maintain adequate WLI include getting help when needed. It is important to recognize that we all need help at times. Maybe you need someone to help with domestic chores to free up some time or you need a short break to decompress after a difficult patient encounter. Whatever it is, do not hesitate to ask for help. It is also important to set and maintain healthy boundaries around your priorities. If you set a boundary around the maximum number of shifts or hours you are willing to work per week, it is important to politely decline when asked to work extra hours. Saying no is a skill and it often comes with backlash but remember that fiercely protecting your boundaries is the only way to not deviate from your goals (Shillcutt, 2022).

Other strategies that may help include separating your work and your home life, such as setting a time to turn off your computer, not answering emails when you are out of work, and scheduling your work tasks exclusively within your work hours. Just to emphasize again, it is important to be present, quality is more important than quantity when it comes to time. Lastly, Nurse E should try not to be too hard on himself; trying his best is enough.

3. How has the COVID-19 pandemic affected work-life integration for healthcare workers?

The COVID-19 pandemic has affected work-life integration for everyone. There were clear disruptions to routine, social support, and daily life in general. Healthcare providers, especially those at the front lines, did not slow down during the global pandemic. They had to work longer hours and put themselves at the highest risk for infection. Nurses experience mental and physical stress at work when facing excessive workload and interpersonal conflict. Nurses working during the COVID-19 pandemic were both exposed to occupational hazards and psychosocial pressures at the same time (Xu et al., 2021).

Healthcare workers are facing multiple psychosocial threats during the COVID-19 pandemic, such as long working hours and high workloads, burnout, and increased psychological distress. Moreover, they experience social isolation to protect family members with reduced social support, which is a pillar of resiliency (Franza et al., 2020). The amount of uncertainty, especially at the beginning of the pandemic, provoked extra fear among healthcare workers who thrive in knowledge and science. Studies show increased compassion fatigue, burnout, and hopelessness among healthcare workers amid the COVID-19 pandemic (Marvaldi et al., 2021). Additionally, because of the COVID-19 pandemic, virtual meetings made it accessible to work from anywhere including home making the separation of work and home life harder. Apart from the work-associated stress, healthcare workers had to juggle child care, remote learning for school-aged kids, protecting aging parents, and other domestic responsibilities. As healthcare workers spent more time at work and had new/increased responsibilities at home their work-life integration was severely affected.

The effects on WLI seen during the COVID-19 pandemic can be extrapolated to future pandemics, natural disasters, wars or any other catastrophic situation that requires healthcare workers to be at the front lines.

4. How can Nurse E set and protect boundaries?

Boundaries are set to protect your time, energy, and well-being. To set effective boundaries, you should start by giving yourself permission to put your needs and wants first. Next, one should explore what are those needs and wants. Writing them down can help with visualization and prioritization. Once your needs are clear, then limits around them can be set. After deciding what your boundaries would be, you have to communicate them using clear and simple language (Shillcutt, 2022). For example, if Nurse E decided that he could only do four shifts per week at maximum. He needs to communicate that clearly with his supervisor.

Communicating your boundaries with others will undoubtedly encounter some backlash. This will take practice, especially if you are used to saying yes to everything previously. One must be firm yet polite when protecting your boundaries. It is imperative to understand that there is no need for apologies when protecting your boundaries. There is no need to be sorry for protecting your time and energy (Shillcutt, 2022). One way that Nurse E could answer when asked to cover an extra shift would be—"I wish I could help but I am already committed for the rest of the week." It is essential to be honest and direct. One should also be consistent with boundaries so that others respect them. If you say no today but yes again next week, they will keep asking.

When setting boundaries, it is also key to be realistic and flexible. There will always be extenuating circumstances that will require adjustments of your boundaries. It may not always be possible to enact one's preferred boundary, depending on the opportunities as well as constraints and/ or demands of the environment (Mellner et al., 2014). Boundaries are beneficial for everyone. They protect the emotional well-being of the individual, make relationships stronger by reducing assumptions, and make caregiving more effective.

5. How can Nurse E carve out some self-care time?

Self-care can be defined as "the self-initiated behavior that one chooses to incorporate to promote good health and general well-being" (Sherman, 2004). Boundaries and scheduling one's time are essential to be able to protect self-care time. Self-care time should be scheduled like any other task. Like with work-life integration, there is not a "one-size-fits-all" approach to self-care. To decide what self-care means to oneself, one should ask oneself, why do I feel depleted? What things make me feel better, more energized, and would help to clear my mind? Regardless of what self-care means for an individual, it is imperative to make it part of one's schedule and consistently honor that time. It may seem tempting to skip self-time when you are busy and overwhelmed with tasks both at work and home. However, that is precisely when you need self-care the most. Nurse E enjoys working out at the cross-fit gym and being outdoors so he could start by spending one hour at the gym before his shifts and jogging outside when he is off service. Whatever it is, he must add it to the schedule and protect this time with strong boundaries. Self-care is a proactive, holistic, and personalized approach to the promotion of health and well-being, in both personal and professional settings (Mills, 2018).

Epilogue

This case illustrates how competing demands at work and in one's personal life can lead to job dissatisfaction and interpersonal conflict (Rössler, 2012). Competing demands, such as life milestones and responsibilities, and a busier work schedule or even a promotion can affect work-life integration negatively (Ahmad, 2022). Work-life integration (WLI) is complex, especially for healthcare workers, and there is no "one-size-fits-all" approach to it. Everyone has different priorities and goals, both at work and in their personal life, and their WLI should be tailored to those. This case demonstrates extenuating circumstances like a global pandemic. However, it is not uncommon for healthcare workers to have longer hours, be asked to cover more shifts, and have less flexibility and more vicarious emotional trauma when compared to other careers (Missouridou, 2017).

To decide what is truly important to oneself, it is imperative to go through the process of setting and prioritizing S.M.A.R.T. goals. Another important strategy to improve WLI is scheduling your home responsibilities, work tasks, and self-care time all in the same calendar to prevent over-commitment. You must also set and protect boundaries around such a calendar. It is essential to be direct, clear, and consistent when protecting your boundaries. Last, but certainly not least, you must set some time for self-care. A stressed, overwhelmed, and fatigued healthcare worker cannot provide high-quality, effective care.

CONCLUSION

To summarize, healthcare careers can bring intellectual challenges and personal gratification, yet a significant amount of healthcare workers report dissatisfaction with their careers. Achieving adequate work-life integration is a complex issue for healthcare workers, during and after training, and requires active work. On the contrary, lack of WLI is associated with healthcare worker burnout with its consequences, especially in physicians. Despite higher levels of resiliency compared to the general population, physicians report higher levels of burnout. Lack of WLI also results in increased family conflict. Successful WLI requires S.M.A.R.T. goal setting, value alignment, scheduling, prioritization, boundary setting, and self-care. There is not a "one-size-fits-all" approach to WLI, everyone has different priorities and interventions should be tailored to these. Satisfactory WLI is not an individual issue and requires organizational/systemic-focused interventions and cultural change. Healthcare workers in direct patient care are conditioned to put patients' needs above their own well-being making WLI challenging. Adequate

WLI offers great benefits to both the individual and the organization. Individuals who report high satisfaction with WLI are more well equipped to offer high-quality-effective care. All strategies discussed in this chapter require flexibility for new needs and life changes/events as well as external, unavoidable, events that affect healthcare delivery such as a pandemic.

REFERENCES

Ahmad, D. A. (2022). The Influence of Interpersonal Conflict, Job Stress, and Work Life Balance on Employee Turnover Intention. *International Journal of Humanities and Education Development*, *4*(2), 1–14. doi:10.22161/jhed.4.2.1

Bravata, D. M., Watts, S. A., Keefer, A. L., Madhusudhan, D. K., Taylor, K. T., Clark, D. M., Nelson, R. S., Cokley, K. O., & Hagg, H. K. (2020). Prevalence, Predictors, and Treatment of Impostor Syndrome: A Systematic Review. *Journal of General Internal Medicine*, *35*(4), 1252–1275. doi:10.100711606-019-05364-1 PMID:31848865

Campbell, K. M., & Rodríguez, J. E. (2019). Addressing the Minority Tax: Perspectives from Two Diversity Leaders on Building Minority Faculty Success in Academic Medicine. *Academic Medicine*, *94*(12), 1854–1857. doi:10.1097/ACM.0000000000002839 PMID:31192803

Clance, P. R., & Imes, S. A. (1978). The imposter phenomenon in high achieving women: Dynamics and therapeutic intervention. *Group Dynamics*, *15*(3), 241–247.

Doran, G. T. (1981). There's a S.M.A.R.T. way to write management's goals and objectives. *Management Review*, *70*(11), 3, 5–36.

Franza, F., Basta, R., & Pellegrino, F. (2020). The Role of Fatigue of Compassion, Burnout and Hopelessness in Healthcare: Experience in the Time of COVID-19 Outbreak. *Psychiatria Danubina*, *32*(1), 10–14. PMID:32890354

Gade, L., & Yeo, H. L. (2019). Work–Life Integration and Time Management Strategies. *Clinics in Colon and Rectal Surgery*, *32*(6), 442–449. doi:10.1055-0039-1693011 PMID:31686996

Haque, O. S., Stein, M. A., & Marvit, A. (2021). Physician, Heal Thy Double Stigma: Doctors with Mental Illness and Structural Barriers to Disclosure. *The New England Journal of Medicine*, *384*(10), 888–891. doi:10.1056/NEJMp2031013 PMID:33705616

Karash, S., Solone, M., Chavez, J., & Shanafelt, T. (2019). Physician Work-Life Integration: Challenges and Strategies for Improvement. *Clinical Obstetrics and Gynecology*, *62*(3), 455–465. doi:10.1097/GRF.0000000000000442 PMID:30950862

Marku, C. (2019). *The Art Of Setting Smart Goals Set Winning Goals and Live a Life of Abundance, Success and Achievement*. Amazon Digital Services LLC.

Marques, V. C., & Berry, G. R. (2021). Enhancing work-life balance using a resilience framework. *Business and Society Review*, *126*(3), 263–281. doi:10.1111/basr.12237

Marvaldi, M., Mallet, J., Dubertret, C., Moro, M. R., & Guessoum, S. B. (2021). Anxiety, depression, trauma-related, and sleep disorders among healthcare workers during the COVID-19 pandemic: A systematic review and meta-analysis. *Neuroscience and Biobehavioral Reviews*, *126*, 252–264. doi:10.1016/j.neubiorev.2021.03.024 PMID:33774085

Maslach, C., Jackson, S. E., & Leiter, M. P. (2017). *Maslach Burnout Inventory Manual* (4th ed.). Mind Garden, Inc.

Mellner, C., Aronsson, G., & Kecklund, G. (2014). Boundary Management Preferences, Boundary Control, and Work-Life Balance among Full-Time Employed Professionals in Knowledge-Intensive, Flexible Work. *Nordic Journal of Working Life Studies*, *4*(4), 7. doi:10.19154/njwls.v4i4.4705

Mills, J., Wand, T., & Fraser, J. A. (2018). Exploring the meaning and practice of self-care among palliative care nurses and doctors: A qualitative study. *BMC Palliative Care*, *17*(1), 63. doi:10.118612904-018-0318-0 PMID:29669559

Missouridou, E. (2017). Secondary Posttraumatic Stress and Nurses' Emotional Responses to Patient's Trauma. *Journal of Trauma Nursing*, *24*(2), 110–115. doi:10.1097/JTN.0000000000000274 PMID:28272184

Murthy, V. H. (2022). Confronting Health Worker Burnout and Well-Being. *The New England Journal of Medicine*, *387*(7), 577–579. doi:10.1056/NEJMp2207252 PMID:35830683

Patel, M., Swift, S., & Digesu, A. (2021). Mental health among clinicians: What do we know and what can we do? *International Urogynecology Journal and Pelvic Floor Dysfunction*, *32*(5), 1055–1059. doi:10.100700192-021-04805-y PMID:33938962

Pitre, C., Ladd, L., & Welch, J. (2017). Negotiating Work-Life Integration. *MedEdPORTAL: the Journal of Teaching and Learning Resources*, *5*(13), 10623. doi:10.15766/mep_2374-8265.10623 PMID:30800824

Rao, T. S., & Indla, V. (2010). Work, family or personal life: Why not all three? *Indian Journal of Psychiatry*, *52*(4), 295–297. doi:10.4103/0019-5545.74301 PMID:21267360

Reith, T. P. (2018). Burnout in United States Healthcare Professionals: A Narrative Review. *Cureus*, *10*(12), e3681. doi:10.7759/cureus.3681 PMID:30761233

Rodriguez, J. E., Campbell, K. M., & Pololi, L. H. (2015). Addressing disparities in academic medicine: What of the minority tax? *BMC Medical Education*, *15*(1), 6. doi:10.118612909-015-0290-9 PMID:25638211

Rössler, W. (2012). Stress, burnout, and job dissatisfaction in mental health workers. *European Archives of Psychiatry and Clinical Neuroscience*, *262*(2), 65–69. doi:10.100700406-012-0353-4 PMID:22926058

Schwartz, S. P., Adair, K. C., Bae, J., Rehder, K. J., Shanafelt, T. D., Profit, J., & Sexton, J. B. (2019). Work-life balance behaviours cluster in work settings and relate to burnout and safety culture: A cross-sectional survey analysis. *BMJ Quality & Safety*, *8*(2), 142–150. doi:10.1136/bmjqs-2018-007933 PMID:30309912

Sexton, J. B., Schwartz, S. P., Chadwick, W. A., Rehder, K. J., Bae, J., Bokovoy, J., Doram, K., Sotile, W., Adair, K. C., & Profit, J. (2017). The associations between work-life balance behaviors, teamwork climate and safety climate: Cross-sectional survey introducing the work-life climate scale, psychometric properties, benchmarking data and future directions. *BMJ Quality & Safety*, *26*(8), 632–640. doi:10.1136/bmjqs-2016-006032 PMID:28008006

Shanafelt, T. D., Boone, S., Tan, L., Dyrbye, L. N., Sotile, W., Satele, D., West, C. P., Sloan, J., & Oreskovich, M. R. (2012). Burnout and Satisfaction with Work-Life Balance Among US Physicians Relative to the General US Population. *Archives of Internal Medicine*, *172*(18), 1377–1385. doi:10.1001/archinternmed.2012.3199 PMID:22911330

Shanafelt, T. D., Dyrbye, L. N., Sinsky, C., Trockel, M., Makowski, M. S., Tutty, M., Wang, H., Carlasare, L. E., & West, C. P. (2022). Imposter Phenomenon in US Physicians Relative to the US Working Population. *Mayo Clinic Proceedings*, *97*(11), 1981–1993. doi:10.1016/j.mayocp.2022.06.021 PMID:36116974

Shanafelt, T. D., West, C. P., Sinsky, C., Trockel, M., Tutty, M., Satele, D. V., Carlasare, L. E., & Dyrbye, L. N. (2019). Changes in Burnout and Satisfaction with Work-Life Integration in Physicians and the General US Working Population Between 2011 and 2017. *Mayo Clinic Proceedings*, *94*(9), 1681–1694. doi:10.1016/j.mayocp.2018.10.023 PMID:30803733

Sherman, D. (2004). Nurses' stress & burnout: How to care for yourself when caring for patients and their families experiencing life-threatening illness. *The American Journal of Nursing*, *104*(5), 52. doi:10.1097/00000446-200405000-00020 PMID:15166716

Shillcutt, S. (2022). *Brave Boundaries: Strategies to Say No, Stand Strong, and Take Control of your time: The Key to Living Empowered*. Health Communications Inc.

SinghR.VolnerK.MarloweD. (2022). *Provider Burnout*. https://www.ncbi.nlm.nih.gov/books/NBK538330/

Wan, W. (2021). *Burned out by the pandemic, 3 in 10 health-care workers consider leaving the profession.* https://www.washingtonpost.com/health/2021/04/22/health-workers-covid-quit/

West, C. P., Dyrbye, L. N., Erwin, P. J., & Shanafelt, T. D. (2016). Interventions to prevent and reduce physician burnout: A systematic review and meta-analysis. *Lancet*, *388*(10057), 2272–2281. doi:10.1016/S0140-6736(16)31279-X PMID:27692469

West, C. P., Dyrbye, L. N., & Shanafelt, T. D. (2018). Physician burnout: Contributors, consequences and solutions. *Journal of Internal Medicine*, *283*(6), 516–529. doi:10.1111/joim.12752 PMID:29505159

West, C. P., Dyrbye, L. N., Sinsky, C., Trockel, M., Tutty, M., Nedelec, L., Carlasare, L. E., & Shanafelt, T. D. (2020). Resilience and Burnout Among Physicians and the General US Working Population. *JAMA Network Open*, *3*(7), e209385. doi:10.1001/jamanetworkopen.2020.9385 PMID:32614425

Xu, H., Stjernswärd, S., & Glasdam, S. (2021). Psychosocial experiences of frontline nurses working in hospital-based settings during the COVID-19 pandemic: A qualitative systematic review. *Int J Nurs Stud Adv*, *3*, 100037. doi:10.1016/j.ijnsa.2021.100037 PMID:34308373

ADDITIONAL READING

Drummond, D. (2016). Prevent Physician Burnout: 4 Work-Life Balance Tools. *Missouri Medicine, 113*(6), 450–454. PMID:30228527

Fridner, A., Belkić, K., Minucci, D., Pavan, L., Marini, M., Pingel, B., Putoto, G., Simonato, P., Løvseth, L. T., & Schenck-Gustafsson, K. (2011). Work environment and recent suicidal thoughts among male university hospital physicians in Sweden and Italy: The health and organization among university hospital physicians in Europe (HOUPE) study. *Gender Medicine, 8*(4), 269–279. doi:10.1016/j.genm.2011.05.009 PMID:21727034

Lacy, B. E., & Chan, J. L. (2018). Physician Burnout: The Hidden Health Care Crisis. *Clinical Gastroenterology and Hepatology, 16*(3), 311–317. doi:10.1016/j.cgh.2017.06.043 PMID:28669661

McFarland, D. C., Hlubocky, F., & Riba, M. (2019). Burnout in Physicians: What is the Role for Psychiatry? *Current Psychiatry Reports, 21*(11), 108. doi:10.100711920-019-1100-6 PMID:31617020

Shanafelt, T. D., Dyrbye, L. N., Sinsky, C., Hasan, O., Satele, D., Sloan, J., & West, C. P. (2016). Relationship Between Clerical Burden and Characteristics of the Electronic Environment with Physician Burnout and Professional Satisfaction. *Mayo Clinic Proceedings, 91*(7), 836–848. doi:10.1016/j.mayocp.2016.05.007 PMID:27313121

Wei, J. L., & Villwock, J. A. (2021). Balance Versus Integration: Work-Life Considerations. *Otolaryngologic Clinics of North America, 54*(4), 823–837. doi:10.1016/j.otc.2021.05.007 PMID:34215359

Chapter 16
Cultivating Wellness and Cultural Humility Through Self-Awareness and Self-Reflection:
The Practice of Physician Cultural Responsibility

Christen DeAnne Johnson
https://orcid.org/0000-0001-8752-0030
Wright State University Boonshoft School of Medicine, USA

EXECUTIVE SUMMARY

When caring for patients of disenfranchised identities, healthcare professionals must be prepared for the complicated emotions they will face in providing equitable care. Through the practice of Physician Cultural Responsibility, one can learn to provide inclusive care and the skills to prevent burnout in doing so. The cases enclosed encourage learners to utilize cultural humility and intercultural communication skills to strengthen the healthcare professional's relationship with, ability to care for, and ability to advocate for the patient. Through discussions of intersectionality, the social determinants of health, and available resources, learners will explore both structural and individual barriers to health equity in two patients of diverse identities. A self-reflection technique is then displayed for the learner to increase their awareness of knowledge gaps, limitations, and both personal and professional biases, as well as protect themselves from burnout through unpacking difficult patient situations.

BACKGROUND

The challenges of caring for disenfranchised communities have been well documented (Fried et. al., 2019; Magnan, 2017). Patients of diverse identities often face trials presented by the social determinants of health or, "the conditions in the environments where people are born, live, learn, work, play, worship, and age that affect a wide range of health, functioning, and quality-of-life outcomes and risks" (U.S.

DOI: 10.4018/978-1-6684-5493-0.ch016

Department of Health and Human Services, 2020). These factors, including access to food and clean air, safe neighborhoods, health care quality, and opportunities for educational attainment and safe occupations dictate 80% of patient's health outcomes and are impacted by societal biases and factors (Fried et. al., 2019; Magnan, 2017). The other 20% of health outcomes could be attributed to the interactions within the exam room which can be impacted by the knowledge, experiences, and options provided by health care workers (Magnan, 2017). Concerns surrounding the care that patients receive can stem from cultural differences, biases, and difficulty with communication that can lead to misunderstandings, and decreases in the quality of care received.

While some of this can be attributed to a lack of resources, knowledge gaps, and even health care worker burnout as rates are at their highest (Amanullah & Ramesh -Shankar, 2020), the social categorization of medicine, or the biases passed through medical training makes providing equitable care for patients of all backgrounds increasingly difficult (Blackie et al, 2019). When matched with the myriad of barriers, environmental and social factors, and administrative frustrations that are known to negatively impact the care of the underserved, health equity can seem unattainable. Further, the quest towards this goal can contribute to moral injury and vicarious trauma, increasing healthcare worker burnout and negatively impacting the care that is received (Nedrow et al, 2012). Preparing healthcare workers with tools to properly manage these challenges is an opportunity to protect patients, decrease health disparities, and support the healthcare workforce.

Defined as, " the physician's attitude of responsibility or ethical duty to patients, colleagues, and themselves to transcend personal biases and preconceived notions and uphold the dignity of all through acknowledging one's limitations, biases, knowledge gaps, and power differential, and committing to the ongoing work of improving one's cultural understanding, skillset, and practice to ensure empathetic, professional, and humanistic exchanges in all facets, " (Johnson, 2022), Physician Cultural Responsibility yields an opportunity for physicians to improve the care for their patients as well as the ways that they care for themselves within and after patient encounters. Arguably, while named Physician Cultural Responsibility, this skillset is fundamental for all health care workers. Physician Cultural Responsibility unites holistic patient care through the practices of cultural humility, intercultural communication, anti-oppression, and advocacy with the key skills that are needed to process one's own emotional challenges associated with the additional stresses faced in the healthcare profession.

Cultural humility is defined by the National Institutes of Health (2007) as, "a lifelong process of self-reflection and self-critique [that] does not require mastery of lists of "different" or peculiar beliefs and behaviors supposedly pertaining to different cultures, rather it encourages [one] to develop a respectful attitude toward diverse points of view". This allows healthcare workers to identify patients' cultural needs as a part of the healthcare plan rather than an obstacle to the care that they would like to provide (Foronda et al, 2016; Masters et. al., 2019; Nazar et. al., 2014; Tervalon and Murray-Garcia, 1998). Further, with intercultural communication skills healthcare workers can strengthen patients' trust of healthcare workers and prevent misunderstandings that complicate and potentially add additional challenges to providing care (Betancourt et. al., 2003; DeVoss et. al., 2002, Tervalon and Murray-Garcia, 1998). Additionally, understanding how intersectionality and the social factors associated with multiple forms of oppression impacts patients' lives and experiences can clarify some of the external barriers that impact patients' needs (Masters et. al., 2019). Likewise, having the tools to impact these systemic factors through advocacy for patients, both within the healthcare system and otherwise, can mitigate some of the barriers that patients face in receiving equitable care (Fried et. al., 2019; Tervalon and Murray-Garcia, 1998).

As each of these individual techniques are useful, alone they are not enough. Best practices suggest a multifactorial approach that will both improve the care that patients of diverse identities receive, improve health outcomes, and improve health disparities (Foronda et al, 2016; Hunter and Thompson, 2019; Masters et. al., 2019). Crenshaw (1991) developed the term intersectionality to describe the layered disenfranchisement that one may experience in 1989. This term lays a foundation to describe the layers of oppression and determinants that impact patient health outcomes. Additionally, the importance of personal identity in the experience of oppression as well as the recognition of oppression from others is key in unpacking the biases that act a barrier to overcoming the barriers to ones needs (Sotto-Santiado et. al., 2022). Without considering one's intersectionality, one is blinded to solely the experiences that they themselves have, which are likely different than their patients and those around them.

Further, a multifactorial approach that provides healthcare workers with the additional skills needed to cope with the difficult demands that health inequities add, can improve their wellness and decrease burnout (Dobie, 2007; Foronda et al, 2016). Burnout or the, "emotional exhaustion, depersonalization, and a sense of reduced personal accomplishment" (West et. al., 2018) is a compound problem that adds to the load that healthcare workers endure. Sources have described this as a consequence of the depletion of personal resources as demands and needs increase. In healthcare, as patient needs and personal obligations grow, individuals' resources decrease. As the complex nature of the source of burnout is not removed, the natural response from the brain is to protect the self and to preserve resources, resulting in the symptoms of burnout (Williams, et. al., 2019). Having the skills of self-awareness and self-reflection is critical to protecting the mental health of health care workers (Dobie, 2007; Foronda et al, 2016). Processing interactions or difficult situations as well as reflecting on personal needs and boundaries is achieved through self-reflection (Dobie, 2007). Further, reflection has been shown to be useful in decreasing one's uncomfortability with encountering alternative or differing viewpoints (Brookfield, 2010), which are ever-present when caring for patients from diverse cultures and identities.

Whether mitigating personal biases, processing the vicarious trauma that occurs in caring for patients who must bear the effects of distressing circumstances, or unpacking the experiences that accompany navigating the challenging social and societal forces that impact the care of patients from diverse identities, utilizing the skills of Physician Cultural Responsibility validates the healthcare workers needs while elevating the importance of the intersectionality or unique combination of dynamics that individual patient displays. Likewise, the Physician Cultural Responsibility framework is a set of critical questions designed to lead health care workers through creating awareness of ones' knowledge gaps, personal biases, and challenges as well as provide space for the self-reflection of emotional needs and areas of support to challenge these ideas and process the difficult situations inherent to this work (Johnson, 2022). The complexity of patients demands an intersectional view of their lives, considering how multiple aspects of societal oppressive sources including biases associated with socioeconomic status, race, sexual orientation, and age impact their interactions with healthcare workers and patient needs. Even the way that patient narratives are written can display these biases (Inoue, 2020).

For the ease of exploring the practice of Physician Cultural Responsibility and its utility in personal experiences, the framework has been incorporated in the following cases where one is watching the healthcare encounter unfold. In the following cases, space has been intentionally left for personal assumptions and biases as well as knowledge gaps to emerge while utilizing the Physician Cultural Responsibility Framework to assist in experiencing the impact of one's own biases on patient care. These will be noted in both patient and healthcare worker identities as well as the language and tone used for the cases. Inherently these cases are multifaceted and very complex aligned with the nature of intersectionality. The questions associated with the framework also ask for reflection into the emotions felt by and needs of the healthcare worker described in the case. While speculative for the following cases, this exercise can assist healthcare workers in examining their needs by learning to utilize the questions asked in their own personal experiences. A personal examination of the biases and emotions personally noted while completing the case can further assist the reflection process and deepen awareness in future patient encounters.

CASE 1: CHRONIC DISEASE OVERSEAS

Goal

This case displays the challenges presented when trying to provide unbiased care to patients from other cultures, highlighting the need for healthcare worker awareness of cultural differences, personal biases, and need as well as displaying reflection techniques from the Physician Cultural Responsibility framework.

Learning Outcomes

1. Describe the Social Determinants of Health that impact the care of patients.
2. Identify biases that impact the care of patients of diverse nationalities.
3. Review the principles of intercultural communication and necessity for interpretation services.
4. Display the impact of cultural differences on patient care outcomes utilizing Physician Cultural Responsibility.
5. Identify the emotional needs and resource to assist with healthcare workers through the practice of self-awareness and self-reflection in Physician Cultural Responsibility.

Case

Mr. B is a 68-year-old male who is presenting to a primary care setting to establish care. He is racially ambiguous and English is not his first language, although he has been living in the United States for the past 6 years. He heard that this place sees patients from all over the world even if they cannot pay. Since his family is now in the US and can no longer send him medication from their home country, he feels this is a good place for him to go. He is dropped off at the office by a close friend and notes, "I am here to see a new doctor".

"Please complete these," says the woman at the front desk as he is handed multiple sheets of paper. Alongside the consent to treat form, are forms asking about his medical history, his current income, and his home life. Mr. B completes the paperwork as best as possible but thinks to himself, "I don't know what any of this means." He saves the income and social screening papers for last as he worries that these may get sent to the immigration officers and his wife's paperwork is not finalized. He considers these answers carefully.

Mr. B is then called back to the desk and the forms are taken from him.

"You didn't finish these."

He begins to feel uncomfortable and states, "Oh, I must have missed them".

The woman at the front desk then asks, "Well how much do you make?".

"Seventy thousand" Mr. B replies. He overheard that was a good salary listening to a conversation at the bank a few days ago. Knowing that he is currently uninsured and working 3 jobs to afford the fees associated with getting his family here, he doesn't want immigration to think he cannot take care of them. The woman at the front desk looks at him and says, "No wonder you skipped these, don't worry about this other one. It's not necessary. We will call you back in a second."

Five minutes later, Mr. B is called to go to a room. They stop by the scale.

"202, not bad sir" the medical assistant says.

Mr. B thinks to himself about how much weight he has gained, "202kg? That cannot be right!" The medical assistant then begins asking him questions and Mr. B again doesn't understand, she seems to be going so fast.

"Do you have any medical problems?"

He replies, "No."

Do you take any medications at this time?"

He states, "No but uh"

"Do you have any concerns for the doctor today?"

He says, "No".

The medical assistant then takes his blood pressure, "189/100 sir, this is an emergency. Do you normally have blood pressures this high? Are you feeling okay? Let me get the doctor!"

Dr. G arrives in minutes. Mr. B hears a knock on the door.

"Hello! I am Dr. G. I heard your blood pressure was dangerously high today. Are you feeling alright?"

Mr. B very nervous and flustered says, "I am fine, what is the issue?"

Dr. G states, "Your blood pressure is high. Let me recheck it"

"I am fine. I am asking for you to explain." Mr. B says while Dr. G is taking his blood pressure. "I came here to get a new doctor. They said I would see Dr. N. I get here, they tell me I have gained 40kg and I'm sick? I don't understand"

"201/110. Sir we need to get you to the hospital to get these down. It sounds like you may not be understanding very well today and we don't want to miss a stroke."

"I am not having a stroke doctor. None of you will listen. I don't even know who you are and you don't know me but you are telling me I am having a stroke and I am just fine."

Dr. G looks at his watch, noting he is now 15 minutes more behind than he was before. "Sir, I recommend we get you some help. If you would prefer to sit and wait for someone else to evaluate you, we can do that. I have another patient waiting on me. If you believe you are fine that is okay".

As Dr. G leaves the room, Mr. B becomes even more frustrated. He came here for help. He wanted to discuss what he could do to lose a little weight, he isn't sleeping the way he once did even though his family is here and he needs his medications. Dr. G sees Dr. N in the hallway and says, "Blood pressure in room 4 is terrible. No records or anything but he's in hypertensive emergency, I mean he acts like he doesn't understand me. I told him he needs eval at the ED because he might be having a stroke and he refused. Good luck. I told my wife I wouldn't be late again and here we go." Dr. N looks through the papers that Dr. G placed on his desk and verifies that the patient states he has no medical problems but was previously on something called Hydrex and Vastator for an unknown amount of time. A google search yields that these medicines come from Haiti. Dr. N also noticed the patient also answered some of the questions incorrectly like when asked how often he exercises, he answered walking.

Within 20 minutes, Dr. N knocks on the door saying "Good afternoon, sir! I am Dr. N and I heard we may have had a little blood pressure trouble today."

Mr. B states, "That's not the only trouble we have. They said I gained 40kg and I'm having a stroke. I don't believe them. I was supposed to see you."

Dr. N then asked Mr. B, "Can we start over? Tell me about yourself."

Mr. B responded, "I don't understand what you want to know."

Dr. N asked, "Where are you from?".

"Haiti" Mr. B responded. "But I've been here for a while."

Dr. N then asked, "Would you like me to get an interpreter for you?".

Mr. B smiled, "Please, French."

With the help of an interpreter on the phone, Dr. N learns that Mr. B was diagnosed with Diabetes, Hyperlipidemia, and Hypertension while he was living in Haiti. He has had more stress with the transition and his wife and children were in Haiti until recently. His wife was previously sending medications to him from the clinic they went to in Haiti but now that she is here he has none left. He also notes that he is concerned about his weight since he was said to have gained 40kg and he knows he hasn't been sleeping well. He has family back home that were impacted by the recent hurricane and he is very stressed as he has not been able to contact them. Dr. N is able to refill Mr. B's medications with comparable medications and discuss considering seeing the mental health professionals to cope with so much change and with his stress. Mr. B also discloses that he and his family do not have insurance and would need assistance. Dr. N is able to refer Mr. B to the Community Health Worker team to assist him with resources, have the team help him to correctly fill out his paperwork for the sliding scale, and do a warm handoff with the dietitian.

Mr. B's blood pressure is 149/92 on repeat. "Looks like those refills should do it. I will see you back in a month and I look forward to seeing your wife and kids as well." Dr. N says.

"Thank you for listening," Mr. B says through the interpreter as he is leaving. "Is there any way that I can only see you from now on? I don't want to come back if I'll have to see Dr. G."

"I'm very sorry that you had that experience, but you can always ask to see who you would like when you make your appointment." Dr. N replied.

QUESTIONS AND ANSWERS

1. Identify the social determinants of health experienced by Mr. B.

In the case above, Mr. B notes concerns about being uninsured and thus did not have access to health care, a doctor that he felt he could trust, or his necessary medications. Likewise, he has a language barrier that could further impact his care without the proper resources, like interpretation services, being utilized. He also notes stresses about economic stability, as he works multiple jobs due to the costs of his family immigrating to the US.

As the social determinants of health are vast, so are the many answers that one may have for this question. The social determinants of health mentioned above are not an exhaustive list of what one may ascertain from this text as additional details are needed from Mr. B. However, in utilizing Physician Cultural Responsibility, healthcare workers can better identify and address these social factors. Rather than prioritizing his social needs based on the values of the healthcare worker, one can identify that Mr. B may have cultural differences that impact the way that he interprets the role of healthcare system in assisting him with these concerns. While considering the social determinants of health experienced by

Mr. B through the lens of Physician Cultural Responsibility, Mr. B's needs can be addressed in a way that honors his cultural values.

2. What biases may Mr. B be facing in this patient encounter?

As patients are intersectional, so are the biases that they may meet. In practicing Physician Cultural Responsibility, this understanding of intersectionality is key is reflecting upon biases that healthcare workers may have and countering them. This can be difficult as biases are not often understood are recognized, even by the person holding them. Implicit bias, or biases held but hidden, are dangerous as they impact decisions, behaviors, interactions, and health outcomes (Feagin & Bennefiled, 2013). Once identified, healthcare workers can actively counter these biases, lessening their impact on the way they care for their patients.

In this case, Mr. B is assumed to speak English as his first language and thus is not given the opportunity to request an interpreter with the initial healthcare workers even though this is detailed in his forms. This creates confusion for the patient and Dr. G as many misunderstandings and misinterpretations result in frustration for both parties. Biases about accents can also lead to patients being treated differently as those with strong accents may be assumed not to speak English and those who have less identifiable accents may be assumed to have English fluency. Further, one's ability to speak a language does not imply their ability to read and write in that language. It is crucial to review demographics with the patient, including preferred language, and to ask if patients need an interpreter, translated forms, or other assistance in their preferred language to assist in providing equitable care (Brisset et al, 2013). Likewise, because of this Mr. B is also assumed to as to be able to pay for his services based on making $70,000 yearly, without insurance or the discussion of family size which could have complicated his care further without the intervention of Dr. N.

Further, biases involving external appearance can lead individuals to assume nationality. Mr. B is noted here to be racially ambiguous then later identified as Haitian. As one may hold stereotypes about what individuals from different countries look, sound, or act like, implicit biases can result in healthcare workers changing behavior towards patients that fit those stereotypes and negatively impacting patient care. As an example, in reading this case and seeing that he was racially ambiguous, one may have read the interaction with Dr. G, and implicitly assigned a nationality to him only to find this to be incongruent to his actual identity. This is significant as these implicit associations can impact one's interaction with the patient, the treatments offered to patients, and thus their health outcomes (Feagin & Bennefiled, 2013).

3. What cultural values or norms are being assumed? Which may be missing? What does the language in this scenario tell us about the assumptions being made?

Mr. B is othered in this scenario. He is seen as one who does not fit and must assimilate to the norms of his surroundings. Within the first paragraph of the case, Mr. B is introduced in a way that sets the expectation that he should speak English better after being in the United States for some time highlighting the expectation of assimilation into the American culture. Shortly after, Mr. B is noted attempting to elevate his finances to hide his current financial situation with concern of his information being shared with immigration. The cultural norms that he may hold remain unknown, however the general American cultural norm has been described to include individualism, or the idea that the self is separate from society (Kirayama et. al., 2010). This is evident in the concerns that Mr. B has associated with policies that would endanger his family if he was to divulge any needs.

Later, in the patient encounter, Dr. G dives into assessment instead of than discussing Mr. B's concerns. Rather than being provided with the opportunity to discuss the plan with Dr. G after openly saying he doesn't understand, it is assumed that Mr. B's mentation is compromised without considering that Mr. B does not speak English as his first language. While this elevated blood pressure does necessitate urgent treatment, Mr. B is treated as though he does not have the health literacy to be able to understand his medical situation. There is no exploration of Mr. B's perceptions, the reasons why he may not agree that this is an emergency or large risk, or addressing his concerns. Mr. B's questions expose misunderstanding as he repeats his weight in pounds with a unit in kilograms but rather than the health care team using this as an opportunity to clarify, Mr. B's questions went unanswered. Further, Dr. G chooses to discuss Mr. B as the "blood pressure in room 4", placing his condition before his humanity which can prevent healthcare workers from remembering to value the person before the problem.

In the encounter with Dr. N, where Physician Cultural Responsibility is displayed, Mr. B is noted to value being heard. Again, while his cultural norms are not explicitly discussed in this case, it is possible that there is an inherent mismatch here which can be overcome. Intercultural communication can exist, regardless of the patient's ethnicity or nationality as two individuals from the same country and racial group can have differing cultural norms (Chiper, 2013; DeVoss et. al., 2002). Considering the facets of communication beyond the words that are used including tone, volume, eye contact and gestures, expectations of the timing of speech, and even the distance between those communicating is important to prevent potential miscommunication (DeVoss et. al., 2002).

In this case, the medical assistant was likely unaware that the speed at which she was communicating was difficult for the patient to answer. Further, open ended questions, rather than those with yes or no answers are more likely to provide the patient with an opportunity to express concerns with understanding the question (Chandra et. al, 2018). When Dr. G arrives, rather than attempting to further explain the concern to the patient in a way that he may understand, his first act is to retake the patient's blood pressure, inviting himself into the patient's personal space. In his haste, concerned about whether the patient was having an emergency, he fails to answer the patient's questions or to recognize the patient has used a unit of measurement that isn't used commonly in the United States and suggests the patient visit the emergency room. Mr. B has now been excluded from making decisions in his care, highlighting the power dynamics which can negatively impact care and relationships with healthcare workers, especially among the confusion created when not considering cultural differences in communication (American Medical Association and American Association of Medical Colleges Center for Health Justice, 2021; DeVoss et al, 2002; Inoue, 2020).

4. Whose stories are being told in this encounter? What more is needed to understand Mr. B's and Dr. G's needs in this situation?

In this case, the story focuses on the inner monologue from the patient and displays the inner turmoil of communication difficulties in the healthcare setting. There is some discussion of Mr. B's life stressors, social determinants of health, needs and values, but much of this is left out of the story, allowing for the reader to assess their own biases. The use of the practice of Physician Cultural Responsibility by Dr. N, assists in giving a more holistic view of his needs and can allow for better care to be provided.

Very little of Dr. G's story is discussed. It is known that Dr. G was not the physician the patient was supposed to see that day. Dr. G notes apprehension about running behind as well as concern about leaving the office on time to fulfill the promise he made to his wife. There is no further backstory to his workload, his family life, or other obligations that may be creating this dynamic. This also provides some insight into the rushed encounter that he had with Mr. B as Dr. G was called in to assist with a perceived emergency that may not have gone to his expectations. We need more information from Dr. G's perspective.

5. What emotions may Dr. G be feeling right now? What is causing them?

Dr. G's emotions aside from concerns surrounding his work obligations and family life are not explicitly stated. It is known that he responded to an emergency, sacrificing his ability to potentially get home in a timely fashion, in an effort to assist a patient that refused to follow his advice. One may see that the stress associated with the abnormal vitals from the patient and Dr. G's personal family obligations could have pushed him outside of personally held values in patient-centered care and shared decision making. Without the urgency of the situation, he may have further discussed the patient's needs but, in this case, decided on a plan and attempted to quickly discussing this with the patient in order to continue with the many other responsibilities that he has at this time.

Healthcare workers often enter the field of healthcare because they like to help others, describing themselves as altruistic people (Burks & Kobus, 2012). However, it is important to note that when under stress, even when one is aware of biases and social determinants of health that impact patient care, one may fall short of their own goals to mitigate these. Work-life balance has been noted as a key driver in the burnout cascade (Shanafelt et. al., 2019; West, et. al., 2018; Williams et. al., 2019).

It is possible the Dr. G is not aware of his burnout symptoms at this time and their impact on patient interactions. This furthers the cycle which can contribute to moral injury and increased burnout. Self-reflection can increase his awareness to his stressors. It is imperative at this point, to begin the discussion of resources to treat burnout. These may include negotiating additional support during clinical hours, decreasing patient load, or seeking emotional support to allow him to prevent the consequences of burnout on his mental health, patient care, and his family obligations.

Epilogue

This case provides an example of the impacts of the social determinants of health, implicit biases associated with nationality and language, and burnout on patient care. The social determinants of health can create additional barriers for even the savviest patients. The skills of intercultural communication are vital in ensuring that these barriers can be overcome. Intercultural communication can mean communication between parties of different nationalities but in reality, each person comes from a different culture and these differences pose space for misunderstandings and miscommunication in every discussion (DeVoss et al, 2002). Individual perspective is deeply rooted in cultural norms and experiences. Healthcare worker burnout can also make those providing care less able to realize these misunderstandings and accommodate patient needs.

The Physician Cultural Responsibility framework questions provide an opportunity to examine the impact of healthcare worker burnout and personal biases on the care provided to Mr. B. This includes the examination of potential viewpoints that are missing, an examination of patient values and culture including how these may be different from the assumed norm, and social factors and intersectionality that impacts patient needs. Just as the medical assistant, in this case, did not specify the unit used for the measurement of Mr. B's weight or an interpreter wasn't offered, Mr. B's care is impacted by the lack of intercultural communication and healthcare worker burnout as well as the social determinants of health that he was facing. As all of the identities that Mr. B held were not explicitly identified, one may note the unwritten story that one may have created for the patient through personal biases as well as the tension created within the case when biases dictate needs rather than patients.

Best practices suggest always offering and utilizing a medical interpretation service for patient encounters where patients may not speak English as their first language. Family members may not provide word-for-word interpretations which can negatively impact care for patients. Likewise, avoiding slang, figures of speech, irony, or sarcasm is important as cultural norms vary (DeVoss et al, 2002). As stressful situations and burnout can change one's usual practice, the utilization of self-awareness and self-reflection techniques can assist healthcare workers in identifying their needs, biases, and emotions. Specifically identifying the emotions that one is feeling, the ways in which personal values or thoughts may be challenged or stretched, and identifying one's own needs can help health care workers to address burnout and to prevent their impact on patient care.

CASE 2: CALLING ON CALL

Goal

This case displays the barriers to unbiased care for patients on the basis of gender identity, highlighting the impact of stereotypes and the social categorization of medicine.

Learning Outcomes

1. Describe the Social Determinants of Health that impact the care of patients.
2. Identify biases that impact the care of patients of various gender identities as well as patients with mental health diagnoses.
3. Identify the barriers to care facing patients with caregiving responsibilities.
4. Assess the impact of the social categorization of medicine on patient care outcomes utilizing Physician Cultural Responsibility.
5. Identify the emotional needs and resource to assist with healthcare workers through the practice of self-awareness and self-reflection in Physician Cultural Responsibility.

Case

Mrs. L is a 52-year-old female who is calling for medical advice after an "episode". She reaches the on-call team after mustering the courage to call. Dr. R is the physician on call. "Dr. R, you have a patient L that called for an "episode" the operator noted.

"What is an episode?" Dr. R asked.

"I'm not sure, that is all she said. Would you like the number?" replied the operator.

"Thanks," said Dr. R as she put her 11-month-old down and picked up a pen to write down the number. Dr. R proceeded to open the patient's chart and review it prior to making the call to see what an episode may include. She read the problem list, noting a history of a miscarriage at 22, sciatica, fibromyalgia, and anxiety. When looking for Mrs. L's last appointment with her primary care doctor, she notices Mrs. L was last seen 8 months ago and her few appointments are scattered between multiple no-shows and late canceled appointments with the psychologist. From the note, it appears that Mrs. L has a normal BMI, eats a healthy diet, and exercises daily with her husband and adult daughter.

"Good evening, Mrs. L. I am Dr. R, the physician on call at your doctor's office. I heard you wanted to discuss an episode earlier?" Dr. R asks after rolling her eyes and confirming that Mrs. L was who answered the phone.

"Yes. I was outside this afternoon in my garden pruning my hydrangeas and I felt like I was going to upchuck. I came in and went to the bathroom, sat there for a while, never puked but my stomach was turning, it hasn't stopped turning either, and I feel all hot and clammy, and…" Mrs. L said before being interrupted.

"Any chest pain Mrs. L?"

"No but I just feel like I'm running but I'm not and I'm all hot and clammy and I don't know what is happening to me because this never…" Mrs. L stated before being interrupted again.

"Mrs. L are you having trouble breathing? What did you eat today" Dr. R asked.

"Uhhh, I ate some potato salad with celery and grapes for lunch before I came out but I really don't feel good so I skipped dinner. I can breathe I think but I just feel like everything is going so fast and I really need to finish my pruning because my sister is coming tomorrow and I can't have her see my garden and my house like this!" Mrs. L replied.

Dr. R replied "Well Mrs. L, looking at your history and your labs in your chart I don't think you are at risk for anything serious. Seems like you take pretty good care of yourself. Potato salad is notorious for causing food poisoning. It sounds like that might be the issue here. Let's have you hydrate tonight and get some rest and if you need we can get you in in the morning to see your PCP. Okay?"

"Okay" Mrs. L replied as she thought to herself, "Maybe I am just crazy. I don't remember getting any labs". Mrs. L ends the call and sits on the bathroom floor just in case she vomits.

Mr. L knocks on the bathroom door 3 hours later, hearing his wife sobbing in the bathroom. "Honey, you alright?"

Mrs. L replies, " I'm not feeling well, doctor said its food poisoning and they'll see me tomorrow but I think this is something else."

Mr. L sighs, "It's 3 o'clock in the morning. I'll grab the trash can if you'll come lay down. You've been in there for hours. Ashley already went to bed"

"I'm so tired, I don't know if I can move," Mrs. L says through her tears. Mrs. L calls the office again and reaches the on-call operator and explains her concern. She puts the phone on her chest and closes her eyes again. "If I could just throw up maybe I would feel better." She whispers to herself.

The phone rings. "Dr. R, you have a patient L that called to discuss her plan of care with you further, looks like she called earlier too" the operator noted.

"You have got to be kidding me. She is fine." Dr. R replied over the audible screams of a baby.

"Would you like the number?" replied the operator.

"No, I have it. Thanks" said Dr. R as she hung up and immediately dialed Mrs. L.

"Mrs. L. Its Dr. R again, what's up?" Dr. R says with her screaming child in the background.

"I haven't thrown up yet but I am so afraid it's something else, I am more tired than I think I've ever been." Mrs. L says choking back tears. "What can I do to make this go away?"

Dr. R sighs, "Mrs. L, is your chest bothering you?"

"No"

"Are you struggling to breathe?"

"No"

"Are you bleeding or having stomach pain so bad you can't sleep?"

"No, I just feel like I'm in danger. I don't feel good, and I'm tired, and I don't know how much longer I can hold on."

"Mrs. L, what do you mean by that? Do you have thoughts of hurting yourself?"

"Heavens no! I just feel like I'm going to die. I have my husband and my daughter to care for. I can't die now"

"Mrs. L, I think you are tired because it is now 3:34 am and you have been feeling off since yesterday. Anxiety can make us feel like we are going to die. I would recommend you take a pill and get some rest. We open in 4 and a half hours and I made you the first appointment I could. Let's try to get some rest, huh? If your chest starts hurting or you have trouble breathing, or you start bleeding, please call 911"

"Okay"

"Okay, I'll see you tomorrow." Dr. R said as she hung up and tried to get her child back to bed.

Mrs. L thought, "if only I could get comfortable", closing her eyes while laying on the bathroom floor. Her husband knocked on the door again, "Honey, what did the doctor say? It's been 3 more hours! Did you fall asleep in there?" No answer. "Ashley, can you check on your mom? My wheelchair won't let me peak in and I don't want to hit her if she's behind the door."

"Mom? Uh Dad she's in here but she won't move and she won't wake up. Mom! Mommy!"

Mr. L called EMS, who arrived within minutes. After leading his daughter to another room, EMS told Mr. L that his wife had suffered a heart attack and they would be rushing her to the hospital. Upon arrival, Mrs. L was sent to the cath lab to have a procedure to reopen the vessels to her heart. It is likely that the heart attack occurred while she was gardening. After 5 long days, she regains consciousness and is on the road to recovery. Mrs. L has never trusted doctors but was cared for by a great team in the hospital and promises to continue her visits with their outpatient cardiology and primary care services. Her husband and her daughter depend on her to do most of the household tasks as well as for transportation so they have had to rely on her sister to assist. When Mrs. L is discharged, she is connected with services including home health care and cardiac rehab as she is now unable to care for herself independently.

QUESTIONS AND ANSWERS

1. Identify the social determinants of health experienced by Mrs. L.?

In the case above, it is noted that Mrs. L has irregular follow up with multiple no-showed appointments present. This can suggest multiple concerns with the social determinants of health including issues with accessing care potentially secondary to transportation, social supports, occupational obligations, financial stresses, or general concerns with the quality of care she has received in the past. While all of these answers are speculated as the case does not directly speak to her concerns initially, she later discloses that she has a mistrust of the medical system. It is also revealed that she is the primary caregiver for both her husband and her adult daughter. Likewise, Mrs. L does not describe anyone else as a support except her sister who lives out of town and was coming to visit per the case, nor is Mrs. L explicitly noted to be working. This may raise questions about caregiver support as well as economic opportunity or stability.

Mrs. L notes that she ate potato salad with celery and grapes for lunch which may or may not be associated with food insecurity. In utilizing the practice of Physician Cultural Responsibility, one can better ascertain whether Mrs. L ate this because this is a normal lunch for her or if this was all that was available to her as cultural differences may place potato salad as a side dish rather than a main course for lunch. It is important to assess the patient's cultural norms here as assumptions that she did not have other options could negatively impact patient rapport. As the social determinants of health are vast, so are the many answers that one may have for this question. The social determinants of health mentioned above are not an exhaustive list of what one may ascertain from this text as additional details are needed from Mrs. L. However, in utilizing Physician Cultural Responsibility, healthcare workers can better identify and address these social factors. While considering the social determinants of health experienced by Mrs. L through the lens of Physician Cultural Responsibility, Mrs. L's needs can be addressed in a way that respects and validates her individual concerns.

2. What biases may Mrs. L be facing in this patient encounter?

Mrs. L is noted to have anxiety and fibromyalgia. The biases against patients with mental health conditions can often leave patients without support from healthcare workers, as they are less likely to take their concerns seriously and attribute these concerns to their mental health diagnoses (Thornicroft et. al., 2007). Biases like these are passed throughout the field of medicine, through the social categorization of medicine, prompting healthcare workers to characterize patients without unfairly (Blackie et. al., 2019). For example, as a patient with fibromyalgia, a painful syndrome that has been associated with mental health diagnoses, Mrs. L may find that many healthcare workers attribute her pain to somatic symptoms associated with her anxiety. As the disorder can be very difficult to treat, the literature notes negative stigma associated with the disorder from healthcare workers that impacts patents, causing feelings of isolation and disbelief while suffering from something that others cannot see (Arfuch et. al., 2022).

This is amplified for people identifying as female. Studies show that female patients' concerns are often attributed to emotions contributing to later diagnosis and poorer outcomes (Samulowitz et al, 2018). In this encounter, Mrs. L could have easily been having symptoms associated with anxiety or gastrointestinal illness, however these symptoms could also be attributed to cardiac crisis in women. It can be noted that the intersectionality of being female, having a mental health diagnosis, and having a highly stigmatized disorder can easily allow for healthcare workers to employ confirmation bias, or prematurely deciding on an answer prior to assessing all possible outcomes. While noting the information that was given, one may examine personal thoughts about the patient's needs as the case progressed, compared to after learning the final outcome.

The dangers of implicit bias can also lurk in unexpected settings. When discussing gender bias, one may consider that Dr. R would be acutely considering these facts as she is also female. However, it is possible for one to have shared identity with another and still harbor biases that impact their care. In this case, Dr. R may have considered the limited history that was presented to her as the on-call physician and prematurely ruled out the patient's risk for cardiac disease based on what as written. She was not aware of the patient's family history. This bias towards her mental health diagnosis may have further anchored her to the patient having a panic attack or food poisoning and overreacting versus potentially having something more serious going on. With Physician Cultural Responsibility, one considers the thought that the patient is overreacting as an opportunity to further explore the patient's needs and motivations behind the reaction present. Mrs. L was never asked if she had experienced panic attacks or if this episode was similar, nor was the option of seeking care sooner to reassure the patient given aside from the specific criteria to seek emergency assistance. Mrs. L attempted to note that she had not experienced this before but was interrupted during the encounter.

3. What cultural values or norms are being assumed? Which may be missing? What does the language in this scenario tell us about the assumptions being made?

Mrs. L notes grave concern about her health in this scenario but it not taken seriously. As noted, the dialogue between Dr. R and Mrs. L suggests Dr. R may have been employing confirmation bias in her medical decision-making. Whether this is centers on the perceived absence of risk factors or is associated with biases associated with Mrs. L's mental health diagnoses and even gender biases remain unclear. Dr. R reviews the chart and seems to be able to reassure Mrs. L, noting that she is healthy and has few risk factors. However, when Mrs. L calls again, asking for further assistance, Dr. R responds that the patient is fine before speaking to her again and attributes the continued symptoms with the patient's mental health. It becomes clear Mrs. L is being evaluated for psychiatric crisis when Dr. R asks if she is having suicidal thoughts and continues to recommend taking medication for the anxiety rather than diving further into why the patient feels as though she may die after Mrs. L denies suicidal ideation.

Likewise, one may have gleaned the matriarchal cultural norm displayed here as both Mrs. L and Dr. R are both female and caring for their families in a way that sacrifices some of their own wellness. It may be worth considering how this case may have been different if these two characters were men and how the assumptions may have changed. One may assume that Dr. R had other options for support to assist with her child during her call shift. Further, one may assume that Mrs. L's sister is supportive and willing or even able to assist with the tasks that Mrs. L is unable to do. It is important to note that so little information is given about the characters' families that these assumptions may prevent one from considering their additional needs for support. While caretakers, like Mrs. L, are noted to have higher risks of cardiovascular disease, increases in depression, and lower wellness overall, Schulz and Sherwood (2009) describe that this is dependent on the needs of those being cared for and the support that the caregiver receives. For example, one may assume that her husband and daughter are not financially contributing to the household since they depend on her for assistance with household tasks and transportation while that may not be the case. In the practice of Physician Cultural Responsibility, healthcare workers can better ascertain what needs that the L family has and how to best support them through identifying what information one is drawing from assumptions and proceeding to ask further questions to ensure alignment with patients needs and values. As personal experience drives perception, the assumptions noted here may not be inclusive of all the assumptions that exist in this case.

4. Whose stories are being told in this encounter? What more is needed to understand Mrs. L's and Dr. R's needs in this situation?

This case is primarily documented from Mrs. L's point of view in her acute distress. She notes feeling very concerned about her health and feeling disbelieved about the severity of her symptoms as she considered if she was "crazy" during her call with Dr. R. This reaffirms the feelings of mistrust for the medical system that she later describes. For the majority of the case, one is unaware that she is caring for those around her and unaware of the impact of caregiving on possibly her multiple calls as well as her difficulties to keep her own appointments. Physician Cultural Responsibility can allow health care workers to validate her concerns through collaboratively building a care plan that meets her needs.

Dr. R's story is overwhelmingly missing. It is known that she is the physician on call, that she is caring for a young child, and she does not know Mrs. L. Further, she reviewed Mrs. L's chart and provided medical advice based on what was available to her. It can be speculated that she is tired as this scenario is occurring in the middle of the night. Dr. R may also be overwhelmed and even frustrated as the child was crying at midnight during the initial call and again at three in the morning. However, little is known about her needs in this situation. The reader is unaware of if she has a support system to help her with childcare or if her support system is sleeping as they may care for the child during the day. It is also unknown what her call experience and thus stress levels have been like within the last 24 hours. Additional information about Dr. R's story may provide additional understanding to the way the encounter unfolded.

5. What emotions may Dr. R be feeling right now? What is causing them?

Dr. R's emotions, while not explicitly noted, can be observed through some of her responses, especially after receiving the second call. In this case, Dr. R seems torn between her own caregiving obligations and the obligations of her work. While speculated, she may be feeling overwhelmed by all of her responsibilities, especially while trying to soothe a small child and having to address seemingly nonemergent calls in the middle of the night. Further, she may be feeling frustrated that she is attempting to help a patient who is not taking her advice but continues to call. In not knowing what support that Dr. R has to assist her and what kind of day she has had, it is possible that she has been handling stressful situations all day, and not having any support of her own to allow her to recharge for her call shift.

Both the presence and the impacts of burnout are higher in female healthcare workers, placing Dr. R at greater risk for its impacts on her health, self-care, and patient outcomes (Shanafelt et. al., 2019; West, et. al., 2018; Williams et. al., 2019). Further, the burnout symptom of exhaustion has been associated with increasing depression (West, et. al., 2018). It has also been noted that probability of medical errors rises alongside one's level of burnout (West, et. al., 2018). This cycle can continue as medical errors can further contribute to depression and burnout symptoms.

Dr. R may be facing, if not already experiencing, burnout. At this point the literature suggests a focus on self-care, managing stress, and assessing the impact of professional obligations on personal wellness to prevent further harm (West, et. al., 2018). In utilizing the practice of Physician Cultural Responsibility, Dr. R can begin self- reflection to address these topics and grow in awareness of her needs at this time. Through naming and validating her emotions, she may be able to better recognize the challenges that she is facing and sources of support to assist her in overcoming them rather than attempting to push through alone. Dr. R may consider looking to her support system, if she has one, to assist her when duties like call require more of her time or consider altering her schedule or work obligations, at least temporarily to address the challenge of caregiving while on call. Further, she may want to seek spaces for personal support to attempt to assist with the symptoms of burnout.

Epilogue

This case provides a close examination of how healthcare worker burnout and biases can impact patient care. Stereotypes especially surrounding patients with mental health diagnoses can create barriers for patients to have their concerns taken seriously. Likewise, gender biases hinder female-identifying patients as their concerns are often thought to be emotionally driven (Samulowitz et al, 2018). Further, as symptoms may differ from those of male patients which are routinely learned and researched in much of the medical literature, female patients have higher rates of delayed diagnosis and poorer outcomes (Samulowitz et al, 2018). The social categorization of medicine allows for these biases to persist and is hazardous to patient outcomes. Healthcare workers must be mindful of biases and differences when caring for patients to prevent missing critical diagnoses as well as have an awareness of the impact of personal biases on patient care outcomes.

The Physician Cultural Responsibility framework questions provide an opportunity to examine the impact of healthcare worker burnout and personal biases on the care provided to Mrs. L. Just as Mrs. L's presentation was very similar to routine and nonemergent ailments, confirmation bias and stereotypes can create dangerous situations that complicate patient care and negatively impact outcomes. This when matched with the influences of the social determinants of health and healthcare worker burnout, can further this harm. Patients who have caregiving roles may also have different risks and need additional support in their health journey. Specifically examining patient needs and becoming aware of the impact of the intersectionality of patients can assist in ensuring that patients receive equitable care.

Utilizing self-awareness and self-reflection focused on the healthcare workers emotions and thoughts can assist healthcare workers in identifying their own biases and needs. It is important to consider that biases can be present even when patients and healthcare workers have shared identities. These assumed similarities can provide space for implicit biases to go unrecognized and unmitigated, potentially creating space for healthcare workers to make assumptions about patients that impact their care.

REFERENCES

Amanullah, S., & Ramesh Shankar, R. (2020). The Impact of COVID-19 on Physician Burnout Globally: A Review. *Health Care*, *8*(4), 421. doi:10.3390/healthcare8040421 PMID:33105757

American Medical Association and American Association of Medical Colleges Center for Health Justice. (2021). *Advancing Health Equity: A guide to language, narrative, and concepts*. American Medical Association.

Arfuch, V. M., Angelats, R. C., Martin, C. A., Goncalves, A. Q., Carrasco-Querol, N., & Gonzalez Serra, G. (2022). Patients' Lived Experience in a Multicomponent Intervention for Fibromyalgia Syndrome in Primary Care: A Qualitative Interview Study. *International Journal of Environmental Research and Public Health*, *19*(20), 13322. Advance online publication. doi:10.3390/ijerph192013322 PMID:36293900

Betancourt, J. R., Green, A. R., Carrillo, J. E., & Ananeh-Firempong, O. II. (2003). Defining Cultural Competence: A practical framework for addressing racial/ethnic disparities in health and health care. *Public Health Reports*, *118*(4), 293–302. doi:10.1016/S0033-3549(04)50253-4 PMID:12815076

Blackie, M., Wear, D., & Zarconi, J. (2019). Narrative Intersectionality in Caring for Marginalized or Disadvantaged Patients. *Academic Medicine, 94*(1), 59–63. doi:10.1097/ACM.0000000000002425 PMID:30134270

Brisset, C., Leanza, Y., & Laforest, K. (2013). Working with interpreters in health care: A systematic review and meta-ethnography of qualitative studies. *Patient Education and Counseling, 91*(2), 131–140. doi:10.1016/j.pec.2012.11.008 PMID:23246426

Brookfield, S. D. (2010). *Theoretical Frameworks for Understanding the Field. In Handbook of Adult and Continuing Education.* SAGE.

Burks, D. J., & Kobus, A. M. (2012). The legacy of altruism in health care: The promotion of empathy, prosociality and humanism. *Medical Education, 2012*(46), 317–325. doi:10.1111/j.1365-2923.2011.04159.x PMID:22324531

Chandra, S., Mohammadnezhad, M., & Ward, P. (2018). Trust and Communication in a Doctor- Patient Relationship: A Literature Review. *Journal of Healthcare Communications, 3*(36), 1–6. doi:10.4172/2472-1654.100146

Chiper, S. (2013) Teaching Intercultural Communication: ICT resources and best practices. *Procedia Social and Behavioral Sciences, 93*, 1641-1645. doi:10.1016/j.sbspro.2013.10.094

Crenshaw, K. (1991). Mapping the Margins: Intersectionality, Identity Politics, and Violence against Women of Color. *Stanford Law Review, 43*(6), 1241–1299. doi:10.2307/1229039

DeVoss, D., Jasken, J., & Hayden, D. (2002). Teaching Intracultural and Intercultural Communication: A critique suggested method. *Journal of Business and Technical Communication, 16*(1), 69–94. doi:10.1177/1050651902016001003

Dobie, S. (2007). Reflections on a Well-Traveled Path: Self-awareness, mindful practice, and relationship centered care as foundations for medical education. *Academic Medicine, 82*(4), 422–427. doi:10.1097/01.ACM.0000259374.52323.62 PMID:17414201

Feagin, J., & Bennefiled, Z. (2013). Systemic racism and US health care. *Social Science & Medicine, 103*, 7–14. doi:10.1016/j.socscimed.2013.09.006 PMID:24507906

Foronda, C., Baptiste, D., Reinholdt, M. M., & Ousman, K. (2016). Cultural Humility: A Concept Analysis. *Journal of Transcultural Nursing, 27*(3), 210–217. doi:10.1177/1043659615592677 PMID:26122618

Fried, J. E., Shipman, S. A., & Sessums, L. L. (2019). Advocacy: Achieving Physician Competency. *Journal of Internal Medicine, 34*(11), 2297–2298. doi:10.100711606-019-05278-y PMID:31420826

Hunter, K., & Thompson, B. (2019). A Scoping review of Social Determinants of Health Curricula in Post-Graduate Medical Education. *Canadian Medical Education Journal, 10*(3), e61–e71. doi:10.36834/cmej.61709 PMID:31388378

Inoue, A. B. (2020). Teaching Antiracist Writing. *Journal of College Reading and Learning, 50*(1), 1–23. doi:10.1080/10790195.2020.1787079

Johnson, C. (2022, February). *Physician Cultural Responsibility* [Unpublished Doctoral Study Manuscript]. Antioch University, Seattle, WA, United States.

Kinayama, S., Karasawa, M., Curhan, K. B., Ryff, C. D., & Markus, H. R. (2010). Independence and interdependence predict health and wellbeing: Divergent patterns in the United States and Japan. *Frontiers in Psychology*, *1*(163), 1–10. doi:10.3389/fpsyg.2010.00163 PMID:21833228

Magnan, S. (2017). *Social Determinants of Health 101 for Health Care: Five Plus Five. In NAM Perspectives*. National Academy of Medicine. doi:10.31478/201710c

Masters, C., Robinson, D., Faulkner, S., Patterson, E., McIlraith, T., & Ansari, A. (2019). Addressing Biases in Patient Care with The 5Rs of Cultural Humility, a Clinician Coaching Tool. *Journal of General Internal Medicine*, *34*(4), 627–630. doi:10.100711606-018-4814-y PMID:30623383

National Institutes of Health. (2007). *Cultural Awareness Glossary of Key Terms*. https://www.niehs.nih.gov/news/events/pastmtg/hazmat/assets/2007/wtp_2007ntec_wruc_latino_tips_glossary_508.pdf

Nazar, M., Kendall, K., Day, L., & Nazar, H. (2015). Decolonising medical curricula through diversity education: Lessons from students. *Medical Teacher*, *37*(4), 385–393. doi:10.3109/0142159X.2014.947938 PMID:25156358

Nedrow, A., Steckler, N. A., Hardman, J. (2012). Physician Resilience and Burnout: Can you make the switch. *Family Practice Management,* 25-30.

Samulowitz, A., Gremyr, I., Eriksson, E., & Hensing, G. (2018). "Brave Men" and "Emotional Women": A theory-guided literature review on gender bias in health care and gendered norms towards patients with chronic pain. *Pain Research & Management*, *2018*, 1–14. doi:10.1155/2018/6358624 PMID:29682130

Schulz, R., & Sherwood, P. R. (2009). Physical and Mental Health Effects of Family Caregiving. *The American Journal of Nursing*, *108*(9), 23–27. doi:10.1097/01.NAJ.0000336406.45248.4c PMID:18797217

Shanafelt, T. D., West, C. P., Sinsky, C., Trockel, M., Tutty, M., Satele, D. V., Carlasare, L. E., & Dyrbye, L. N. (2019). Changes in Burnout and Satisfaction With Work-Life Integration in Physicians and the General US Working Population Between 2011 and 2017. *Mayo Clinic Proceedings*, *94*(9), 1681–1694. doi:10.1016/j.mayocp.2018.10.023 PMID:30803733

Sotto-Santiado, A., Poll-Hunter, N., Trice, T., Buenconsejo-Lum, L., Golden, S., Howell, J., Jacobs, N., Lee, W., Mason, H., Ogunyemi, D., Crespon, W., & Lamba, S. (2022, January). A Framework for Developing Antiracist Medical Educators and Prationer-Scholars. *Academic Medicine*, *97*(1), 41–47. Advance online publication. doi:10.1097/ACM.0000000000004385

Tervalon, M., & Murray-Garcia, J. (1998). Cultural Humility Versus Cultural Compentence: A critical distinction in defining physician training outcomes in multicultural education. *Journal of Health Care for the Poor and Underserved*, *9*(2), 117–125. doi:10.1353/hpu.2010.0233 PMID:10073197

Thornicroft, G., Rose, D., & Kassam, A. (2007). Discrimination in health care against people with mental illness. *International Review of Psychiatry (Abingdon, England)*, *19*(2), 113–122. doi:10.1080/09540260701278937 PMID:17464789

U.S. Department of Health and Human Services. (in press). *Disparities: Healthy People 2030*. U.S. Department of Health and Human Services, Office of Disease Prevention and Health Promotion.

West, C. P., Dyrbye, L. N., & Shanafelt, T. D. (2018). Physician burnout: Contributors, consequences and solutions. *Journal of Internal Medicine*, *283*(6), 516–529. doi:10.1111/joim.12752 PMID:29505159

Williams, E. S., Rathert, C., & Buttigieg, S. C. (2019). The Personal and Professional Consequences of Physician Burnout: A Systematic Review of the Literature. *Medical Care Research and Review: MCRR*, *77*(5), 371–386. doi:10.1177/1077558719856787 PMID:31216940

Wright, A. A., & Katz, I. T. (2018). Beyond Burnout— Redesigning Care to Restore Meaning and Sanity for Physicians. *The New England Journal of Medicine*, *378*(4), 309–311. doi:10.1056/NEJMp1716845 PMID:29365301

Chapter 17
Curiosity, Humility, and Accountability:
Key Elements to Advance a Culture of Diversity, Equity, and Inclusion in Health Professions Education

Monica Yepes-Rios
https://orcid.org/0000-0001-8270-8608
Cleveland Clinic Foundation, USA

Monica Chavan
https://orcid.org/0000-0001-6480-2190
Case Western Reserve University School of Medicine, USA

Maria Claudia Moncaliano
https://orcid.org/0000-0003-3671-0533
Case Western Reserve University School of Medicine, USA

Amy L. Wilson-Delfosse
Case Western Reserve University School of Medicine, USA

Yael Mauer
Cleveland Clinic Foundation, USA

Colleen Croniger
https://orcid.org/0000-0002-8300-0983
Case Western Reserve University School of Medicine, USA

Jason V. Lambrese
Cleveland Clinic Foundation, USA

Lia Logio
https://orcid.org/0000-0002-5686-9237
Case Western Reserve University School of Medicine, USA

EXECUTIVE SUMMARY

Health professions educators have the opportunity and responsibility to teach and stimulate scientific knowledge and curiosity in a context that eliminates bias towards minoritized communities and informs emerging understanding of race in research and healthcare. Through the key elements of curiosity, humility, and accountability, the authors propose methods to change the narrative that may otherwise perpetuate biases and inappropriate presentations of race as purely biological rather than a social

DOI: 10.4018/978-1-6684-5493-0.ch017

construct. The evolution of scientific discovery has brought to question our understanding and teaching of race in health, clinical decision-making, and health outcomes. Through case presentations, the authors invite the reader to reflect on their teaching materials and apply methods to 1) decrease bias in case presentations and 2) explain racial health disparities in the context of longstanding structural racism. A Q&A section will draw on resources to advance health equity in health professions education.

BACKGROUND

Health professions education has struggled to eliminate bias based on race and other demographic identifiers. Just as such biases have been historically woven into the legal, financial, and housing industries, health professions education has been impacted by systemic racism. Consequently, newly trained health professionals are graduating from programs with curricula that may fail to acknowledge the inherent biases and may have gaps addressing diversity, equity, and inclusion which have been unconsciously incorporated into their core teachings. Examples of these limitations include course materials that use gender-specific language for sexual health topics, textbooks and diagrams that exclusively use light skin tones as models and representations of skin diseases, and epidemiologic data that indicates individuals of a particular racial or ethnic demographic have a propensity for a particular disease. Evidence has shown that these limitations perpetuate unconscious biases amongst health professionals, leading to race essentialism (Herd et al., 2021; Rhodes & Moty, 2020) and can negatively impact health outcomes (Amutah et al., 2021).

Reexamining the inherent biases in health professions curricula is a necessary step to begin to address how biases perpetuate health disparities amongst marginalized groups. Medical, physician assistant, dental, nursing, and other health professions students benefit from curricula that directly and intentionally address the patient diversity that trainees will see in future clinical practice. Patients often have intersectional identities with complex and individualized social determinants of health, which should not be simplified to race or socioeconomic status alone. Health professions students must be trained to see beyond their own unconscious biases and recognize the limits of their own lived experiences. Only then can students begin to identify inherent biases built into the healthcare system and understand the challenges patients face in overcoming them.

By nature of current events and internet-based grassroots movements for social justice, today's health professions students are more aware of their own biases and of historic injustices towards marginalized groups in healthcare (Brooks, 2015). Yet health professions educators are uniquely positioned to encouragae trainees to consider how that *awareness* can translate to *clinical practices and professional actions* which can directly address disparities and gaps in care for patients historically marginalized (Cuellar et al., 2008). Health professions educators not only have a responsibility to instruct students in the basic science and technical aspects needed for their future careers, but also have an ethical duty to mentor them on how to become effective and altruistic practitioners and caregivers ("Beyond the Curriculum: Academic Nursing's Responsibility for Excellence in Diversity, Equity, and Inclusion.," 2021). The spirit of service is inherent to clinical practice; society places health professionals in an important and powerful role to serve as patient advocates. With such power comes the responsibility to train health profession students to be mindful of both their individual impact on patients and their ability to become agents of systemic change at the population health level.

A major challenge to large scale improvements and change in health professions curricula is the fact that current educational models have numerous components, each of which is usually overseen by dozens, if not hundreds, of faculty members (Carter & Phillips, 2021). At many institutions, the preclinical component of the curriculum is split into several distinct units, each with a team of faculty leaders who oversee a subsection that is specific to their clinical specialty (McOwen et al., 2020). Attempting to address bias in every aspect of a curriculum at once would be a massive project. It is therefore necessary to institute a culture of change (Parkhurst et al., 2017), wherein the work to address bias in a curriculum is divided across many individuals and becomes a collective and continuous quality improvement effort. This effort would enable multiple approaches and perspectives to address different identities and their intersectionality, and encourage self-reflection from faculty and students alike (Haley & Brown, 2022). Establishing a culture of self-reflection and self-critique in the effort to address unconscious biases within ourselves and our health professions curricula requires administrators to promote three core values for their entire education community: curiosity, humility, and accountability.

Curiosity

Faculty and students together must establish a culture of learning and foster a growth mindset. No person's singular lived experience is sufficient to fully understand systemic racism and historic injustices towards groups historically underrepresented in medicine (URiM). To be curious, teachers and trainees alike must be encouraged to ask questions, learn from one another, and develop a genuine interest in exploring viewpoints and perspectives to which they have not previously been exposed.

Humility

Educators and students must be able to self-reflect and identify gaps in their knowledge and experience. Additionally, a culture of forgiveness must be cultivated to allow those who err to earnestly apologize, be met with forgiveness, and be supported in their genuine attempts to improve. When an individual or an institution demonstrates humility by admitting a mistake this should result in a show of grace from the community. Institutions should be humble enough to admit imperfections and strive for improvement by encouraging faculty and students to speak up in the face of injustice.

Accountability

Each member of an educational community must be held to a high standard of accountability, expected to acknowledge their mistakes. Quality improvement is the responsibility of the community at large, not a lone individual. Both faculty and students must continually evaluate a curriculum to identify areas for improvement and commit to advancing diversity, equity, and inclusion (Schwartz et al., 2020). This requires a level of individual and institutional accountability that must be intentionally created and continually upheld by educators including creating psychological safety in the learning environment (McClintock et al., 2021).

Building a culture that emphasizes curiosity, humility, and accountability requires intentionality on the part of all members at an educational institution – administrators, faculty, staff, and students. At our institutions, students are a driving force in providing feedback on educational content and processes, highlighting aspects of the curriculum that should be prioritized for evaluation of unintended bias. Students and faculty collaborate to create and implement tools to address unconscious bias within our curriculum and amongst educators and learners (Chavan et al., 2022). In addition, numerous faculty members have been recruited to examine the curriculum with respect to an array of potential biases including sexism, racism, ageism, ableism, religion, and discrimination based on ethnicity, sexual orientation, or religion. In building this infrastructure we have set the stage for future efforts to address other aspects of discrimination that have not yet been considered.

One of the most prominent aspects of our institution's preclinical medical curriculum is the "Case Inquiry" model, our version of problem-based small group learning (PBL) (Margolius et al., 2020; Parkhurst et al., 2017). Historically, the patients featured in these cases had pre-selected demographic information including age, gender, race, and home address. These identifiers inadvertently primed students to limit their differential diagnoses and may have contributed to over-ascription of disease pathology to non-biologic factors such as a patient's race. In the first case described below, we will discuss the development of a tool to randomize patient demographic identifiers to provide students the opportunity to see beyond non-biologic factors, – such as social determinants of health – which may impact disease presentation, progression, and clinical management.

In promoting conversations about social determinants of health focusing on addressing unconscious bias, we have also found that trainees new to our programs require instruction on how to exhibit the curiosity, humility, and accountability considered to be core values of our campus culture. In the second case, we will explore how gaps in health professions education further reinforce biases that lead to race essentialism, or the belief that a genetic or biological essence defines all members of a racial category (Herd et al., 2021; Rhodes & Moty, 2020). As educators we must go beyond attributing demographic information to incidence and outcomes of disease, and instead teach students how to investigate the true factors contributing to patient health. We hope this chapter encourages other institutions to use similar tools to promote diversity, equity, and inclusion within health professions training programs.

CASE 1: PROMOTING CONSIDERATION OF DIVERSE POPULATIONS WHILE AVOIDING IMPLICIT BIAS IN LEARNING CASES

Goal

This case explores an approach to augment student exposure to diverse patient identities through small group learning cases (e.g., PBL) while also encouraging faculty and students to be curious, humble, and accountable.

Learning Outcomes

1. Compare and contrast the benefits and potential harms of intentional *versus* random assignment of patient identities in case-based learning approaches.
2. Describe one way that students and faculty can collaborate in the development of curricula.
3. Consider how faculty can be supported to express curiosity and humility while also maintaining accountability in the training of students to care for diverse populations.

Case

Clark Roberts is a second-year medical student who is interested in improving the medical education curriculum at his school. He makes an appointment with Dr. India Quinn, the director of problem-based learning (PBL) and during this meeting asks if Dr. Quinn could make the patients in the PBL cases more diverse. Clark did an audit of the cases in the first-year curriculum and found that race, ethnicity, and sexual orientation were only described for very few of the over 40 cases he encountered during his first year. Clark suggests that Dr. Quinn could start by adding some diversity around LGBTQ+ to just one of the current cases. Dr. Quinn acknowledges that the PBL cases need revision to better represent diversity and is grateful to Clark for sharing the responsibility to improve their curriculum.

Dr. Quinn works with one of the case authors to add diversity around sexual orientation. The author assigns the patient in the case as a gay, white male who has contracted HIV. In a subsequent feedback session with the students, the faculty learned that the addition of sexual orientation to the case was not well received. The students explained that assigning this patient as gay with HIV and developing AIDS was fraught with bias. The faculty member who wrote the case was accused of stereotyping gay men. The method used to assign sexual orientation lacked objectivity and needed to be corrected.

Questions and Answers

1. The medical students were unhappy about the patient with HIV in the PBL case being described as a gay male. What special healthcare concerns of the LGBTQ+ community may have led the students to be concerned about this characterization of this patient?

Although men who have sex with men are at risk for acquiring HIV, there are many other health concerns that need to be considered when working with LGBTQ+ patients. By only commenting on the patient's HIV status, his other health concerns are unrecognized; this runs the risk of reinforcing the notion that HIV is the primary concern when working with gay male patients, framing the patient in this PBL case as stereotypical and one-dimensional. LGBTQ+ patients have difficulty accessing competent healthcare or may avoid the healthcare system due to prior negative experiences, leading to missed opportunities for prevention and disengagement from the healthcare system; other times, LGBTQ+ patients are denied care due to the biases of healthcare providers. By focusing only on the patient's HIV status, this case runs the risk of further contributing to this problem, as students may overemphasize a gay male patient's HIV risk, alienating the patient. LGBTQ+ patients report being blamed for their healthcare status as well as needing to teach their physicians about their health needs (Makadon, 2006; Streed et al., 2021).

2. Why might the PBL case authors have characterized the patient in this HIV case as being a gay male?

When working with any sexually active patient, it is prudent to consider their HIV risk, need for testing, and possible counseling on pre-exposure prophylaxis. Although literature does support an increased risk of HIV in men who have sex with men, healthcare providers should also consider other healthcare needs, including vaccination recommendations (such as Hepatitis A virus, Hepatitis B virus, Human papilloma virus), mental health screening (for depression, suicidal ideation, and substance use), and anal cancer screening. Moreover, there is a risk that students would then ignore HIV risk in other patient populations. Instead, focusing on the link between patient and health outcome is necessary; anyone who engages in unprotected receptive anal sexual intercourse is at risk for contracting HIV, regardless of their sexual orientation. Unfortunately, literature demonstrates that first-year medical students carry both explicit and implicit bias towards LGBTQ+ individuals, though increasing exposure to LGBTQ+ patients in medical school has been shown to improve knowledge and empathy when working with this population (Burke et al., 2015; Sanchez et al., 2006; Vogan et al., 2014; Wilkin, 2015).

3. Clark Roberts demonstrated a significant commitment to improving the medical education curriculum. What are the potential benefits of students and faculty working together to co-produce the medical education program?

We ultimately want future healthcare providers to partner with their patients to determine the best approach to health. It is unreasonable to think, then, that if we continue to implement health professions education using the traditional hierarchical model where students just do what their teachers tell them to do, we will miss an opportunity to role model the kind of collaboration that will make for the best provider-patient relationship. This coproduction of the education model may be particularly important in medical education where there may be a temptation to believe that the physician always has the answers. Joining faculty and student perspectives in the design of curricula to prepare students to care for diverse patient populations may be especially valuable as students and faculty bring the expertise of their lived experiences and societal perspectives (Englander et al., 2020).

Dr. Quinn explains to the students that it was not the intention of the faculty to stereotype gay men and has the humility to admit that they need a better approach. She partners with Clark to assemble a curriculum development team made up of stakeholders that include faculty, staff, and students who represent diversity themselves. The team does a literature review focused on how to best represent diversity in learning cases. Through the literature review, they learn that to prepare them to care for diverse populations, students need exposure to patients representing these populations throughout their curricula. They find that undergraduate medical education programs often lack diversity in a variety of areas, including skin tone, sexual orientation, and gender identity (Bellicoso et al., 2021; Ebede & Papier, 2006; Pratt-Chapman, 2020). With this new understanding, the stakeholders develop a new method to add diversity to all the PBL cases in the pre-clerkship curriculum while avoiding the risk of introducing implicit bias in the assignment of patient identities. The new method includes the creation of patient identification cards, inspired by the demographics section of an electronic health record (Croniger et al., n.d.) and is designed to represent the overall demographic frequencies recorded in the 2020 US Census (*2010 Census of Population Housing*, n.d.). Each card includes the patient's age, sex assigned at birth, gender identity, sexual orientation, racial identity, and zip code (a proxy for socio-economic status). To avoid implicit bias in the assignment of patient identities, each of the domains of identity are randomly assigned to the patient in each PBL case. To make the patients more realistic, the curriculum development team decides to include a photo of the patient. Learning from previous experience, the team piloted the case ID cards with a group of students prior to widespread dissemination.

Figure 1. PBL Patient Identification Card

Demographics

Name: Emily Parker
Preferred Name: Mx. Parker
Age: 30 y/o
Sex at Birth: Female

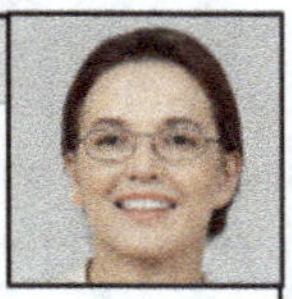

Social Information

Gender Identity: Agender
Pronouns: They/Them/Theirs
Sexual Orientation: Queer
Racial Identity: White
Ethnicity: Declined to Answer

Address

City: Cleveland State: OH
Zip Code: 44106
Country: USA

With this new plan in place, the faculty are ready to implement diversity in their cases. The first patient is Mx. Parker who identifies as agender, queer, and uses gender-neutral pronouns. Mx. Parker presents with hyperthyroidism that is treated and turns to hypothyroidism when they are lost to follow-up. In addition to the patient ID cards, resources on care for agender patients are included. As is the custom in this PBL program, the faculty meet weekly to prepare for the cases of the coming week. They receive a facilitator guide with information about the foundational science in the case and a description of the demographics, including definitions for each patient ID card. Upon review of the patient ID card for Mx. Parker, the faculty are confused. One person says that when they read the case, they thought there were grammatical errors in the use of the they/them/their pronouns, and they wonder how to pronounce "Mx." Another facilitator questioned if the use of "queer" was not an offensive term. And yet a third faculty member expressed confusion about the term "agender." Dr. Quinn, the director of this PBL program, appreciated the curiosity of the facilitators and their willingness to openly acknowledge and express their questions and confusions which led to a robust discussion that better prepared faculty to facilitate the case of Mx. Parker in a respectful and inclusive manner. At the facilitator meeting the following week, the faculty expressed that some students stumbled over the use of the gender-neutral pronouns for Mx. Parker, but appreciated the opportunity to practice this language together within the safe environment of their small groups.

4. Why is it important that faculty develop the skills of cultural competence and cultural humility in the classroom setting and with their students?

This case illustrates how cultural competence and cultural humility inform the faculty's planning and management of a health professions education session. Cultural competence provides a framework of inquiry for health professionals and educators to gain understanding of populations served, and best practices to manage and advance their healthcare. Cultural competence, however, can run the risk of creating stereotypes that can reinforce biases. Cultural humility invites faculty and students to be flexible, maintain awareness of biases, and strive for self-reflection and lifelong learning. Under this paradigm, students and educators can be humble in recognizing and accepting gaps in knowledge, curious to learn more, and held accountable to each other in the pursuit of lifelong learning.

Case Conclusion

Feedback from the students about this comprehensive approach to introduce patient diversity to the PBL cases was generally positive, however the number of underrepresented identities was increased so that students would encounter these patients with a frequency that allowed more reasonable exposure for educational purposes.

Epilogue

Dr. India Quinn transformed the representation of diversity in the PBL pre-clerkship curriculum by collaborating with a diverse group of stakeholders to share accountability for designing an unbiased approach to integrate diversity in their PBL cases. This approach also provided a valuable opportunity for faculty to work together to learn about aspects of diversity that they may not have previously appreciated.

CASE 2: RECOGNIZING AND ADDRESSING RACE ESSENTIALISM

Goal

This case explores the concept of race essentialism, and the role of health professions education in perpetuating or changing the narrative to address it and improve patient care and health outcomes.

Learning Outcomes

1. Define race essentialism.
2. Consider how humility and accountability in health professions education can change the narrative of race essentialism.
3. Describe interventions to mitigate race essentialism.

Case

A health professions student gives an oral presentation on a patient with a recent diagnosis of heart disease. The patient has long standing hypertension with suboptimal control and quit smoking 3 years ago. The patient self-identifies as Black, with a strong family history of hypertension and early cardiovascular deaths. The student reports she recently attended a didactic session on hypertensive heart disease and recalls that Black and Hispanic patients have worse cardiovascular outcomes than their white counterparts. In her interaction with the patient, she discussed medication management and attributed the patient's disease state and projected outcome to her race and ethnicity.

As a preceptor, you see the opportunity to discuss racial and ethnic health disparities with the student and set out to explore with her what social and structural factors affect Black patients' health and outcomes. You also take note to discuss with the course director how to include these discussions in didactic presentations and avoid perpetuating a narrative of race essentialism.

Questions and Answers

1. Discuss how the statement "Black and Hispanic patients have worse cardiovascular outcomes" infers race essentialism.

The statement *"Black and Hispanic patients have worse cardiovascular outcomes,"* runs the risk of introducing bias by assuming that all Black and all Hispanic patients have an inherent genetic or biological characteristic that predisposes them to worse cardiovascular outcomes. Race essentialism posits that racial categories are expressions of discrete, fixed, uniform, and defining characteristics that are shared by all members of a group, are informative about them, and differentiate them from everyone else (Herd et al., 2021; Rhodes & Moty, 2020). In other words, it proposes that members of a racial or ethnic group are biologically similar to each other and different to others in meaningful ways.

The American Society of Human Genetics, founded on years of research, has affirmed that humans are not divided into biologically distinct categories but rather express a gradient of genetic variation explained by longstanding patterns of migration (McChesney KY, 2015). The Human Genome Project in 2003 demonstrated that humans are 99.9% identical at the DNA level (*Humans-Are-999-Genetically-Identical*, n.d.; Yudell et al., 2016) and informed that 'race' is not a genetic or biological construct. Mounting evidence supports that race is not a reliable proxy for meaningful genetic differences, yet when race is included in health professions literature, it is often presumed to be representative of a biological construct. Thus, when race is reported to correlate with health outcomes, one needs to question *how* race is understood to affect those outcomes.

2. If not race essentialism, what else could account for race-reported health outcomes?

Public health reports and the health professions literature frequently describe well-established disparities in health and health outcomes for Blacks, Hispanics, Native Americans and other minority groups in the US (*CDC Health Disparities & Inequalities Report*, n.d.). The trends in disparities by race and ethnicity have remained relatively stagnant despite the U.S. Department of Health and Human Services goal of Healthy People 2020 to *"achieve health equity, eliminate disparities, and improve the health of all groups"*(*Healthy People 2020 Overview of Health Disparities. Healthy People 2020 Final Review.*, n.d.). It becomes imperative to teach the next generation of health professionals to not only be aware of such disparities, but to be curious and question why disparities exist and empower them to be agents of change. According to the National Academy of Medicine (*Social-Determinants-of-Health-101-for-Health-Care-Five-plus-Five*, n.d.), 80% of a person's health is related to the social determinants of health, the conditions where people live, work, and play. A National Institute of Minority Health and Health Disparities' framework (*National Institute on Minority Health and Health Disparities*, n.d.) proposes that health outcomes are determined by domains of influence such as biological, behavioral, environmental, sociocultural, and healthcare systems, at the individual, family, community, and population health levels. The complexity of the matrix underscores the multiple and intersecting elements that affect any population's health and health outcomes. The relative contributions of social stability, education, neighborhood conditions (such as crime rate or safe green spaces), access to healthy food, health insurance status and community engagement are all key social determinants of cardiovascular outcomes, and disproportionately affect minority communities (Jilani et al., 2021). Furthermore, racial health disparities reflect additional, longstanding lived experiences and limited socioeconomic attainment of marginalized Black communities, set in motion by decades-old redlining. Structural racism explains the accumulation of multiple reinforcing systems of discrimination, that in turn reinforce discriminatory practices and beliefs. Race thus becomes a proxy of lived experiences, an identity imposed by society and system structures. The trauma of discrimination further compounds stress as a risk factor for health conditions such as hypertension and cardiovascular disease (Baiden et al., 2022; Forde et al., 2020). Understanding the relative contribution of the social determinants of health and health outcomes has only more recently entered research analysis of health outcomes. As an example, a neighborhood disadvantage index (NDI) that accounts for several measures of socioeconomic status, was a strong predictor of cardiovascular disease outcomes, explaining 32% of census-tract variation in cardiovascular event rates, compared to only 10% accounted for by a traditional pooled cohort equation risk model. This narrative needs to be included in health professions education, lest the absence of it erroneously lead students to reduce health disparities to race essentialism.

3. What are the implications of the biases introduced by race essentialism in students' understanding of health outcomes?

Race essentialism, the understanding that patients from different races are biologically different in meaningful ways, as well as implicit racial bias, are deeply rooted in medical education (Sabin, 2022), passed down from clinicians to students through lectures, textbooks, and bedside teaching. The psychology literature demonstrates that essentialist thinking can lead to dehumanization and increased racial prejudice, and thus affect patient care (Jones, 2001; Tsai, 2022). With an essentialist understanding, clinicians provide biased care, tailored to presumed biological differences. These include the development of differential diagnoses that may utilize race "corrections" for kidney and lung function, racialized risk calculators such as the Fracture Risk Assessment (FRAX) score for osteoporosis and Atherosclerosis Cardiovascular Disease (ASCVD), as well as a treatment plan that may be based on a racialized management algorithm (Tsai, 2022). The interpersonal and systemic consequences of biased care are profound. For instance, as Blacks are thought to have a higher muscle mass than Whites (Cerdeña et al., 2020) a Black patient may not be eligible for a kidney transplant based on her calculated GFR, when a White patient with identical kidney function would. The perception that Black people have a higher threshold of pain may lead to underestimating and undertreating them patients for pain (Jones, 2001). In maternal health, Black and Hispanic women receive significantly lower rates of epidural analgesia (Rust et al., 2004), and biases that can contribute to racial disparities in care (Saluja & Bryant, 2021). A

2017 literature review found health care providers' implicit racial bias to be associated with diagnostic uncertainty, negative clinical interactions, less patient-centeredness, poor provider communication, and stigmatization of Black patients as less adherent (Sabin, 2022). Furthermore, essentialist teachings regarding patients' outcomes limit the students' curiosity to ask critical questions regarding the role of social determinants of health and social experience on health. Similarly, they diminish students' sense of accountability and responsibility to address health gaps. Teaching students to understand implicit bias with the Implicit Association Test holds promise to decrease student's biases (van Ryn et al., 2015).

4. How can health professions educators avoid perpetuating the narrative of race essentialism and advance health equity?

Health professions students learn of racial and ethnic health disparities through the literature or presentations during their training. This creates a window of opportunity for health professions educators to address the reasons underlying the health disparities and engage the curiosity of students in questioning why such disparities exist. One of the challenges for educators is the lack in the health professions literature of a consistent requirement to address the upstream causes of health disparities (Lett et al). While efforts are under way to remediate this (Aifah et al., 2021; Breathett et al., 2021), educators must at present demonstrate the humility and curiosity to recognize and address the shortcomings in the literature. Researchers can for example incorporate experiential elements that are not addressed in their study design and explore how these could have impacted an association with race (Lett et al., 2022).

An explanation of how study participants are identified and how racial and ethnic categories are selected can inform steps towards accurate reporting, mitigating essentialist elements (Flanagin et al., 2021). Dr. Jones urges epidemiologists to invest in elucidating the causes of race-associated disparities to interpret rather than simply reporting race-associated differences, acknowledging race as a social construct and the diversity within racial groups, recognize the present-day and perpetuated systemic racism, while engaging marginalized communities to raise questions and advocate for change (Jones, 2001). Setting high quality standards of research design and communicating limitation and potential biases can redirect health professions educators to convey that level of uncertainty and curiosity in their teaching. Another tool for health professions educators is the application of the literature on implicit bias.(Gonzalez et al., 2021). Educators can create a safe environment and invite students to question assumptions and approach the learning through a new lens. Reflective practice can invite students, through guiding questions, to remain curious and question assumptions made in health disparities reports. In planning a didactic session, educators can apply tools to raise their own awareness about bias and race essentialism before teaching students. A checklist proposed by Amy Carouso, prompts an educator to systematically approach the demographic descriptors in a case presentation, and pause and reflect on potential biases introduced (*The Informed Patient. A Podcast Connecting You With Health, Science and Medicine*, n.d.). The checklist will alert the educator presenting the case of a "Black woman with poorly controlled hypertension and heart disease" to consider why race and gender are mentioned on the heading of the case, and if by doing so, they may inadvertently introduce bias and increase the risk that trainees will conceptualize Black women as inherently at risk of poorly controlled cardiovascular disease, as was the case with our student. An additional slide or paragraph may further explain social determinants of health: socioeconomic status, education, access to safe green spaces, affordable nutritious foods, and consistent healthcare and medications, as well as stressors and trauma, all contributors to the observed health disparities (Havranek et al., 2015; Williams et al., 2019). A system of accountability can be set in motion with faculty development, student feedback, and continuous review of curricular modifications and improvements.

Case Conclusion

Health professions students are frequently presented with data on racial health disparities without context of the root causes, creating the risk of promoting race essentialism. An educator teaching on hypertension health disparities can add a slide about the structural and social determinants of health that may contribute to those disparities. The presentation can highlight the association of hypertension with access to healthy affordable foods (*USDA Mapping Food Deserts in the US*, n.d.) and the stress of structural racism (Havranek et al., 2015; Williams et al., 2019) among others. Ideally, students will take home a message that averts race essentialism.

Epilogue

Essentialist beliefs assume that certain phenotypic or cultural characteristics can predict or determine health outcomes. Race essentialism leads to inappropriate generalizations, legitimization of existing social hierarchies, and acceptance and further promotion of racial inequality. Race essentialism introduces bias in health professions education, which risks promoting further health inequities. As we train the next generation of healthcare professionals, we have the gift and responsibility to teach and stimulate scientific knowledge in a context that informs emerging understanding of racism in research and science and places our students in a position to be agents of change. Through this case discussion, we have invited health educators to articulate how to move away from using race as a genetic or biological construct, tools to pause and augment the content of their teaching to create a narrative that avoids race essentialism and bias.

REFERENCES

Aifah, A., Onakomaiya, D., Rakhra, A., & Ogedegbe, G. (2021). Uprooting race-based assumptions in biomedical journal articles. *Trends in Molecular Medicine*, *27*(9), 830–832. doi:10.1016/j.molmed.2021.06.003

Amutah, C., Greenidge, K., Mante, A., Munyikwa, M., Surya, S. L., Higginbotham, E., Jones, D. S., Lavizzo-Mourey, R., Roberts, D., Tsai, J., & Aysola, J. (2021). Misrepresenting Race—The Role of Medical Schools in Propagating Physician Bias. *The New England Journal of Medicine*, *384*(9), 872–878. https://doi.org/10.1056/NEJMms2025768

Baiden, D., Parry, M., Nerenberg, K., Hillan, E. M., & Dogba, M. J. (2022). Connecting the Dots: Structural Racism, Intersectionality, and Cardiovascular Health Outcomes for African, Caribbean, and Black Mothers. *Health Equity*, *6*(1), 402–405. doi:10.1089/heq.2021.0077

Bellicoso, E., Quick, S. O., Ayoo, K. O., Beach, R. A., Joseph, M., & Dahlke, E. (2021). Diversity in Dermatology? An Assessment of Undergraduate Medical Education. *Journal of Cutaneous Medicine and Surgery*, *25*(4), 409–417. https://doi.org/10.1177/12034754211007430

Beyond the curriculum: Academic nursing's responsibility for excellence in diversity, equity, and inclusion. (2021). *Journal of Professional Nursing* , *37*(2), A1–A2. doi:10.1016/j.profnurs.2021.02.006

Breathett, K., Spatz, E. S., Kramer, D. B., Essien, U. R., Wadhera, R. K., Peterson, P. N., Ho, P. M., & Nallamothu, B. K. (2021). The Groundwater of Racial and Ethnic Disparities Research: A Statement From Circulation: Cardiovascular Quality and Outcomes. *Circulation: Cardiovascular Quality and Outcomes*, *14*(2), e007868. https://doi.org/10.1161/CIRCOUTCOMES.121.007868

Brooks, K. C. (2015). A piece of my mind. A silent curriculum. *Journal of the American Medical Association*, *313*(19), 1909–1910. https://doi.org/10.1001/jama.2015.1676

Burke, S. E., Dovidio, J. F., Przedworski, J. M., Hardeman, R. R., Perry, S. P., Phelan, S. M., Nelson, D. B., Burgess, D. J., Yeazel, M. W., & van Ryn, M. (2015). Do Contact and Empathy Mitigate Bias Against Gay and Lesbian People Among Heterosexual First-Year Medical Students? A Report From the Medical Student CHANGE Study. *Academic Medicine*, *90*(5), 645–651. https://doi.org/10.1097/ACM.0000000000000661

Carter, B. M., & Phillips, B. C. (2021). Revolutionizing the Nursing Curriculum. *Creative Nursing*, *27*(1), 25–30. https://doi.org/10.1891/CRNR-D-20-00072

CDC Health Disparities & Inequalities Report. (n.d.). https://www.cdc.gov/minorityhealth/chdireport.html#:~:text=The%20CDC%20Health%20Disparities%20and%20Inequalities%20Report%20%E2%80%93,income%2C%20education%2C%20disability%20status%20and%20other%20social%20characteristics

Census of Population Housing. (2011). USC B: 2010 Census of Population and Housing. U.S. Department of Commerce EaSA.

Cerdeña, J. P., Plaisime, M. V., & Tsai, J. (2020). From race-based to race-conscious medicine: How anti-racist uprisings call us to act. *Lancet*, *396*(10257), 1125–1128. https://doi.org/10.1016/S0140-6736(20)32076-6

Chavan, M., Moncaliano, M., & Clarke, A. (2022). Preparing Trainees to Care for Diverse Patient Populations: Medical Students as Leaders in Curriculum Development. *Academic Medicine*, *97*(8), 1100–1101. https://doi.org/10.1097/ACM.0000000000004472

Croniger, C.M., Qua, K., Rowland Seymour, A., Podugu, P., Laseter, J., Linz, M.O., & Wilson-Delfosse, A. (n.d.). *Preparing Students to Deliver Care to Diverse Populations*. Academic Press.

Cuellar, N. G., Brennan, A. M. W., Vito, K., & de Leon Siantz, M. L. (2008). Cultural competence in the undergraduate nursing curriculum. *Journal of Professional Nursing* , *24*(3), 143–149. https://doi.org/10.1016/j.profnurs.2008.01.004

Ebede, T., & Papier, A. (2006). Disparities in dermatology educational resources. *Journal of the American Academy of Dermatology*, *55*(4), 687–690. https://doi.org/10.1016/j.jaad.2005.10.068

Englander, R., Holmboe, E., Batalden, P., Caron, R. M., Durham, C. F., Foster, T., Ogrinc, G., Ercan-Fang, N., & Batalden, M. (2020). Coproducing Health Professions Education: A Prerequisite to Coproducing Health Care Services? *Academic Medicine*, *95*(7), 1006–1013. https://doi.org/10.1097/ACM.0000000000003137

Flanagin, A., Frey, T., & Christiansen, S. L. (2021). Updated Guidance on the Reporting of Race and Ethnicity in Medical and Science Journals. *Journal of the American Medical Association*, *326*(7), 621–627. https://doi.org/10.1001/jama.2021.13304

Forde, A. T., Sims, M., Muntner, P., Lewis, T., Onwuka, A., Moore, K., & Diez Roux, A. V. (2020). Discrimination and Hypertension Risk Among African Americans in the Jackson Heart Study. *Hypertension, 76*(3), 715–723. doi:10.1161/HYPERTENSIONAHA.119.14492

Gonzalez, C. M., Lypson, M. L., & Sukhera, J. (2021). Twelve tips for teaching implicit bias recognition and management. *Medical Teacher*, *43*(12), 1368–1373. https://doi.org/10.1080/0142159X.2021.1879378

Haley, C. M., & Brown, B. P. (2022). Implementation of diversity, equity, and inclusion dialogue for second-year dental students. *Journal of Dental Education*, *86*(5), 599–604. https://doi.org/10.1002/jdd.12862

Havranek, E. P., Mujahid, M. S., Barr, D. A., Blair, I. V., Cohen, M. S., Cruz-Flores, S., Davey-Smith, G., Dennison-Himmelfarb, C. R., Lauer, M. S., Lockwood, D. W., Rosal, M., & Yancy, C. W. (2015). Social Determinants of Risk and Outcomes for Cardiovascular Disease: A Scientific Statement From the American Heart Association. *Circulation*, *132*(9), 873–898. https://doi.org/10.1161/CIR.0000000000000228

Healthy People 2020 Overview of Health Disparities. Healthy People 2020 Final Review. (n.d.). doi:10.15620/cdc:111173

Herd, P., Mills, M. C., & Dowd, J. B. (2021). Reconstructing Sociogenomics Research: Dismantling Biological Race and Genetic Essentialism Narratives. *Journal of Health and Social Behavior*, *62*(3), 419–435. https://doi.org/10.1177/00221465211018682

Humans-are-999-genetically-identical. (n.d.). https://www.pbs.org/video/humans-are-999-genetically-identical-1lggn4/

Jilani, M. H., Javed, Z., Yahya, T., Valero-Elizondo, J., Khan, S. U., Kash, B., Blankstein, R., Virani, S. S., Blaha, M. J., Dubey, P., Hyder, A. A., Vahidy, F. S., Cainzos-Achirica, M., & Nasir, K. (2021). Social Determinants of Health and Cardiovascular Disease: Current State and Future Directions Towards Healthcare Equity. *Current Atherosclerosis Reports*, *23*(9), 55. https://doi.org/10.1007/s11883-021-00949-w

Jones, C. P. (2001). Invited commentary: "race," racism, and the practice of epidemiology. *American Journal of Epidemiology*, *154*(4), 299–304. https://doi.org/10.1093/aje/154.4.299

Lett, E., Asabor, E., Beltrán, S., Cannon, A. M., & Arah, O. A. (2022). Conceptualizing, Contextualizing, and Operationalizing Race in Quantitative Health Sciences Research. *Annals of Family Medicine*, *20*(2), 157–163. https://doi.org/10.1370/afm.2792

Makadon, H. J. (2006). Improving health care for the lesbian and gay communities. *The New England Journal of Medicine*, *354*(9), 895–897. https://doi.org/10.1056/NEJMp058259

Margolius, S. W., Papp, K. K., Altose, M. D., & Wilson-Delfosse, A. L. (2020). Students perceive skills learned in pre-clerkship PBL valuable in core clinical rotations. *Medical Teacher*, *42*(8), 902–908. https://doi.org/10.1080/0142159X.2020.1762031

McChesney, K. Y. (2015). *Teaching Diversity: The Science You Need to Know to Explain Why Race Is Not Biological.* doi:10.1177/2158244015611712

McClintock, A. H., Fainstad, T. L., & Jauregui, J. (2021). Creating Psychological Safety in the Learning Environment: Straightforward Answers to a Longstanding Challenge. *Academic Medicine*, *96*(11S), S208–S209. https://doi.org/10.1097/ACM.0000000000004319

McOwen, K. S., Whelan, A. J., & Farmakidis, A. L. (2020). Medical Education in the United States and Canada, 2020. *Academic Medicine* , *95*(9S), S2–S4. doi:10.1097/ACM.0000000000003497

National Institute on Minority Health and Health Disparities. (n.d.). https://www.nimhd.nih.gov/about/overview/research-framework/nimhd-framework.html

Parkhurst, D. C., Kayingo, G., & Fleming, S. (2017). Redesigning Physician Assistant Education to Promote Cognitive Diversity, Inclusion, and Health Care Equity. *The Journal of Physician Assistant Education: the Official Journal of the Physician Assistant Education Association*, *28*(Suppl 1), S38–S42. https://doi.org/10.1097/JPA.0000000000000128

Pratt-Chapman, M. L. (2020). Implementation of sexual and gender minority health curricula in health care professional schools: A qualitative study. *BMC Medical Education*, *20*(1), 138. https://doi.org/10.1186/s12909-020-02045-0

Rhodes, M., & Moty, K. (2020). What is social essentialism and how does it develop? *Advances in Child Development and Behavior*, *59*, 1–30. https://doi.org/10.1016/bs.acdb.2020.05.001

Rust, G., Nembhard, W. N., Nichols, M., Omole, F., Minor, P., Barosso, G., & Mayberry, R. (2004). Racial and ethnic disparities in the provision of epidural analgesia to Georgia Medicaid beneficiaries during labor and delivery. *American Journal of Obstetrics and Gynecology*, *191*(2), 456–462. https://doi.org/10.1016/j.ajog.2004.03.005

Sabin, J. A. (2022). Tackling Implicit Bias in Health Care. *The New England Journal of Medicine*, *387*(2), 105–107. https://doi.org/10.1056/NEJMp2201180

Saluja, B., & Bryant, Z. (2021). How Implicit Bias Contributes to Racial Disparities in Maternal Morbidity and Mortality in the United States. *Journal of Women's Health, 30*(2), 270–273. doi:10.1089/jwh.2020.8874

Sanchez, N. F., Rabatin, J., Sanchez, J. P., Hubbard, S., & Kalet, A. (2006). Medical students' ability to care for lesbian, gay, bisexual, and transgendered patients. *Family Medicine*, *38*(1), 21–27.

Schwartz, S. B., Smith, S. G., & Johnson, K. R. (2020). ADEA Faculty Diversity Toolkit: A Comprehensive Approach to Improving Diversity and Inclusion in Dental Education. *Journal of Dental Education*, *84*(3), 279–282. https://doi.org/10.1002/jdd.12143

Social-determinants-of-health-101-for-health-care-five-plus-five. (n.d.). https://nam.edu/social-determinants-of-health-101-for-health-care-five-plus-five/

Streed, C. G. J., Lunn, M. R., Siegel, J., & Obedin-Maliver, J. (2021). Meeting the Patient Care, Education, and Research Missions: Academic Medical Centers Must Comprehensively Address Sexual and Gender Minority Health. *Academic Medicine*, *96*(6), 822–827. https://doi.org/10.1097/ACM.0000000000003703

The Informed Patient. (n.d.). *A podcast connecting you with health, science and medicine*. https://www.upstate.edu/informed/2022/051322-caruso-brown-podcast.php

Tsai, J. (2022). How Should Educators and Publishers Eliminate Racial Essentialism? *AMA Journal of Ethics*, *24*(3), E201–E211. https://doi.org/10.1001/amajethics.2022.201

USDA mapping food deserts in the US. (n.d.). https://www.ers.usda.gov/amber-waves/2011/december/data-feature-mapping-food-deserts-in-the-us/accessed

van Ryn, M., Hardeman, R., Phelan, S. M., Burgess, D. J., Dovidio, J. F., Herrin, J., Burke, S. E., Nelson, D. B., Perry, S., Yeazel, M., & Przedworski, J. M. (2015). Medical School Experiences Associated with Change in Implicit Racial Bias Among 3547 Students: A Medical Student CHANGES Study Report. *Journal of General Internal Medicine*, *30*(12), 1748–1756. https://doi.org/10.1007/s11606-015-3447-7

Vogan, C. L., McKimm, J., Da Silva, A. L., & Grant, A. (2014). Twelve tips for providing effective student support in undergraduate medical education. *Medical Teacher*, *36*(6), 480–485. https://doi.org/10.3109/0142159X.2014.907488

Wilkin, T. (2015). Clinical Practice. Primary Care for Men Who Have Sex with Men. *The New England Journal of Medicine*, *373*(9), 854–862. https://doi.org/10.1056/NEJMcp1401303

Williams, D. R., Lawrence, J. A., & Davis, B. A. (2019). Racism and Health: Evidence and Needed Research. *Annual Review of Public Health*, *40*, 105–125. https://doi.org/10.1146/annurev-publhealth-040218-043750

Yudell, M., Roberts, D., DeSalle, R., & Tishkoff, S. (2016). Science and Society. Taking race out of human genetics. *Science*, *351*(6273), 564–565. https://doi.org/10.1126/science.aac4951

Chapter 18
Increasing Diversity in Medical Education:
A Case Study

Margaret A. Hadinger
https://orcid.org/0000-0002-7908-7668
OnlineMedEd, USA

Judith Natale Sabino
Lehigh Valley Health Network, USA

Eric J. Gertner
Lehigh Valley Health Network, USA

Joseph J. Napolitano
Lehigh Valley Health Network, USA

María de los A. Ortiz Reyes
Ortiz, Lord, Hope and Associates, Puerto Rico & University of Puerto Rico at Río Piedras, Puerto Rico

EXECUTIVE SUMMARY

A health professions learning environment that includes diverse learners enhances learning and attitudes and builds learners' confidence and ability to work with patients from all cultures – and these benefits extend to all students. Impacts extend to patients via increased access to care for the underserved, increased patient adherence, and other positive outcomes. This chapter presents a case study of a health network that sought to increase diversity and attract learners from groups traditionally underrepresented in medicine. The authors discuss strengths, weaknesses, and challenges related to strategies implemented. The epilogue contextualizes progress made and describes a third nursing strategy currently being undertaken.

DOI: 10.4018/978-1-6684-5493-0.ch018

BACKGROUND

Importance of Physician Diversity

While a variety of factors contribute to health care disparities, the mismatch between the race/ethnicity of the US population and the physicians who serve it has detrimental impacts on patient care outcomes. This mismatch bears out in basic demographics; racial and ethnic diversity[1] continues to increase in the US (US Census, 2020) but diversity in the physician workforce has not kept pace. Most recent data reflects that most active physicians are still White (56.2%) and male (64.1%) (Association of American Medical Colleges, 2019). Further, while diversity among medical school applicants, matriculants, and graduates continues to grow, the representation of individuals from certain groups - specifically Black or African American applicants, matriculants, and graduates – continues to lag behind other groups (Association of American Medical Colleges, 2019).

Race and ethnicity impacts health disparities; racial and ethnic minorities and the poor – particularly Hispanic and non-Hispanic Black groups - continue to have shorter life expectancy and widened health disparity as compared to non-Hispanic White groups (2022 National Healthcare Quality and Disparities Report, 2022).

As others have argued, a healthcare workforce which includes colleagues who represent the cultures of the communities it serves is vital for the delivery of high quality, equitable and culturally responsive care that meets each patient's unique needs and preferences (Institute of Medicine, 2004; Gonzaga et al., 2020; Boatright et al., 2018; Castillo-Page, 2006). Thus, diversifying the physician workforce is one strategy shown to help address disparities and improve patient care outcomes. Physician diversity contributes to increased access to health care services for the underserved and to expanded options for patient care (Castillo-Page, 2006) as, in general, physicians representing racial and ethnic minority groups, as well as female physicians, are more likely to treat patients of low socioeconomic status, patients covered by Medicaid, and patients who are uninsured (Cantor et al., 1996; Komaromy et al., 1996; Moy & Bartman, 1995).

Further, although recent studies suggest that the connection between race-concordance and patient-physician communication is not totally clear or fully understood (Shen et al., 2018), previous studies suggest a positive correlation between physician diversity and physician-patient communication. Physician-patient communication in turn has been linked to higher patient satisfaction, higher adherence rates and better health outcomes (Betancourt et al., 2003). Other studies have demonstrated that race-concordant patient–physician relationships are generally favored among all racial and ethnic groups (Castillo-Page, 2006); race-concordant physicians are more participatory (Cooper-Patrick et al., 1999; Cooper et al., 2003); race concordance is positively associated with patient satisfaction (Cooper-Patrick et al., 1999); race concordant visits are longer and more positively rated by patients (Cooper et al., 2003); and racially and ethnically concordant patient–physician relationships have higher levels of trust (Tarn et al., 2005) and respect (Malat, 2001).

Diversity in the Learning Environment

Similarly, a learning environment which includes individuals from racial-minority members positively impacts learning (Antonio et al., 2004; Nemeth & Wachtler, 1983). In medical education specifically, research has shown that cross-cultural interactions are associated with higher self-reported levels of preparedness for care of patients from diverse backgrounds (Niu et al., 2012). Relatedly, the educational benefits of diversity extend to both minority and non-minority students; White medical students within the highest quintile for student body racial and ethnic diversity have been shown to be more likely to rate themselves as highly prepared to care for minority patients and were more likely to have strong attitudes endorsing access to care compared to their counterparts at schools with less diversity (Saha et al., 2008). Further, medical students have reported valuing diversity in their class as an integral component of their education (Hung et al., 2007; Whitla et al., 2003). The converse has also been demonstrated; medical students believe that being in a student body that is not ethnically diverse hinders the quality of medical education (Hung et al., 2007).

Recognizing both the need to diversify the physician workforce and the educational benefits of diversity in medical education, the Association of American Medical Colleges (AAMC, 2022), the Liaison Committee on Medical Education (LCME, 2022; Barzansky et al., 2021), the Accreditation Council on Graduate Medical Education (ACGME, 2022), and other similar national bodies have affirmed that future physicians must learn and train in an environment characterized by diversity and inclusion if they are to be prepared to practice.

Recruiting for Diversity

Recruiting and onboarding students, residents, fellows and other trainees from backgrounds that are traditionally underrepresented in medicine is thus a priority for both undergraduate- and graduate-level medical education programs.

Programs that are successful in recruiting efforts are characterized by the ability to foster intellectual discussions based on various lived experiences, expand health care delivery to traditional as well as under resourced communities, provide opportunities for authentic conversations about racial equity, and reduce the negative consequences of implicit bias and inequities.

Organizational Approaches to Diversity, Equity, Inclusion, and Belonging

In addition to recruitment, several organizational factors are essential to fostering diversity, equity, inclusion and belonging (DEIB) in health care networks, including establishing and sustaining strategies to recruit and retain learners from traditionally underrepresented groups (American Hospital Association, 2022).

Effective DEIB organizational elements begin with broad leadership commitment, not only within medical education, but across the health system (Gertner et al., 2010; Gonzaga et al., 2020; Gonzaga et al., 2022). This commitment provides necessary focus given to recruitment and retention efforts among competing priorities, provides sufficient financial and in-kind resources to meet established goals and aligns recruitment strategies with other organizational initiatives. Engaged leaders across organizational levels and departments can speak to and demonstrate the value of these initiatives to organizational mission and operational success. All other factors flow from leadership prioritization of and commitment to diversity efforts.

Organizations must allocate financial resources to meet short- and long-term deliverables. Philanthropic funding can be used to pilot innovative programs such as recruitment strategies and foster relationships with external partners that can establish and strengthen recruitment pipelines. Ongoing operational funds must be built into budgets in order to maximize and sustain pilot initiatives and build on relationships needed to achieve recruitment goals. With insufficient funding support, initial gains can be lost.

Further, sufficient infrastructure and staffing (including protected time and expertise) are essential to DEIB-related organizational change. For example, personnel should be dedicated to implementing recruitment tactics such as promoting diversity initiatives with potential candidates, using current data to prioritize tactics and tracking data over time to measure the outcomes; creating standard applicant screening rubrics, structured interview formats, providing implicit bias and other training for interviewers, expanding interview and ranking teams to include multiple perspectives, and establish retention strategies for incoming residents from underrepresented groups. Also essential are strengthened partnerships that build and sustain talent pipelines and provide welcome and integration for learners, residents and colleagues from underrepresented backgrounds who move into the organization's community.

Organizations must also incorporate effective strategic planning, change and project management tools to achieve expected outcomes to improve the likelihood of sustained and widespread organizational success (Shea, 2020). Specifically related to recruitment, efforts to attract candidates from underrepresented groups must be linked to and included within the organization's strategic plan to ensure they are effectively prioritized by all stakeholders throughout the organization and over time, particularly when considering other important priorities. For this to occur, success metrics must be clearly defined and agreed upon, grounded in evidence, and use the experience of past recruitment efforts as their foundation. Process and outcome data must be regularly monitored to assure alignment to expected goals and provide direction for needed modifications. Institutions should further challenge themselves to establish meaningful goals and to collect outcome data that are relevant for specific stakeholders, and - in the case of heath care - patients themselves.

Finally, regular communication with key stakeholders about the progress of initiatives is critical for sustained transformation. Recruitment of individuals from underrepresented groups is often first sparked as a priority due to a request from the community for greater diversity in the ethnic composition of the organization's workforce. This initial impetus for change must be translated into a value statement that can be internalized as a driving force within the organization. Further, continuous communication is essential to ensure that recruitment goals remain prioritized at the highest levels of the organization and are critical for accountability related to established goals. Communication is necessary to ensure that roadblocks are addressed as they are encountered. Ideally, communication should contain not only outcome and process updates but also personal stories from recruited learners. Their experiences through the process can inform improvements and foster sustained departmental and organizational commitment.

ONE CASE STUDY: TWO STRATEGIES

Goal

This case portrays two strategies implemented over the course of a decade at a large academic community health network interested in increasing not only the diversity of its residency and fellowship programs, and ultimately, its physician workforce, but also to improve its understanding of the health care needs and health care behaviors of its own growing Hispanic/Latino/Latina/Latinx community through collaboration and partnership with colleagues in Puerto Rico.

Learning Outcomes

1. Identify strategies used to attract candidates historically underrepresented in medicine in which candidates learn about an institution and its physician training programs, as well as about the region in which they are located.
2. Describe factors organizations should consider when creating strategies to attract candidates from underrepresented groups.
3. Describe the role of cultural humility in implementing strategies targeting diverse candidates.

Case

The context for this case spans two regions: Pennsylvania and Puerto Rico.

The case centers on the activities of a large academic community health network in Pennsylvania. Historically, and similar to other communities across nationally, the demographics of the health network's physician workforce and its physician training programs did not fully reflect the demographic changes occurring in the region. This reflected the larger challenges faced by the network, to care for patients, both recent arrivals as well as established residents, who came from backgrounds and cultures often with different health beliefs and experiences related to the health care system.

In 2007, the local service area of the population served by the health network was multicultural. In the region's largest city, 37.3% of the population identified as Hispanic or Latino with close to 60% of them having roots in Puerto Rico. Over time, the demographics of the community continued to change. By 2021, 54% of city residents identified at Hispanic or Latino and 17% identified as Black or African American (not Hispanic or Latino), 4% identified as Asian, 2% as American Indian or Alaskan Native and 22% identified as some other race (US Census, 2020).

The health network has a long history of medical and dental residency and fellowship training programs but did not historically track and therefore did not have metrics related to the diversity of its trainees. The importance of trainee diversity became a focus in the early 2000s as the health network elevated diversity, equity and inclusion to the level of network priorities.

During this period, like other organizations nationally, the health network was early in its diversity equity and inclusion journey. Prior to 2006, the health care organization met the cultural needs of patients through staff education and contracted telephone interpretation services. Following a retreat which aimed to enhance the patient experience, an organizational assessment was conducted, and a subsequent strategic plan was written and approved to comprehensively improve the delivery of culturally appropriate services. It would be a few years before the implementation of the strategic plan and appointment of dedicated staff for this work would emerge.

The health network historically benefited from financial support from both an external philanthropic foundation as well as internal funds set aside to support innovation in education, expansion of diversity initiatives, and other priorities. Additionally, the health network invested in and demonstrated commitment to the development of a comprehensive department of education. The department had responsibility for coordinating innovation- and education-focused projects funded by external grants, including this particular project.

Equally central to this case is the territory of Puerto Rico, which shares direct ties with Pennsylvania via the migration patterns of island residents and those living in the US mainland. As others have noted, understanding migration patterns is critical to understanding challenges inherent to these patterns and proposing strategies for addressing them aligned to the specific socio-economic conditions of Puerto Rico within a global perspective (Ortiz Reyes & Sepúlveda Arroyo, 2020).

Puerto Rico has been designated a US territory since 1898 and has both Spanish and English as official languages. Puerto Rico is a US Commonwealth: Puerto Ricans are US citizens, but residents of the island do not have the right to vote in national elections. US federal and state laws apply on the island. Since 2006 and after Hurricanes Maria and Fiona, the island has undergone difficult economic constraints, increasing the number of Puerto Ricans who emigrated to the US. US Census Bureau data show that from mid-2010 to 2016 more people left the island for the US mainland, than migrated to Puerto Rico; the largest gap between inward and outward migration of the previous three decades (Velázquez-Estrada, 2016). This increasing loss fueled the islands' first sustained population decline in its history.

Most current data as of 2014 indicates that in approximately 12 Puerto Rican municipalities (mostly in the center of the island), between 60% and 68% of the population lives below the poverty line (Cordero Guzmán, 2016). The search for better economic opportunities was the most common explanation given by island-born Puerto Ricans who relocated in the mainland from 2006-2015. Of these 40% indicated job-related reasons for moving stateside, 39% gave family-related reasons and 9% reported housing as a reason to leave Puerto Rico.

Strategy 1 – Enhancing Cooperation with, Learning from, and Representation of Hispanic and Spanish-speaking Perspectives

Overview

In the early 2000's, health network and community leadership collaborated to more fully address the need to provide more culturally and linguistically appropriate care to the Hispanic/Latino/Latina/Latinx and Spanish-speaking patient population it serves. Since a majority of the local Hispanic/Latino/Latina/Latinx population identified at Puerto Rican, collaboration with Puerto Rico became this project's focus. In furtherance of this goal, in 2005 the health network developed and implemented a multi-pronged project. It is important to note that the primary goal of this project was not to recruit candidates for the health network, but rather to establish and grow a meaningful exchange with colleagues in Puerto Rico and within our own community in order to improve our understanding of the health care needs and behaviors of Puerto Ricans living in our region that would result in a desire of learners to seek experiences in this community. Project leadership applied the guiding principle that the health network act as a partner with the community looking to improve collective understandings on how best to mutually serve populations in both the health network's region and in Puerto Rico. The project was modeled on the successful cooperative model of teacher exchange that was in place between multiple schools in Puerto Rico and a college local to the health network.

Project leadership focused the project on building relationships with counterparts in the medical schools in Puerto Rico for multiple reasons. First, at that time there were three medical schools accredited by the Liaison Committee on Medical Education (LCME), meaning that students and graduates from those schools were eligible for medical student rotations and training experiences similar to any other US medical student or graduate. Second, as mentioned, the project built on the foundation of existing positive relationships between multiple schools in Puerto Rico and a college local to the health network. Project leadership actively engaged representatives both in Puerto Rico and at the local college to help make connections and for consultation in developing the project.

An exchange component of the project was modelled after one in which the project lead participated during residency that saw students from Brazil coming to the US for rotations and residency, and students and residents from the US going to Brazil for rotations in tropical medicine and infectious diseases. The project included funding for consultant and visiting professor visits to the health network, a Spanish for medical professionals' course, and a cultural experience in Puerto Rico for a group of health network physicians and support staff.

Two tactics aimed at attracting Hispanic/Latino/Latina/Latinx and Spanish-speaking medical students, including: 1) health network visits to the medical schools located in Puerto Rico during their annual residency fairs and 2) scholarships for fourth-year medical students from the Puerto Rican medical schools to complete clinical rotations and scholarships for first- and second-year students to complete two-week summer internships with the health network.

The project was embedded in the wider work of the health network's cultural awareness and patient-centered experience initiatives and was led by a physician and coordinated by an education administrator. Funding to support this project was provided by an external philanthropic foundation for the first three years; in a final fourth year of the project, visits to the Puerto Rican medical school residency fairs and scholarships for fourth-year summer internships continued through operational resources provided by the health network. This continuation of funding was an intentional design of the project and was a commitment made by the health network prior to receiving external grant support.

Outcomes

The project resulted in numerous outcomes. Most broadly, the cultural learnings that resulted from the meaningful exchanges and conversations between colleagues proved invaluable to the individual participants. For example, health network providers gained insight into nuances related to the treatment of Puerto Rican children in Pennsylvania, for example, an understanding that parents in Puerto Rico were accustomed to seeking and receiving acute care for their children in the emergency department rather than their pediatrician's office.

Specifically related to the goal of attracting of Hispanic/Latino/Latina/Latinx and Spanish-speaking medical students, this project provided scholarships to a total of 14 fourth-year medical students over the course of four years, and additionally provided eight first- and second-year medical students with two-week paid summer internships. Over 100 students requested more information about residency opportunities at the health network - exceeding initial project goals - and that number remained steady at one-year post-grant funding. Over the course of four years, the number of students from the Puerto Rican medical schools applying to the health network's residency programs tripled. A total of four students ultimately matched to residency programs within the health network during this time. In addition to meeting students at the school residency fairs, health network personnel used these visits to strengthen relationships with school leaders. Additionally, interest in collaboration with Puerto Rican schools expanded to include nursing leadership from a local community college in Pennsylvania.

Learnings

The health network presence at the school residency fairs preceded the start of this project, beginning in 2002; as a result, the project benefited from existing relationships with school leaders and a history of health network presence at school events. The project also benefited from strong leadership engagement from key departmental leaders – including a Latina department chair of medicine – as well as passionate project leaders. The success of the project was largely attributable to the positive relationships cultivated with leadership at the medical schools in Puerto Rico. The project benefited from the participation of a physician graduate of a Puerto Rican medical school who both during his residency at the health network and afterwards as an attending helped liaise with school leadership and built rapport with medical students.

Despite its demonstrated success in achieving goals, the sustainability of this project proved challenging. Although visits to Puerto Rico continued for some years after the end of the initial project grant period, the other strategies ended when grant funding ceased, as did tracking of metrics related to recruitment of medical students specifically from the Puerto Rican medical schools.

Strategy 2 – Underrepresented in Medicine (UriM) Pipeline Development

Overview

In 2021, the health network's graduate medical education leadership, in partnership with the health network's chief diversity liaison and a partner from a secondary school, launched another multi-pronged project that again aimed to increase the cross-cultural skills of its providers and enhance the recruitment of trainees from underrepresented groups in its residency training programs and physician workforce.

First, this effort targeted recruitment of medical students from groups underrepresented in medicine (URiM) interested in completing medical school rotations at the health network. Financial assistance was allocated for these students and approved for direct scholarship payments to selected students, free dormitory lodging, and a meal stipend for the duration of their rotations at the health network. During its first year, the project team developed promotional information, a student application, and a selection process for identifying scholarship recipients; scholarships were first awarded in year two of the project.

Second, the project sought to increase the depth of knowledge about DEIB among GME faculty, staff, and other learners by funding speakers and consultants with content and lived expertise and/or experience in these domains. The goal was to create and promote faculty and learner participation in a yearlong schedule of DEIB-focused sessions.

Finally, the project aimed to deepen the pipeline of health professional students by providing scholarship funds for URiM high school students from local high schools interested in participating in a dual-enrollment program sponsored in part by the health network.

This project was embedded in the wider work of the health network's cultural awareness committee, GME committee, and multicultural physician committees. The project was co-led by the health network's designated institutional official and its chief diversity liaison, in collaboration with six residency and one fellowship program director and a career and technical school leader (for the high school dual-enrollment strategy). Funding to support this project was provided by an internal health network grant.

Outcomes

At the time of publication of this chapter, this project is in its second year, and the first-year scholarships were awarded to qualifying UriM medical students. Six students were awarded scholarships and no scholarships for high school students were provided as of this book's publication. While no additional consultant speakers/educational sessions on topics related to DEIB at the network level were yet funded by the project, speakers and sessions on these topics have been completed within individual departments. It is expected that in subsequent years of the project additional scholarships will be awarded and educational sessions will be provided.

Learnings

This project offered multiple opportunities for learning. Time is always a limited resource, and the project team benefited from the ability to dedicate nearly a full first year of the grant to planning. This time was needed to develop the full project team, to identify and engage key stakeholders throughout the health network, to define a process for disbursing scholarship funds to students, and to clearly define success metrics. The project also re-surfaced a challenge that without allocating ("carving out" or "building in" or "paying") time for project leadership and team participation, team members are strapped to "add on" project responsibilities in addition to responsibilities outlined in formal job descriptions. This causes organizational and personal stress, as team members are challenged to find time to meet and to advance project goals they deem important but may not be seen as valuable within the formal organizational structure and priorities.

Timing of such projects is important. This project launched with the support of internal grant funding that was available for the first time and was focused on advancing DEIB and education efforts within the health network. The project capitalized on momentum focusing on attracting a more diverse workforce that was growing within the network. Additionally, timing matters when offering scholarships to students – either high school or medical students; the timing of when scholarship details were finalized and communicated to eligible students impacted how many students were notified and could ultimately apply.

Training and consensus on key objectives are similarly critical. The project team quickly realized that although we all had enhanced diversity as a goal, each team member had a slightly different notion of what "diversity" meant and how it should be measured and defined. An entire project team meeting was spent reviewing the literature and definitions of "underrepresentation" that existed at that time in medical education and defining the criteria that would be used to select students for the scholarships. The team reviewed institutional, community, and national demographic data to identify groups most underrepresented with the institution's medical education programs. Ultimately, as lack of diversity in terms of race and ethnicity - specifically from Hispanic, Black/African-American, and Native American groups - represented the most critical area for immediate improvement, the team decided to focus solely on diversity in terms of learner self-reported race and ethnicity for the initial roll-out of the scholarship. The team focused its efforts to promote the scholarship to Hispanic, Black/African-American, and Native American learners specifically, with the hopes of seeing an increase in the number of individuals from these groups entering the institution's medical education programs.

The project underwent a significant transition at the end of year 1 in which the project lead left the health network for other employment. The project continued under the leadership of an interim project lead and with the commitment of the project team, and a new project lead was designated within four months, however any change in leadership of such a project can disrupt momentum, can increase stress and workload for remaining project team members, and may impact timelines.

QUESTIONS AND ANSWERS

1. What factors should organizations consider when creating strategies to attract candidates from underrepresented backgrounds?

First and foremost, organizations seeking to attract candidates from underrepresented backgrounds must measure the outcomes and impacts of their initiatives and make necessary adjustments to meet established goals. Next, organizations must work to identify and address implicit biases that can be inherent in recruiting processes. This may include requiring unconscious bias training for all individuals involved in the recruitment and selection process and may include considering elements of holistic review in GME and hiring decisions. Learners from traditionally underrepresented groups may feel that they do not fit the usual profile for a program, including academic rigor, test scores, and even level of fluency in English. However, if an organization places sufficient value on increasing its diversity to reflect the needs of its community, strong leadership advocacy may be necessary to promote this broader and more inclusive acceptance criterion (without reducing academic rigor or performance standards) while taking care to create a culture of inclusion within the program overall.

Importantly, organizations must solicit, value, and include perspectives from individuals from the underrepresented backgrounds they seek to attract, including individuals currently participating in their training programs, patients, and individuals in the communities they serve. These partners often can be the strongest advocates for the organization and for the needs to broaden the number of diverse candidates, especially where genuine collaborative relationships and trust are well established.

Organizations must also consider the potential impacts of different licensing, accreditation, and other requirements when seeking to attract candidates from different states, territories, or countries. Each state in the United States has specific requirements for the issuance of a license to any health care provider and these can vary from state to state. These prerequisites include, but are not limited to, appropriate academic preparation and criminal background clearance. Most states require additional criteria for those outside of the continental US, such as demonstration of English proficiency. These criteria have been changed, modified, or even temporarily suspended in extreme crisis environments such as during the initial COVID era.

2. With the strategies described in this chapter, some but not all intended project goals were achieved. What could the health network have done differently to achieve desired results?

This case highlighted two different strategies implemented over a period of two decades. Although the strategies differed in several ways, both were challenged by sustainability.

Vital with any grant-funded initiative is the priority that must be placed on development of a plan for sustainability, to ensure that strategies implemented during the life cycle of a grant are continued or converted in some way into the future. Planning for sustainability might have been better incorporated into the initial grants for both projects, with project teams and organizational leaders held accountable to specific milestones related to sustainability plans incorporated throughout the initial grant life cycles.

Additionally, both strategies integrated existing health network resources. In the first strategy, funding was allocated for time for project leaders to dedicate to the grant's work; in the second, funding was not allocated for time. In both instances, using existing resources meant that resources were often challenged to find time to dedicate to grant work; with the second grant wherein, funding was not allocated for time, this proved even more challenging, specifically for physician project team members.

With both strategies, the health network might have prioritized the strategies at a higher level to ensure both their prioritization and their sustainability. However, the difficult challenge persists: health networks are tasked with numerous priorities and have limited resources to achieve them. Overall, strategies that may have helped in this case are incorporation and alignment of the projects into health network strategic planning and regular reporting of metrics to the highest level of the health network. These would help ensure project team accountability to established goals and would help surface challenges – including resource constraints – at the highest levels of the organization.

3. What additional strategies might the health network have implemented, or might it implement in the future?

The health network has committed resources to the development of so-called "pipeline" programs for youth in the region to pursue health care careers. In the past, specific focus has been on support of underserved urban schools, with a large percentage of Hispanic/Latino/Latina/Latinx and Spanish-speaking youth in the community. This focus should continue, as local youth are more likely to choose to stay and practice close to home, and Hispanic/Latino/Latina/Latinx and Spanish-speaking youth represent a demographic underrepresented within the health network workforce.

The health network should also focus on continuation of relationships, specifically relationships with the Puerto Rican medical schools, as well as Hispanic/Latino/Latina/Latinx and Spanish-speaking organizations and leaders locally. These efforts require time, continuity of personnel, and warm hand-off/succession planning when leadership changes occur.

4. What is the role of health network leadership in the success or failure of strategies such as those implemented by this health network?

Leadership buy-in is critical to the initiation, continuation, sustainability, and success of such strategies. In both strategies described within this chapter, key leaders within the health network initiated, supported, guided, and provided funding in support of the strategies. This included support of project teams as they sought and secured grant funding, allowing project team members time to dedicate to the strategies, and championing the strategies at the highest levels of the organization. However, diversity must be valued and nurtured at all levels of an organization for it to be sustained and for it to grow. Bringing top candidates to the institution for consideration is helpful, but there also needs to be agreement and appreciation of the unique value of these learners at all levels to ensure these candidates are then accepted into the various educational programs over time.

Leaders who actively value and champion inclusion and equity are critical. Although diversity initiatives can and do start from the ground up, having top organizational leadership driving for change can put a spotlight on these initiatives, help identify initial funding, provide political leverage when needed, and add organizational awareness of how diversity initiatives fit with wider institutional goals. Also important to consider is the propensity to unequally place the responsibility of DEIB efforts on minority faculty and staff; leaders should actively ensure that organizational DEIB efforts do not add to the "minority tax" that is often felt by those representing the very groups they are trying to support (Faucett et al., 2022; Rodríguez, Campbell, & Pololi, 2015).

As mentioned previously, sustainability is key to lasting impact. Leaders must ensure diversity programs align with institutional values and culture, and with strategic plans. Further, leadership support is necessary to ensure that funding is operationalized or included within standing budgets so that programs with demonstrated success need not cease when initial funding ceases. Sustained support – including budget support – can be challenging when considered against other priorities, thus it critical that DEIB efforts be woven into the fabric of an organization and considered as an element within all other organizational initiatives.

5. What role does cultural humility play when implementing strategies such as those discussed?

Cultural humility - the process of self-reflection and discovery to understand oneself and then others in order to build honest and trustworthy relationships (Tervalon & Murray-García, 1998) - is critical when implementing strategies such as those described in this chapter (Diaz, Navarro, & Chen, 2020).

Beyond consideration of race and ethnicity, cultural humility is critical when dealing with all learners, as it is also when dealing with all patients. Valuing differences and working effectively together with people with differing characteristics and identities related to hearing ability, sexual orientation, socioeconomic status, English language ability, country of origin, immigration status, age, gender, ability, veteran status, and others all requires a sense of curiosity, willingness to learn, and willingness to view the "other" as valued. Equally essential is an appreciation of the unlimited variation that occurs within groups, and the impact of intersectional identities on individuals as well as groups.

Humility extends to program leaders as well, as they consider the framework, strategies, and metrics of their interventions. No one person will have all the answers for how to develop and implement strategies such as those described in this chapter. Studying the literature and understanding what has worked in different contexts is important, but just as important is listening to and valuing the lived experience of members of all groups the organization is striving to attract. This valuing of diverse perspectives could mean including URiM members on the project team or in other stages of program planning, conducting focus groups of current URiM trainees and employed staff, and hosting listening sessions with patient and community members.

Further, organizations must consider the impact of strategies such as those described here on the communities wherein they are working to attract candidates. Most importantly, organizations must consider the impact of recruiting URiM away from their communities, specifically the potential for "brain drain" of individuals from areas that are in critical need of health care providers to those that are more well-resourced (Saravia & Miranda, 2004; Diallo, 2004). This is especially important during periods of health care employment crisis and in areas that experience acute health care provider shortages. As much as possible, efforts to attract learners should be viewed as a partnership, between their home communities, the organization and its community, and the learner. The continued success of any individual diversity program is based on the success of each stakeholder, and efforts to build and grow the relationships in many ways, beyond recruitment alone, can leave a more lasting, sustained legacy.

6. How can candidates from underrepresented backgrounds optimize opportunities available to them?

The demonstrated need for increased diversity in medicine and the most recent focus on this as a national priority means that a plethora of opportunities are available for individuals from underrepresented backgrounds interested in pursuing careers in health care. Numerous resources also exist for individuals to find trusted information on how to navigate educational and training options, as well as opportunities for funding, mentorship, and forms of support. However, many historical challenges to representation exist still today; one of these challenges is identifying and making sense of all the opportunities available. Thus seeking out trusted sources of information and mentorship is critical (Hadinger, 2017). Medical schools – particularly offices of admission, student affairs, and diversity – can be particularly helpful in providing accurate and timely information about opportunities. National organizations - such as the Association for American Medical Schools (AAMC), the American Osteopathic Association (AOA), the American Medical Association (AMA), and the Accreditation Council on Graduate Medical Education (ACGME), among others - and student leadership organizations - such as the Student National Medical Association (SNMA) and the Latino Medical Student Association (LMSA), among others – are also good sources for information applicable at each step of the medical education process. Individuals can actively seek and capitalize on opportunities for mentorship, whenever possible from those with insight and commitment towards supporting underrepresented students, which could include individuals with similar backgrounds who have navigated through their own health care education journeys, as well as others. When applying for positions or opportunities, candidates should ask for feedback. Medical students who have opportunities to visit organizations as they complete rotations should seek to get to know the region, not just the hospital or other location being visited. Candidates should ask questions and look for an organization where they feel they will best fit in and be successful.

Epilogue

In the ensuing two decades since the initial project described herein was undertaken, the health network's commitment to delivering cross-cultural, linguistically-appropriate care has grown in scope and depth to the extent that these elements are now considered integral to operations and the care delivery process. The health network's commitment to diversifying its workforce is just one example of this organizational cultural shift.

For example, several graduate medical education programs are employing strategies such as expanding program promotion strategies (including social media) to diverse audiences, using holistic review when evaluating applicants, and standardizing interview questions and selection matrices to recruit residents from underrepresented backgrounds.

All network residency programs are incorporating more content on equity, inclusion and belonging through DEIB task forces, didactic education, and mentoring programs. This work is aligned with network-level initiatives related to recruitment, professional development, staff education and implementation of additional colleague resource groups (Gurchiek, 2019).

Future work could include expanding metrics beyond representation to determine correlation of DEIB efforts with data on patient outcomes.

Most recently, in response to the challenges experienced by health care organizations globally brought on by the COVID-19 pandemic and ensuing market forces, in 2021 the health network's interest in re-cruiting health professionals from geographically diverse regions was rekindled and re-focused on the recruitment of nursing students, graduate nurses, and nursing professionals. Strategies to attract nurses included re-invigorating connections previously established with health professions schools in Puerto Rico. Both the original educational administrator from the health network and the on-site consultant in Puerto Rico were engaged in planning, and lessons learned from previous efforts related to medical students were considered in the development of this new nursing-focused recruitment. Results of this most recent effort are pending at the time of this publication. In addition, the health network continues to support multiple regional initiatives encouraging local youth to pursue careers in health care and considers these as part of the mid- and long-term workforce development pipeline.

As this chapter goes to print, the role of race in higher education admissions is being considered by the US Supreme Court as it considers two cases – *Students for Fair Admissions v. President and Fellows of Harvard College* and *Students for Fair Admissions v. University of North Carolina* - with decisions on both expected in mid-2023. The cases center on appeals from a student group challenging the use of race as a factor in undergraduate college admissions.

The decisions are expected to have far-reaching impacts not only college admissions and admissions at selective primary and secondary schools, but employment as well – and by extension, in medical education and medical workforces.

In its amicus brief, the Association of American Medical Colleges and 45 other health organizations asked the Court not to disrupt the current admissions processes of health professions schools because decisions in favor of the plaintiff might limit schools' ability to use race as a factor in admissions and this is expected to have immediate, dramatic, adverse implications on diversity in higher education and on patient care (AAMC, 2022).

Regardless the decisions in these cases – and others that may follow them - what is clear from the research is that racial concordance positively impacts patient outcomes, and that educational diversity positively impacts learning. Even more broadly, principles of cultural competency and humility will remain critically important into the future.

REFERENCES

Accreditation Council on Graduate Medical Education. (2022). *Common program requirements*. https://prep.acgme.org/what-we-do/accreditation/common-program-requirements/

American Hospital Association, Institute for Diversity and Health Equity. (2022). *Health equity, diversity and inclusion measures for hospital and health system dashboards*. https://ifdhe.aha.org/health-equity-diversity-inclusion-measures-hospitals-and-health-system-dashboards

Antonio, A. L. (2004). Effects of racial diversity on complex thinking in college students. *Psychological Science, 15*, 507–510.

Association of American Medical Colleges. (2019). *Diversity in Medicine: Facts and Figures 2019.* https://www.aamc.org/data-reports/workforce/report/diversity-medicine-facts-and-figures-2019

Association of American Medical Colleges. (2022). *Advancing diversity, equity, and inclusion in medical education*. https://www.aamc.org/about-us/equity-diversity-inclusion/advancing-diversity-equity-and-inclusion-medical-education

Association of American Medical Colleges. (2022). *AAMC leads amicus brief in support of consideration of race in higher education admissions*. https://www.aamc.org/news-insights/press-releases/aamc-leads-amicus-brief-support-consideration-race-higher-education-admissions

Association of American Medical Colleges, Group on Diversity and Inclusion. (2022). https://www.aamc.org/career-development/affinity-groups/gdi#:~:text=How%20the%20AAMC%20Defines%20Diversity%20and%20Inclusion.%20Diversity.,identity%2C%20sexual%20orientation%2C%20religion%2C%20geography%2C%20disability%20and%20age

Barzansky, B., Hash, R. B., Catanese, V., & Waechter, D. (2021). What is the role of accreditation in achieving medical school diversity? *The Journal of Ethics*, *23*(12), E946–E952. doi:10.1001/amajethics.2021.946

Betancourt, J. R., Green, A. R., Carrillo, J. E., & Ananeh-Firempong, O., II. (2003). Defining cultural competence: a practical framework for addressing racial/ethnic disparities in health and health care. *Public Health Reports, 118*(4), 293–302. doi:10.1093/phr/118.4.293

Boatright, D., Branzetti, J., Duong, D., Hicks, M., Moll, J., Perry, M., Pierce, A., Samuels, E., Smith, T., Angerhofer, C., & Heron, S. (2018). Racial and ethnic diversity in academic Emergency Medicine: How far have we come? Next steps for the future. *Academic Emergency Medicine Education and Training, 2*(Suppl 1), S31–S39. doi:10.1002/aet2.10204

Cantor, J., Miles, E., Baker, L., & Barker, D. (1996). Physician service to the underserved: Implications for affirmative action. *Inquiry*, *33*, 167–181.

Castillo-Page, L. (2006). *Diversity in the physician workforce: Facts & figures 2006.* Association of American Medical Colleges. https://www.aamc.org/morediversity

Cooper, L. (2003). Patient-centered communication, ratings of care and concordance of patient and physician race. *Annals of Internal Medicine*, *139*(11), 907–915.

Cooper-Patrick, L. (1999). Race, gender and partnership in the patient-physician relationship. *Journal of the American Medical Association*, *282*(6), 583–589.

Cordero Guzmán, H. (2016). *The production and reproduction of poverty in Puerto Rico; A socio-economic and demographic analysis with data from Puerto Rico Community Survey*. Interamerican University.

Diallo, K. (2004). Data on the migration of health-care workers: Sources, uses, and challenges. *Bulletin of the World Health Organization*, *82*(8), 601–607.

Diaz, T., Navarro, J. R., & Chen, E. H. (2020). An institutional approach to fostering inclusion and addressing racial bias: Implications for diversity in academic medicine. *Teaching and Learning in Medicine*, *32*(1), 110–116. https://doi.org/10.1080/10401334.2019.1670665

Faucett, E. A., Brenner, M. J., Thompson, D. M., & Flanary, V. A. (2022). Tackling the minority tax: A roadmap to redistributing engagement in diversity, equity, and inclusion initiatives. *Otolaryngology - Head and Neck Surgery*, *166*(6), 1174–1181. https://doi.org/10.1177/01945998221091696

Gertner, E. J., Sabino, J. N., Mahady, E., Deitrick, L. M., Patton, J. R., Grim, M. K., Geiger, J. F., & Salas-Lopez, D. (2010). Developing a culturally competent health network: A planning framework and guide. *Journal of Healthcare Management*, *55*(3), 190–204.

Gomez, L. E., & Bernet, P. (2019). Diversity improves performance and outcomes. *Journal of the National Medical Association*, *111*(4), 383–392. https://doi.org/10.1016/j.jnma.2019.01.006

Gonzaga, A., Appiah-Pippim, J., Onumah, C. M., & Yialamas, M. A. (2020). A framework for inclusive graduate medical education recruitment strategies: Meeting the ACGME standard for a diverse and inclusive workforce. *Academic Medicine*, *95*(5), 710–716. https://doi.org/10.1097/ACM.0000000000003073

Gonzaga, A. M., Marbin, J., & Terhune, K. (2022). Evidence-based inclusive graduate medical education recruitment strategies. *Journal of Graduate Medical Education*, *14*(1), 115–116. https://doi.org/10.4300/JGME-D-21-01134.1

Guiton, G., Chang, M. J., & Wilkerson, L. (2007). Student body diversity: Relationship to medical students' experiences and attitudes. *Academic Medicine*, *82*(Suppl), S85–S88. doi:10.1097/ACM.0b013e31813ffe1e

Gurchiek, K. (2019). *ERGs to effect change, spark innovation*. Society for Human Resource Management (SHRM). https://www.shrm.org/resourcesandtools/hr-topics/behavioral-competencies/global-and-cultural-effectiveness/pages/use-ergs-to-affect-change-spark-innovation.aspx

Hadinger, M. A. (2017). Underrepresented minorities in medical school admissions: A qualitative study. *Teaching and Learning in Medicine*, *29*(1), 31–41. https://doi.org/10.1080/10401334.2016.1220861

Hung, R. (2007). Student perspectives on diversity and the cultural climate at a US medical school. *Academic Medicine*, *82*(2), 184–192.

Komaromy, M. (1996). The role of Black and Hispanic physicians in providing health care for underserved populations. *The New England Journal of Medicine*, *334*(2), 1305–1310.

Liaison Committee on Medical Education. (2022). *Functions and structure of a medical school*. https://lcme.org/publications/

Malat, J. (2001). Social distance and patients' rating of healthcare providers. *Journal of Health and Social Behavior*, *42*(4), 360–372.

Moy, E., & Bartman, B. (1995). Physician race and care of minority and medically indigent patients. *Journal of the American Medical Association*, *273*(19), 1515–1520.

National Healthcare Quality and Disparities Report. (2022). Agency for Healthcare Research and Quality. AHRQ Pub. No. 22(23)-0030.

Niu, N. N., Syed, Z. A., Krupat, E., Crutcher, B. N., Pelletier, S. R., & Shields, H. M. (2012). The impact of cross-cultural interactions on medical students' preparedness to care for diverse patients. *Academic Medicine*, *87*(11), 1530–1534.

Ortiz Reyes, M., & Sepúlveda Arroyo, L. (2020). The impact of recent demographic changes and migration patterns on education in Puerto Rico. In M. Slowey, H. Schuetze, & T. Zubrzycki (Eds.), *Inequality, Innovation and Reform in Higher Education* (pp. 59–69). Springer Nature Switzerland AG.

Rodríguez, J. E., Campbell, K. M., & Pololi, L. H. (2015). Addressing disparities in academic medicine: What of the minority tax? *BMC Medical Education*, *15*, 6. https://doi.org/10.1186/s12909-015-0290-9

Saha, S., Guiton, G., Wimmers, P. F., & Wilkerson, L. (2008). Student body racial and ethnic composition and diversity-related outcomes in US medical schools. *Journal of the American Medical Association*, *300*(10), 1135–1145. https://doi.org/10.1001/jama.300.10.1135

Saravia, N. G., & Miranda, J. F. (2004). Plumbing the brain drain. *Bulletin of the World Health Organization*, *82*(8), 608–615.

Shea, G., & Solomon, C. A. (2020). *Leading successful change, revised and updated edition: 8 keys to making change work*. Wharton School Press.

Shen, M. J., Peterson, E. B., Costas-Muñiz, R., Hernandez, M. H., Jewell, S. T., Matsoukas, K., & Bylund, C. L. (2018). The Effects of Race and Racial Concordance on Patient-Physician Communication: A Systematic Review of the Literature. *Journal of Racial and Ethnic Health Disparities*, *5*(1), 117–140. https://doi.org/10.1007/s40615-017-0350-4

Smedley, B. D., Stith Butler, A., & Bristow, L. R. (Eds.). (2004). In the nation's compelling interest: Ensuring diversity in the health-care workforce. National Academies Press (US).

Tarn, D. M., & … . (2005). Trust in one's physician: The role of ethnic match, autonomy, acculturation, and religiosity among Japanese and Japanese Americans. *Annals of Family Medicine*, *3*(4), 339–347.

Tervalon, M., & Murray-García, J. (1998). Cultural humility versus cultural competence: A critical distinction in defining physician training outcomes in multicultural education. *Journal of Health Care for the Poor and Underserved*, *9*(2), 117–125. doi:10.1353/hpu.2010.0233

US Census Bureau. (2020). *2020 Census*. https://www.census.gov/programs-surveys/decennial-census/decade/2020/2020-census-main.html

Velázquez-Estrada, A. (2016). *Perfil del migrante 2014*. Instituto de Estadísticas de Puerto Rico. https://estadisticas.pr/files/Publicaciones/Perfil_del_Migrante_2014_0.pdf

Whitla, D. K., Orfield, G., Silen, W., Teperow, C., Howard, C., & Reede, J. (2003). Educational benefits of diversity in medical school: A survey of students. *Academic Medicine*, *78*(5), 460–466. https://doi.org/10.1097/00001888-200305000-00007

ENDNOTE

1 Definitions of diversity abound. The Association of American Medical Colleges defines diversity as: "[Embodying] inclusiveness, mutual respect, and multiple perspectives and serves as a catalyst for change resulting in health equity. In this context, we are mindful of all aspects of human differences such as socioeconomic status, race, ethnicity, language, nationality, sex, gender identity, sexual orientation, religion, geography, disability and age" (AAMC Group on Diversity and Inclusion, 2022). In this context, it is critical to remember that race and ethnicity are but elements to consider within a larger spectrum of many characteristics and identities that make individuals unique. Nonetheless, race and ethnicity continue to provide a starting point upon which more expansive definitions of diversity, research, and initiatives can build.

Compilation of References

AAMC. (2022). Retrieved from Matriculating Student Questionnaire (MSQ): https://www.aamc.org/data-reports/students-residents/report/matriculating-student-questionnaire-msq

Accreditation Council on Graduate Medical Education. (2022). *Common program requirements.* https://prep.acgme.org/what-we-do/accreditation/common-program-requirements/

Ackerman-Barger, K., & Jacobs, N. N. (2020). The Microaggressions Triangle Model: A Humanistic Approach to Navigating Microaggressions in Health Professions Schools. *Academic Medicine, 95*(12S), S28–S32. doi:10.1097/ACM.0000000000003692 PMID:32889926

ADA Amendments Act of 2008. (2008). 42 U.S.C. § 12101 et seq. Retrieved July 22, 2022 from https://www.ada.gov/pubs/adastatute08.htm

Adams, M., Bell, L. A., & Griffin, P. (Eds.). (2007). Teaching for diversity and social justice (2nd ed.). Routledge/Taylor & Francis Group. doi:10.4324/9780203940822

Agaronnik, N. D., El-Jawahri, A., & Iezzoni, L. I. (2022). Implications of physical access barriers for breast cancer diagnosis and treatment in women with mobility disability. *Journal of Disability Policy Studies, 33*(1), 46–54. doi:10.1177/10442073211010124 PMID:35875606

Agaronnik, N. D., Pendo, E., Campbell, E. G., Ressalam, J., & Iezzoni, L. I. (2019). Knowledge of practicing physicians about their legal obligations when caring for patients with disability. *Health Affairs, 38*(4), 545–553. doi:10.1377/hlthaff.2018.05060 PMID:30933590

Agency for Healthcare Research and Quality (AHRQ). (2015). Health literacy universal precautions toolkit (2nd ed.). AHRQ. https://www.ahrq.gov/professionals/quality-patient-safety/quality-resources/tools/literacy-toolkit/index.html

Agrawal, P., Madsen, T. E., Lall, M., & Zeidan, A. (2020). Gender disparities in academic emergency medicine: Strategies for the recruitment, retention, and promotion of women. *AEM Education and Training, 4*(S1), S67–S74. doi:10.1002/aet2.10414 PMID:32072109

AHA. (2011). *Improving Health Equity Through Data Collection and Use: A Guide For Hospital Leaders.* AHA.

Ahmad, D. A. (2022). The Influence of Interpersonal Conflict, Job Stress, and Work Life Balance on Employee Turnover Intention. *International Journal of Humanities and Education Development, 4*(2), 1–14. doi:10.22161/jhed.4.2.1

AHRQ. (2012). *Improving Patient Safety Systems for Patients with Limited English Proficiency. A Guide for Hospitals.* AHRQ. https://www.ahrq.gov/sites/default/files/publications/files/lepguide.pdf

AHRQ. (2017). *Patients With Limited English Proficiency.* Agency for Healthcare Research and Quality. https://www.ahrq.gov/teamstepps/lep/index.html

Aifah, A., Onakomaiya, D., Rakhra, A., & Ogedegbe, G. (2021). Uprooting race-based assumptions in biomedical journal articles. *Trends in Molecular Medicine*, *27*(9), 830–832. doi:10.1016/j.molmed.2021.06.003

Al Shamsi, H., Almutairi, A. G., Al Mashrafi, S., & Al Kalbani, T. (2020). Implications of language barriers for health-care: A systematic review. *Oman Medical Journal*, *35*(2), e122. doi:10.5001/omj.2020.40 PMID:32411417

AlFaris, E., Irfan, F., Qureshi, R., Naeem, N., Alshomrani, A., Ponnamperuma, G., Al Yousufi, N., Al Maflehi, N., Al Naami, M., Jamal, A., & van der Vleuten, C. (2016). Health professions' students have an alarming prevalence of depressive symptoms: Exploration of the associated factors. *BMC Medical Education*, *16*(1), 279. doi:10.118612909-016-0794-y PMID:27769235

Alinor, M. (2022). Research: The Real-Time Impact of Microaggressions. *Harvard Business Review*. Retrieved from https://hbr.org/2022/05/research-the-real-time-impact-of-microaggressions

Alvord, L. A. (2013). Medical School Accommodations for Religious and Cultural Practices. *The Virtual Mentor*, *15*(3), 198–201. doi:10.1001/virtualmentor.2013.15.3.ecas3-1303 PMID:23472807

Amanullah, S., & Ramesh Shankar, R. (2020). The Impact of COVID-19 on Physician Burnout Globally: A Review. *Health Care*, *8*(4), 421. doi:10.3390/healthcare8040421 PMID:33105757

American Foundation for the Blind. (2006). *ADA Checklist: Health Care Facilities and Service Providers*. AFB. https://www.afb.org/blindness-and-low-vision/your-rights/advocacy-resources/ada-checklist-health-care-facilities-and#%5B1%5D

American Hospital Association, Institute for Diversity and Health Equity. (2022). *Health equity, diversity and inclusion measures for hospital and health system dashboards*. https://ifdhe.aha.org/health-equity-diversity-inclusion-measures-hospitals-and-health-system-dashboards

American Medical Association and American Association of Medical Colleges Center for Health Justice. (2021). *Advancing Health Equity: A guide to language, narrative, and concepts*. American Medical Association.

American Medical Association. (2021). *AMA seeks more help for medical students, residents with disabilities*. AMA. https://www.ama-assn.org/education/medical-school-diversity/ama-seeks-more-help-medical-students-residents-disabilities

American Medical Association. (2022). *AMA Guides to the Evaluation of Permanent Impairment*. AMA. https://ama-guides.ama-assn.org/books/book/8/AMA-Guides-to-the-Evaluation-of-Permanent

American Osteopathic Association. (2019). *Accreditation of Colleges of Osteopathic Medicine: COM Continuing Accreditation Standards*. Commission on Osteopathic College Accreditation. Microsoft Word - 2019 COM Continuing Accreditation Standards Rev 2-20.

Americans With Disabilities Act of 1990, Pub. L. No. 101-336, 104 Stat. 328 (1990).

Americans with Disabilities Act of 1990. (1990). 42 U.S.C. § 12101 et seq. Retrieved July 22, 2022 from https://www.ada.gov/pubs/adastatute08.htm

Amutah, C., Greenidge, K., Mante, A., Munyikwa, M., Surya, S. L., Higginbotham, E., Jones, D. S., Lavizzo-Mourey, R., Roberts, D., Tsai, J., & Aysola, J. (2021). Misrepresenting Race—The Role of Medical Schools in Propagating Physician Bias. *The New England Journal of Medicine*, *384*(9), 872–878. https://doi.org/10.1056/NEJMms2025768

Anderson, P. M., & Vanderbilt, A. A. (2018). Bridging the gap between physician and medical student education: Using the Train the Trainer model to improve cultural competence training in the clerkship years of medical school. *Advances in Medical Education and Practice*, *9*, 495–498. doi:10.2147/AMEP.S163485 PMID:29983602

Andresen, E. M., Peterson-Besse, J. J., Krahn, G. L., Walsh, E. S., Horner-Johnson, W., & Iezzoni, L. I. (2013). Pap, mammography, and clinical breast examination screening among women with disabilities: A systematic review. *Women's Health Issues*, *23*(4), e205–e214. doi:10.1016/j.whi.2013.04.002 PMID:23816150

Antonio, A. L. (2004). Effects of racial diversity on complex thinking in college students. *Psychological Science*, *15*, 507–510.

Arfuch, V. M., Angelats, R. C., Martin, C. A., Goncalves, A. Q., Carrasco-Querol, N., & Gonzalez Serra, G. (2022). Patients' Lived Experience in a Multicomponent Intervention for Fibromyalgia Syndrome in Primary Care: A Qualitative Interview Study. *International Journal of Environmental Research and Public Health*, *19*(20), 13322. Advance online publication. doi:10.3390/ijerph192013322 PMID:36293900

Association of American Medical Colleges & Liaison Committee on Medical Education. (2003). *Functions and structure of a medical school: standards for accreditation of medical education programs leading to the MD degree*. Liaison Committee on Medical Education.

Association of American Medical Colleges, Group on Diversity and Inclusion. (2022). https://www.aamc.org/career-development/affinity-groups/gdi#:~:text=How%20the%20AAMC%20Defines%20Diversity%20and%20Inclusion.%20Diversity.,identity%2C%20sexual%20orientation%2C%20religion%2C%20geography%2C%20disability%20and%20age

Association of American Medical Colleges. (2015). *Helping Medical Schools Assist Students with Disabilities*. AAMC. https://www.aamc.org/professional-development/affinity-groups/gsa/webinars/assist-students-with-disabilities

Association of American Medical Colleges. (2019). *Diversity in Medicine: Facts and Figures 2019*. https://www.aamc.org/data-reports/workforce/report/diversity-medicine-facts-and-figures-2019

Association of American Medical Colleges. (2020). *The state of women in academic medicine: The pipeline and pathways to leadership*. https://store.aamc.org/the-state-of-women-in-academic-medicine-2018-2019-exploring-pathways-to-equity.html

Association of American Medical Colleges. (2022). *AAMC leads amicus brief in support of consideration of race in higher education admissions*. https://www.aamc.org/news-insights/press-releases/aamc-leads-amicus-brief-support-consideration-race-higher-education-admissions

Association of American Medical Colleges. (2022). *Advancing diversity, equity, and inclusion in medical education*. https://www.aamc.org/about-us/equity-diversity-inclusion/advancing-diversity-equity-and-inclusion-medical-education

Axelson, R. D., Solow, C. M., Ferguson, K. J., & Cohen, M. B. (2010). Assessing implicit gender bias in Medical Student Performance Evaluations. *Evaluation & the Health Professions*, *33*(3), 365–385. doi:10.1177/0163278710375097 PMID:20801977

Ayyala, R. S., Artunduaga, M., Morin, C. E., & Coley, B. D. (2022). Leveraging diversity, equity and inclusion for promoting wellness in the radiology workplace. *Pediatric Radiology*, *52*(9), 1–6. doi:10.100700247-022-05292-z PMID:35088132

Baah, F. O., Teitelman, A. M., & Riegel, B. (2019). Marginalization: Conceptualizing patient vulnerabilities in the framework of social determinants of health—An integrative review. *Nursing Inquiry*, *26*(1), e12268. doi:10.1111/nin.12268 PMID:30488635

Baiden, D., Parry, M., Nerenberg, K., Hillan, E. M., & Dogba, M. J. (2022). Connecting the Dots: Structural Racism, Intersectionality, and Cardiovascular Health Outcomes for African, Caribbean, and Black Mothers. *Health Equity*, *6*(1), 402–405. doi:10.1089/heq.2021.0077

Balakrishnan, V., Roper, J., Cossey, K., Roman, C., & Jeanmonod, R. (2016). Misidentification of English language proficiency in triage: Impact on satisfaction and door-to-room time. *Journal of Immigrant and Minority Health*, *18*(2), 369–373. doi:10.100710903-015-0174-4 PMID:25750135

Balboni, M. J., Bandini, J., Mitchell, C., Epstein-Peterson, Z. D., Amobi, A., Cahill, J., Enzinger, A. C., Peteet, J., & Balboni, T. (2015). Religion, Spirituality, and the Hidden Curriculum: Medical Student and Faculty Reflections. *Journal of Pain and Symptom Management*, *50*(4), 507–515. doi:10.1016/j.jpainsymman.2015.04.020 PMID:26025271

Balboni, M. J., Sullivan, A., Enzinger, A., Epstein-Peterson, Z. D., Tseng, Y. D., Mitchell, C., Niska, J., Zollfrank, A., VanderWeele, T. J., & Balboni, T. A. (2014). Nurse and physician barriers to spiritual care provision of the end of life. *Journal of Pain and Symptom Management*, *48*(3), 400–410. doi:10.1016/j.jpainsymman.2013.09.020 PMID:24480531

Barwise, A., Jaramillo, C., Novotny, P., Wieland, M. L., Thongprayoon, C., Gajic, O., & Wilson, M. E. (2018). Differences in Code Status and End-of-Life Decision Making in Patients With Limited English Proficiency in the Intensive Care Unit. *Mayo Clinic Proceedings*, *93*(9), 1271–1281. doi:10.1016/j.mayocp.2018.04.021 PMID:30100192

Barzansky, B., Hash, R. B., Catanese, V., & Waechter, D. (2021). What is the role of accreditation in achieving medical school diversity? *The Journal of Ethics*, *23*(12), E946–E952. doi:10.1001/amajethics.2021.946

Bates, T. (1997). *Race, Self-Employment, and Upward Mobility: An Illusive American Dream*. The Johns Hopkins University Press.

Battalova, A., Bulk, L., Nimmon, L., Hole, R., Krupa, T., Lee, M., Mayer, Y., & Jarus, T. (2020, November). "I Can Understand Where They're Coming From": How Clinicians' Disability Experiences Shape Their Interaction With Clients. *Qualitative Health Research*, *30*(13), 2064–2076. doi:10.1177/1049732320922193 PMID:32449447

Becker, G., & Newsom, E. (2003). Socioeconomic Status and Dissatisfaction with Health Care Among Chronically Ill African Americans. *American Journal of Public Health*, *93*(5), 742–748. doi:10.2105/AJPH.93.5.742 PMID:12721135

Begley, C., Basu, R., Lairson, D., Reynolds, T., Dubinsky, S., Newmark, M., Barnwell, F., Hauser, A., & Hesdorffer, D. (2011). Socioeconomic status, health care use, and outcomes: Persistence of disparities over time. *Epilepsia*, *52*(5), 957–964. doi:10.1111/j.1528-1167.2010.02968.x PMID:21320113

Bellicoso, E., Quick, S. O., Ayoo, K. O., Beach, R. A., Joseph, M., & Dahlke, E. (2021). Diversity in Dermatology? An Assessment of Undergraduate Medical Education. *Journal of Cutaneous Medicine and Surgery*, *25*(4), 409–417. https://doi.org/10.1177/12034754211007430

Bell, S. K., Dong, J., Ngo, L., McGaffigan, P., Thomas, E. J., & Bourgeois, F. (2022). Diagnostic error experiences of patients and families with limited English-language health literacy or disadvantaged socioeconomic position in a cross-sectional US population-based survey. *BMJ Quality & Safety*, bmjqs-2021-013937. Advance online publication. doi:10.1136/bmjqs-2021-013937 PMID:35121653

Bell, T., & Zarzaur, B. (2013). Insurance status is a predictor of failure to rescue in trauma patients at both safety net and non-safety net hospitals. *The Journal of Trauma and Acute Care Surgery*, *75*(4), 728–733. doi:10.1097/TA.0b013e3182a53aaa PMID:24064890

Benda, N. C., Wesley, D. B., Nare, M., Fong, A., Ratwani, R. M., & Kellogg, K. M. (2022). Social determinants of health and patient safety: An analysis of patient safety event reports related to limited English-proficient patients. *Journal of Patient Safety*, *18*(1), e1–e9. doi:10.1097/PTS.0000000000000663 PMID:32168283

Berger, G., Conroy, S., Peerson, A., & Brazil, V. (2014). Clinical supervisors and cultural competence. *The Clinical Teacher*, *11*(5), 370–374. doi:10.1111/tct.12170 PMID:25041671

Berk, R. A. (2017). Microaggressions trilogy: Part 1. Why do microaggressions matter? *Journal of Faculty Development, 31*(1), 63.

Betancourt, J. R., Green, A. R., Carrillo, J. E., & Ananeh-Firempong, O., II. (2003). Defining cultural competence: a practical framework for addressing racial/ethnic disparities in health and health care. *Public Health Reports, 118*(4), 293–302. doi:10.1093/phr/118.4.293

Betancourt, J. R., Green, A. R., Carrillo, J. E., & Ananeh-Firempong, O. II. (2003). Defining Cultural Competence: A practical framework for addressing racial/ethnic disparities in health and health care. *Public Health Reports, 118*(4), 293–302. doi:10.1016/S0033-3549(04)50253-4 PMID:12815076

Beyond the curriculum: Academic nursing's responsibility for excellence in diversity, equity, and inclusion. (2021). *Journal of Professional Nursing , 37*(2), A1–A2. doi:10.1016/j.profnurs.2021.02.006

Bhatt, N., & Gentile, J. (2021). Interviewing Techniques for Patients with Intellectual Disability. *Journal of Mental Health Disorders, 1*(1), 10–14.

Blackburn, R. (2006). The Global Pension Crisis: From Gray Capitalism to Responsible Accumulation. *Politics & Society, 34*(2), 135–186. doi:10.1177/0032329206288150

Blackie, M., Wear, D., & Zarconi, J. (2019). Narrative Intersectionality in Caring for Marginalized or Disadvantaged Patients. *Academic Medicine, 94*(1), 59–63. doi:10.1097/ACM.0000000000002425 PMID:30134270

Blume, A. W., Lovato, L. V., Thyken, B. N., & Denny, N. (2012). The relationship of microaggressions with alcohol use and anxiety among ethnic minority college students in a historically White institution. *Cultural Diversity & Ethnic Minority Psychology, 18*(1), 45–54. https://doi.org/10.1037/a0025457

Boatright, D., Branzetti, J., Duong, D., Hicks, M., Moll, J., Perry, M., Pierce, A., Samuels, E., Smith, T., Angerhofer, C., & Heron, S. (2018). Racial and ethnic diversity in academic Emergency Medicine: How far have we come? Next steps for the future. *Academic Emergency Medicine Education and Training, 2*(Suppl 1), S31–S39. doi:10.1002/aet2.10204

Bodner, E. (2009). On the origins of ageism among older and younger adults. *International Psychogeriatrics, 21*(6), 1003–1014. doi:10.1017/S104161020999055X PMID:19619389

Boone, L. (2020). *Classism.* Salem Press Encyclopedia.

Boscolo-Hightower, A., Rafton, S. A., Tolman, M., Zhou, C., & Ebel, B. E. (2014). Identifying families with limited English proficiency using a capture-recapture approach. *Hospital Pediatrics, 4*(1), 16–22. doi:10.1542/hpeds.2013-0040 PMID:24435596

Bravata, D. M., Watts, S. A., Keefer, A. L., Madhusudhan, D. K., Taylor, K. T., Clark, D. M., Nelson, R. S., Cokley, K. O., & Hagg, H. K. (2020). Prevalence, Predictors, and Treatment of Impostor Syndrome: A Systematic Review. *Journal of General Internal Medicine, 35*(4), 1252–1275. doi:10.100711606-019-05364-1 PMID:31848865

Breathett, K., Spatz, E. S., Kramer, D. B., Essien, U. R., Wadhera, R. K., Peterson, P. N., Ho, P. M., & Nallamothu, B. K. (2021). The Groundwater of Racial and Ethnic Disparities Research: A Statement From Circulation: Cardiovascular Quality and Outcomes. *Circulation: Cardiovascular Quality and Outcomes, 14*(2), e007868. https://doi.org/10.1161/CIRCOUTCOMES.121.007868

Bright, M. A., Kleinman, L., Vogel, B., & Shenkman, E. (2018). Visits to Primary Care and Emergency Department Reliance for Foster Youth: Impact of Medicaid Managed Care. *Academic Pediatrics, 18*(4), 397–404. doi:10.1016/j.acap.2017.10.005 PMID:29081362

Brisset, C., Leanza, Y., & Laforest, K. (2013). Working with interpreters in health care: A systematic review and meta-ethnography of qualitative studies. *Patient Education and Counseling, 91*(2), 131–140. doi:10.1016/j.pec.2012.11.008 PMID:23246426

Brookfield, S. D. (2010). *Theoretical Frameworks for Understanding the Field. In Handbook of Adult and Continuing Education*. SAGE.

Brooks, K. C. (2015). A piece of my mind. A silent curriculum. *Journal of the American Medical Association, 313*(19), 1909–1910. https://doi.org/10.1001/jama.2015.1676

Brottman, M. R., Char, D. M., Hattori, R. A., Heeb, R., & Taff, S. D. (2020). Toward Cultural Competency in Health Care: A Scoping Review of the Diversity and Inclusion Education Literature. *Academic Medicine, 95*(5), 803–813. doi:10.1097/ACM.0000000000002995 PMID:31567169

Brown, M. E. L., Hunt, G. E. G., Hughes, F., & Finn, G. M. (2020). 'Too male, too pale, too stale': A qualitative exploration of student experiences of gender bias within medical education. *BMJ Open, 10*(8), e039092. doi:10.1136/bmjopen-2020-039092 PMID:32792453

Bulk, L. Y., Easterbrook, A., Roberts, E., Groening, M., Murphy, S., Lee, M., Ghanouni, P., Gagnon, J., & Jarus, T. (2017). 'We are not anything alike': Marginalization of health professionals with disabilities. *Disability & Society, 32*(5), 615–634. doi:10.1080/09687599.2017.1308247

Bulk, L. Y., Tikhonova, J., Gagnon, J. M., Battalova, A., Mayer, Y., Krupa, T., Lee, M., Nimmon, L., & Jarus, T. (2020). Disabled healthcare professionals' diverse, embodied, and socially embedded experiences. *Advances in Health Sciences Education: Theory and Practice, 25*(1), 111–129. doi:10.100710459-019-09912-6 PMID:31538268

Burke, S. E., Dovidio, J. F., Przedworski, J. M., Hardeman, R. R., Perry, S. P., Phelan, S. M., Nelson, D. B., Burgess, D. J., Yeazel, M. W., & van Ryn, M. (2015). Do Contact and Empathy Mitigate Bias Against Gay and Lesbian People Among Heterosexual First-Year Medical Students? A Report from the Medical Student CHANGE Study. *Academic Medicine, 90*(5), 645–651. doi:10.1097/ACM.0000000000000661 PMID:25674910

Burke, S. E., Dovidio, J. F., Przedworski, J. M., Hardeman, R. R., Perry, S. P., Phelan, S. M., Nelson, D. B., Burgess, D. J., Yeazel, M. W., & van Ryn, M. (2015). Do Contact and Empathy Mitigate Bias Against Gay and Lesbian People Among Heterosexual First-Year Medical Students? A Report From the Medical Student CHANGE Study. *Academic Medicine, 90*(5), 645–651. https://doi.org/10.1097/ACM.0000000000000661

Burks, D. J., & Kobus, A. M. (2012). The legacy of altruism in health care: The promotion of empathy, prosociality and humanism. *Medical Education, 2012*(46), 317–325. doi:10.1111/j.1365-2923.2011.04159.x PMID:22324531

Burton, N. (2020, March 6). Why Asians in masks should not be the "face" of the coronavirus. *Vox*. https://www.vox.com/identities/2020/3/6/21166625/coronavirus-photos-racism

Butler, J. (1999). *Gender Trouble: Feminism and the Subversion of Identity*. Routledge.

Butler, R. N. (1969). Age-ism: Another form of bigotry. *The Gerontologist, 9*(4), 243–246. doi:10.1093/geront/9.4_Part_1.243 PMID:5366225

Campbell, K. M., & Rodríguez, J. E. (2019). Addressing the Minority Tax: Perspectives from Two Diversity Leaders on Building Minority Faculty Success in Academic Medicine. *Academic Medicine, 94*(12), 1854–1857. doi:10.1097/ACM.0000000000002839 PMID:31192803

Cano-Ibáñez, N., Zolfaghari, Y., Amezcua-Prieto, C., & Khan, K. S. (2021). Physician-Patient Language Discordance and Poor Health Outcomes: A Systematic Scoping Review. *Frontiers in Public Health*, *9*, 629041. doi:10.3389/fpubh.2021.629041 PMID:33816420

Cantor, J., Miles, E., Baker, L., & Barker, D. (1996). Physician service to the underserved: Implications for affirmative action. *Inquiry*, *33*, 167–181.

Capodilupo, C. M., Nadal, K. L., Corman, L., Hamit, S., Lyons, O. B., & Weinberg, A. (2010). The manifestation of gender microaggressions. In *Microaggressions and marginality: Manifestation, dynamics, and impact* (pp. 193–216). John Wiley & Sons Inc.

Carmona, R. H., & McCabe, J. (2005). Improving the health and wellness of persons with disabilities: A call to action. *American Journal of Public Health*, *95*(11), 1883–1883. doi:10.2105/AJPH.95.11.1883 PMID:16254229

Carr, P. L., Ash, A. S., Friedman, R. H., Szalacha, L., Barnett, R. C., Palepu, A., & Moskowitz, M. M. (2000). Faculty perceptions of gender discrimination and sexual harassment in academic medicine. *Annals of Internal Medicine*, *132*(11), 889–896. doi:10.7326/0003-4819-132-11-200006060-00007 PMID:10836916

Carr, P. L., Gunn, C. M., Kaplan, S. A., Raj, A., & Freund, K. M. (2015). Inadequate progress for women in academic medicine: Findings from the National Faculty Study. *Journal of Women's Health*, *24*(3), 190–199. doi:10.1089/jwh.2014.4848 PMID:25658907

Carter, B. M., & Phillips, B. C. (2021). Revolutionizing the Nursing Curriculum. *Creative Nursing*, *27*(1), 25–30. https://doi.org/10.1891/CRNR-D-20-00072

Casey, L. S., Reisner, S. L., Findling, M. G., Blendon, R. J., Benson, J. M., Sayde, J. M., & Miller, C. (2019). Discrimination in the United States: Experiences of lesbian, gay, bisexual, transgender, and queer Americans. *Health Services Research*, *54*(S2), 1454–1466. doi:10.1111/1475-6773.13229 PMID:31659745

Castillo-Page, L. (2006). *Diversity in the physician workforce: Facts & figures 2006*. Association of American Medical Colleges. https://www.aamc.org/morediversity

CDC Health Disparities & Inequalities Report. (n.d.). https://www.cdc.gov/minorityhealth/chdireport.html#:~:text=The%20CDC%20Health%20Disparities%20and%20Inequalities%20Report%20%E2%80%93,income%2C%20education%2C%20disability%20status%20and%20other%20social%20characteristics

Census of Population Housing. (2011). USC B: 2010 Census of Population and Housing. U.S. Department of Commerce EaSA.

Centers for Disease Control and Prevention. (2020). *Autism Case Training: A Developmental-Behavioral Pediatrics Curriculum*. CDC. https://www.cdc.gov/ncbddd/actearly/autism/curriculum/class.html

Centers for Disease Control and Prevention. (January 14, 2022). *Autism and Developmental Disabilities Monitoring (ADDM) Network*. CDC. https://www.cdc.gov/ncbddd/autism/addm.html

Centers for Medicare and Medicaid Services Office of Minority Health. (2022). *Improving Communication Access For Individuals Who Are Blind Or Have Low Vision*. CMS. https://www.cms.gov/files/document/omh-visual-sensory-disabilities-brochure-508c.pdf

Cerdeña, J. P., Plaisime, M. V., & Tsai, J. (2020). From race-based to race-conscious medicine: How anti-racist uprisings call us to act. *Lancet*, *396*(10257), 1125–1128. https://doi.org/10.1016/S0140-6736(20)32076-6

Cerisier, K. (2019). Connecting Chronically Ill, Uninsured Patients Who Use the Emergency Department as a Medical Home: A Process Improvement Project. *Journal of Emergency Nursing: JEN*, *45*(3), 249–253. doi:10.1016/j.jen.2018.08.011 PMID:30293814

Chandra, S., Mohammadnezhad, M., & Ward, P. (2018). Trust and Communication in a Doctor- Patient Relationship: A Literature Review. *Journal of Healthcare Communications*, *3*(36), 1–6. doi:10.4172/2472-1654.100146

Chatterjee, P., Warner, L. N., Basil, M. C., Christopher, M., Manning, K., Fisher, H. N., Rexrode, K. M., Solomon, S. R., Kakoza, R. M., & Yialamas, M. A. (2021). "Make the Implicit Explicit": Measuring Perceptions of Gender Bias and Creating a Gender Bias Curriculum for Internal Medicine Residents. *Advances in Medical Education and Practice*, *12*, 49–52. doi:10.2147/AMEP.S292166 PMID:33488136

Chavan, M., Moncaliano, M., & Clarke, A. (2022). Preparing Trainees to Care for Diverse Patient Populations: Medical Students as Leaders in Curriculum Development. *Academic Medicine*, *97*(8), 1100–1101. https://doi.org/10.1097/ACM.0000000000004472

Cheah, C. S. L., Wang, C., Ren, H., Zong, X., Cho, H. S., & Xue, X. (2020). Covid-19 racism and Mental Health in Chinese American families. *Pediatrics*, *146*(5). https://doi.org/10.1542/peds.2020-021816

Children's Bureau. (2020). *The AFCARS report: Preliminary FY 2019 estimates as of June 23, 2020 -No. 27.* U.S. Department of Health and Human Services, Administration for Children and Families. https://www.acf.hhs.gov/cb/resource/afcars-report-27

Chiper, S. (2013) Teaching Intercultural Communication: ICT resources and best practices. *Procedia Social and Behavioral Sciences, 93*, 1641-1645. doi:10.1016/j.sbspro.2013.10.094

Chomsky, N. (2017). *Requiem for the American Dream: The 10 Principles of Concentration of Wealth & Power. Seven Stories Press.*

Chonody, J. M., & Teater, B. (2016). Why do I dread looking old?: A test of social identity theory, terror management theory, and the double standard of aging. *Journal of Women & Aging*, *28*(2), 112–126. doi:10.1080/08952841.2014.950533 PMID:26716474

Cho, S., Crenshaw, K. W., & McCall, L. (2013). Toward a Field of Intersectionality Studies: Theory, Applications, and Praxis. *Signs (Chicago, Ill.)*, *38*(4), 785–810. doi:10.1086/669608

Christov-Moore, L., Simpson, E. A., Coude, G., Grigaityte, K., Iacoboni, M., & Ferrari, P. F. (2014). Empathy: gender effects in brain and behavior. *Neurosci Biobehav Rev, 46*(Pt 4), 604-627. doi:10.1016/j.neubiorev.2014.09.001

Clance, P. R., & Imes, S. A. (1978). The imposter phenomenon in high achieving women: Dynamics and therapeutic intervention. *Group Dynamics*, *15*(3), 241–247.

CMS. (2016). *A practical Guide to Implementing the National CLAS Standards.* National Committee for Quality Assurance. https://www.cms.gov/About-CMS/Agency-Information/OMH/Downloads/CLAS-Toolkit-12-7-16.pdf

Cogin, J., & Fish, A. (2009). Sexual harassment—A touchy subject for nurses. *Journal of Health Organization and Management*, *23*(4), 442–462. doi:10.1108/14777260910979326 PMID:19862867

Cohen, A. L., Rivara, F., Marcuse, E. K., McPhillips, H., & Davis, R. (2005). Are language barriers associated with serious medical events in hospitalized pediatric patients? *Pediatrics*, *116*(3), 575–579. doi:10.1542/peds.2005-0521 PMID:16140695

Commission on Dental Accreditation. (2021). *Accreditation Standards for Dental Education Programs*. CODA. https://coda.ada.org/~/media/CODA/Files/2022_predoc_standards.pdf?la=en

Cooper, L. (2003). Patient-centered communication, ratings of care and concordance of patient and physician race. *Annals of Internal Medicine, 139*(11), 907–915.

Cooper-Patrick, L. (1999). Race, gender and partnership in the patient-physician relationship. *Journal of the American Medical Association, 282*(6), 583–589.

Cordero Guzmán, H. (2016). *The production and reproduction of poverty in Puerto Rico; A socio-economic and demographic analysis with data from Puerto Rico Community Survey.* Interamerican University.

Couto, M. C. P. de P., & Wentura, D. (2017). Implicit Ageism. In *Ageism.* The MIT Press., doi:10.7551/mitpress/10679.003.0006

Crenshaw, K. (1991). Mapping the Margins: Intersectionality, Identity Politics, and Violence against Women of Color. *Stanford Law Review, 43*(6), 1241–1299. doi:10.2307/1229039

Croniger, C.M., Qua, K., Rowland Seymour, A., Podugu, P., Laseter, J., Linz, M.O., & Wilson-Delfosse, A. (n.d.). *Preparing Students to Deliver Care to Diverse Populations.* Academic Press.

Cuellar, N. G., Brennan, A. M. W., Vito, K., & de Leon Siantz, M. L. (2008). Cultural competence in the undergraduate nursing curriculum. *Journal of Professional Nursing , 24*(3), 143–149. https://doi.org/10.1016/j.profnurs.2008.01.004

Cuffee, Y. L., Hargraves, J. L., Rosal, M., Briesacher, B. A., Schoenthaler, A., Person, S., Hullett, S., & Allison, J. (2013). Reported racial discrimination, trust in physicians, and medication adherence among inner-city African Americans with hypertension. *American Journal of Public Health, 103*(11), e55–e62. https://doi.org/10.2105/AJPH.2013.301554

Cutilli, C. C. (2020). Excellence in Patient Education: Evidence-Based Education that "Sticks" and Improves Patient Outcomes. *The Nursing Clinics of North America, 55*(2), 267–282. doi:10.1016/j.cnur.2020.02.007 PMID:32389259

Davies, N. (2011). Reducing inequalities in healthcare provision for older adults. Nursing standard (Royal College of Nursing (Great Britain): 1987), 25(41), 49–58. doi:10.7748/ns2011.06.25.41.49.c8573

de Bruijne, M. C., van Rosse, F., Uiters, E., Droomers, M., Suurmond, J., Stronks, K., & Essink-Bot, M. L. (2013). Ethnic variations in unplanned readmissions and excess length of hospital stay: A nationwide record-linked cohort study. *European Journal of Public Health, 23*(6), 964–971. doi:10.1093/eurpub/ckt005 PMID:23388242

De Hert, S. (2020). Burnout in healthcare workers: Prevalence, impact and preventative strategies. *Local and Regional Anesthesia, 13,* 171–183. doi:10.2147/LRA.S240564 PMID:33149664

De Marco, M., Thorburn, S., & Zhao, W. (2008). Perceived discrimination during prenatal care, labor, and delivery: An examination of data from the Oregon Pregnancy Risk Assessment Monitoring System, 1998-1999, 2000, and 2001. *American Journal of Public Health, 98*(10), 1818–1822. doi:10.2105/AJPH.2007.123687 PMID:18703444

De Moissac, D., & Bowen, S. (2019). Impact of language barriers on quality of care and patient safety for official language minority Francophones in Canada. *Journal of Patient Experience, 6*(1), 24–32. doi:10.1177/2374373518769008 PMID:31236448

DeJong, G., Palsbo, S. E., & Beatty, P. W. (2002). The organization and financing of health services for persons with disabilities. *The Milbank Quarterly, 80*(2), 261–301. doi:10.1111/1468-0009.t01-1-00004 PMID:12101873

Devi, N. J., Kumari, A., & Murty, D. (2016). The impact of orientation program for first M.B.B.S students in the transformation of perceptual learning into experiential learning-An insight. *IOSR Journal of Dental and Medical Sciences, 15*(6), 40–45. doi:10.9790/0853-1506084045

DeVoss, D., Jasken, J., & Hayden, D. (2002). Teaching Intracultural and Intercultural Communication: A critique suggested method. *Journal of Business and Technical Communication, 16*(1), 69–94. doi:10.1177/105065190201600100З

Diallo, K. (2004). Data on the migration of health-care workers: Sources, uses, and challenges. *Bulletin of the World Health Organization, 82*(8), 601–607.

Diamond, L. C., Schenker, Y., Curry, L., Bradley, E. H., & Fernandez, A. (2009). Getting by: Underuse of interpreters by resident physicians. *Journal of General Internal Medicine, 24*(2), 256–262. doi:10.100711606-008-0875-7 PMID:19089503

Diamond, L., Izquierdo, K., Canfield, D., Matsoukas, K., & Gany, F. (2019). A Systematic Review of the Impact of Patient-Physician Non-English Language Concordance on Quality of Care and Outcomes. *Journal of General Internal Medicine, 34*(8), 1591–1606. doi:10.100711606-019-04847-5 PMID:31147980

Diaz, T., Navarro, J. R., & Chen, E. H. (2020). An institutional approach to fostering inclusion and addressing racial bias: Implications for diversity in academic medicine. *Teaching and Learning in Medicine, 32*(1), 110–116. https://doi.org/10.1080/10401334.2019.1670665

Dickens, C., Lambert, B. L., Cromwell, T., & Piano, M. R. (2013). Nurse overestimation of patients' health literacy. *Journal of Health Communication, 18*(sup1), 62–69. doi:10.1080/10810730.2013.825670 PMID:24093346

Dimant, O. E., Cook, T. E., Greene, R. E., & Radix, A. E. (2019). Experiences of Transgender and Gender Nonbinary Medical Students and Physicians. *Transgender Health, 4*(1), 209–216. doi:10.1089/trgh.2019.0021 PMID:31552292

Disability Inclusion Overview. (2022, April 14). World Bank. Retrieved December 8, 2022, from https://www.worldbank.org/en/topic/disability

Dismantle. (2022). Retrieved from Merriam-Webster: https://www.merriam-webster.com/dictionary/dismantle

Divi, C., Koss, R. G., Schmaltz, S. P., & Loeb, J. M. (2007). Language proficiency and adverse events in US hospitals: A pilot study. *International Journal for Quality in Health Care, 19*(2), 60–67. doi:10.1093/intqhc/mzl069 PMID:17277013

Dobie, S. (2007). Reflections on a Well-Traveled Path: Self-awareness, mindful practice, and relationship centered care as foundations for medical education. *Academic Medicine, 82*(4), 422–427. doi:10.1097/01.ACM.0000259374.52323.62 PMID:17414201

Doebrich, A., Quirici, M., & Lunsford, C. (2020). COVID-19 and the need for disability conscious medical education, training, and practice. *Journal of Pediatric Rehabilitation Medicine, 13*(3), 393–404. doi:10.3233/PRM-200763 PMID:33252100

Doran, G. T. (1981). There's a S.M.A.R.T. way to write management's goals and objectives. *Management Review, 70*(11), 3, 5–36.

Dos Santos, T. (1970). The Concept of Social Classes. *Science and Society, 34*(2), 166–193.

Doximity. (2017). *Language Barriers in U.S. Health Care: Understanding communication trends between U.S. physicians and patients.* Doximity. https://s3.amazonaws.com/s3.doximity.com/press/Doximity%20Language%20in%20U.S.%20Health%20Care%20Report.pdf

Drouin, J., & Rivet, C. (2003). Training medical students to communicate with a linguistic minority group. *Academic Medicine, 78*(6), 599–604. doi:10.1097/00001888-200306000-00009 PMID:12805039

Dumont, L. (1981). Homo Hierarchicus: The Caste System and Its Implications (2nd ed.). University of Chicago Press.

Dunn, L. B., Iglewicz, A., & Moutier, C. (2008). A conceptual model of medical student well-being: Promoting resilience and preventing burnout. *Academic Psychiatry, 32*(1), 44–53. doi:10.1176/appi.ap.32.1.44 PMID:18270280

Duong, L. M., Singh, S. D., Buchanan, N., Phillips, J. L., & Gerlach, K. (2012). Evaluation of primary/preferred language data collection. *Journal of Registry Management*, *39*(3), 121–132. PMID:23443456

Dyrbye, L. N., Shanafelt, T. D., Johnson, P. O., Johnson, L. A., Satele, D., & West, C. P. (2019). A cross-sectional study exploring the relationship between burnout, absenteeism, and job performance among American nurses. *BMC Nursing*, *18*(1), 1–8. doi:10.118612912-019-0382-7 PMID:31768129

Dyrbye, L. N., West, C. P., Satele, D., Boone, S., Tan, L., Sloan, J., & Shanafelt, T. D. (2014). Burnout among US medical students, residents, and early career physicians relative to the general US population. *Academic Medicine*, *89*(3), 443–451. doi:10.1097/ACM.0000000000000134 PMID:24448053

Ebede, T., & Papier, A. (2006). Disparities in dermatology educational resources. *Journal of the American Academy of Dermatology*, *55*(4), 687–690. https://doi.org/10.1016/j.jaad.2005.10.068

Ehie, O., Muse, I., Hill, L., & Bastien, A. (2021). Professionalism: Microaggression in the healthcare setting. *Current Opinion in Anaesthesiology*, *34*(2), 131–136. doi:10.1097/ACO.0000000000000966 PMID:33630771

El-Abidi, K., Moreno-Poyato, A. R., Toll Privat, A., Corcoles Martinez, D., Aceña-Domínguez, R., Pérez-Solà, V., & Mané, A. (2021). Determinants of mechanical restraint in an acute psychiatric care unit. *World Journal of Psychiatry*, *11*(10), 854–863. doi:10.5498/wjp.v11.i10.854 PMID:34733647

Elgendi, M. M., Stewart, S. H., MacKay, E. J., & Deacon, S. H. (2021). Two aspects of psychological functioning in undergraduates with a history of reading difficulties: Anxiety and self-efficacy. *Annals of Dyslexia*, *71*(1), 84–102. doi:10.100711881-021-00223-3 PMID:33786751

Ellaway, R. H., Cooper, G., Al-Idrissi, T., Dubé, T., & Graves, L. (2014). Discourses of student orientation to medical education programs. *Medical Education Online*, *19*(1), 23714. doi:10.3402/meo.v19.23714 PMID:24646440

Encyclopaedia Britannica. (n.d.). Macroeconomics. In *The Britannica Dictionary*. https://www.britannica.com/dictionary/macroeconomics

Englander, R., Holmboe, E., Batalden, P., Caron, R. M., Durham, C. F., Foster, T., Ogrinc, G., Ercan-Fang, N., & Batalden, M. (2020). Coproducing Health Professions Education: A Prerequisite to Coproducing Health Care Services? *Academic Medicine*, *95*(7), 1006–1013. https://doi.org/10.1097/ACM.0000000000003137

Equality. (2022). In T. Grant (Ed.), *The Britannica Dictionary*. Retrieved from https://www.britannica.com/dictionary/equality

Evans, C. R., Williams, D. R., Onnela, J. P., & Subramanian, S. V. (2018) A multilevel approach to modeling health inequalities at the intersection of multiple social identities. *Social Science & Medicine*, *203*, 64-73. doi:10.1016/j.socscimed.2017.11.011

Eymard, A. S., & Douglas, D. H. (2012). Ageism among health care providers and interventions to improve their attitudes toward older adults: An integrative review. *Journal of Gerontological Nursing*, *38*(5), 26–35. doi:10.3928/00989134-20120307-09 PMID:22420518

Ezzell, B. (2002). Laws of Racial Identification and Racial Purity in Nazi Germany and the United States: Did Jim Crow Write the Laws That Spawned the Holocaust. Southern University Law Review, 30, 1-14.

Fairygodboss. (2019). Ageism in the workplace. *Fairygodboss*. https://d207ibygpg2z1x.cloudfront.net/image/upload/v1564675149/files/Ageism_in_the_Workplace.pdf

Faucett, E. A., Brenner, M. J., Thompson, D. M., & Flanary, V. A. (2022). Tackling the minority tax: A roadmap to redistributing engagement in diversity, equity, and inclusion initiatives. *Otolaryngology - Head and Neck Surgery, 166*(6), 1174–1181. https://doi.org/10.1177/01945998221091696

Feagin, J., & Bennefiled, Z. (2013). Systemic racism and US health care. *Social Science & Medicine, 103*, 7–14. doi:10.1016/j.socscimed.2013.09.006 PMID:24507906

Feaster, B., McKinley-Grant, L., & McMichael, A. J. (2021). Microaggressions in medicine. *Cutis, 107*(5), 235–237. doi:10.12788/cutis.0249 PMID:34288848

Fields, W. W., Asplin, B. R., Larkin, G. L., Marco, C. A., Johnson, L. A., Yeh, C., Ghezzi, K. T., & Rapp, M. (2001). The Emergency Medical Treatment and Labor Act as a Federal Health Care Safety Net Program. *Academic Emergency Medicine, 8*(11), 1064–1069. doi:10.1111/j.1553-2712.2001.tb01116.x PMID:11691669

Fischer, A., Conigliaro, J., Allicock, S., & Kim, E. J. (2021). Examination of social determinants of health among patients with limited English proficiency. *BMC Research Notes, 14*(1), 299. doi:10.118613104-021-05720-7 PMID:34353369

Flanagin, A., Frey, T., & Christiansen, S. L. (2021). Updated Guidance on the Reporting of Race and Ethnicity in Medical and Science Journals. *Journal of the American Medical Association, 326*(7), 621–627. https://doi.org/10.1001/jama.2021.13304

Flores, G., Abreu, M., Barone, C. P., Bachur, R., & Lin, H. (2012). Errors of medical interpretation and their potential clinical consequences: A comparison of professional versus ad hoc versus no interpreters. *Annals of Emergency Medicine, 60*(5), 545–553. doi:10.1016/j.annemergmed.2012.01.025 PMID:22424655

Flores, O., Seminario, S. S., Contreras, E., & Perez, P. (2016). Actitud terapéutica de los tutores y residentes de cuarto año de Medicina Familiar y Comunitaria de Girona frente a las infiltraciones periarticulares. *Atencion Primaria, 48*(6), 421–422. doi:10.1016/j.aprim.2015.09.007 PMID:26817805

Fnais, N., Soobiah, C., Chen, M. H., Lillie, E., Perrier, L., Tashkhandi, M., Straus, S. E., Mamdani, M., Al-Omran, M., & Tricco, A. C. (2014). Harassment and discrimination in medical training: A systematic review and meta-analysis. *Academic Medicine, 89*(5), 817–827. doi:10.1097/ACM.0000000000000200 PMID:24667512

Foley, G. N., & Gentile, J. P. (2010). Nonverbal communication in psychotherapy. *Psychiatry (Edgmont (Pa.: Township)), 7*(6), 38–44.

Fong, K. (2020). Getting Eyes in the Home: Child Protective Services Investigations and State Surveillance of Family Life. *American Sociological Review, 85*(4), 610–638. doi:10.1177/0003122420938460

Forde, A. T., Sims, M., Muntner, P., Lewis, T., Onwuka, A., Moore, K., & Diez Roux, A. V. (2020). Discrimination and Hypertension Risk Among African Americans in the Jackson Heart Study. *Hypertension, 76*(3), 715–723. doi:10.1161/HYPERTENSIONAHA.119.14492

Foronda, C., Baptiste, D., Reinholdt, M. M., & Ousman, K. (2016). Cultural Humility: A Concept Analysis. *Journal of Transcultural Nursing, 27*(3), 210–217. doi:10.1177/1043659615592677 PMID:26122618

Frajerman, A., Morvan, Y., Krebs, M. O., Gorwood, P., & Chaumette, B. (2019). Burnout in medical students before residency: A systematic review and meta-analysis. *European Psychiatry, 55*, 36–42. doi:10.1016/j.eurpsy.2018.08.006 PMID:30384110

Franza, F., Basta, R., & Pellegrino, F. (2020). The Role of Fatigue of Compassion, Burnout and Hopelessness in Healthcare: Experience in the Time of COVID-19 Outbreak. *Psychiatria Danubina, 32*(1), 10–14. PMID:32890354

Fredman, S. (2016). Directorate-General for Justice and Consumers, Intersectional discrimination in EU gender equality and non-discrimination law. *Publications Office*. https://data.europa.eu/doi/10.2838/241520

Fried, J. E., Shipman, S. A., & Sessums, L. L. (2019). Advocacy: Achieving Physician Competency. *Journal of Internal Medicine*, *34*(11), 2297–2298. doi:10.100711606-019-05278-y PMID:31420826

Furunes, T., & Mykletun, R. J. (2010). Age discrimination in the workplace: Validation of the Nordic Age Discrimination Scale (NADS). *Scandinavian Journal of Psychology*, *51*(1), 23–30. doi:10.1111/j.1467-9450.2009.00738.x PMID:19694986

Gade, L., & Yeo, H. L. (2019). Work–Life Integration and Time Management Strategies. *Clinics in Colon and Rectal Surgery*, *32*(6), 442–449. doi:10.1055-0039-1693011 PMID:31686996

Galinato, J., Montie, M., Shuman, C., Patak, L., & Titler, M. (2016). Perspectives of Nurses on Patients With Limited English Proficiency and Their Call Light Use. *Global Qualitative Nursing Research*, *3*. doi:10.1177/2333393616637764 PMID:28393085

Garcia Farina, E., Rowell, J., Revette, A., Haakenstad, E. K., Cleveland, J. L. F., Allende, R., Hassett, M., Schrag, D., & McCleary, N. J. (2022). Barriers to Electronic Patient-Reported Outcome Measurement Among Patients with Cancer and Limited English Proficiency. *JAMA Network Open*, *5*(7), e2223898. doi:10.1001/jamanetworkopen.2022.23898 PMID:35867056

Gerchow, L., Burka, L. R., Miner, S., & Squires, A. (2021). Language barriers between nurses and patients: A scoping review. *Patient Education and Counseling*, *104*(3), 534–553. doi:10.1016/j.pec.2020.09.017 PMID:32994104

Gertner, E. J., Sabino, J. N., Mahady, E., Deitrick, L. M., Patton, J. R., Grim, M. K., Geiger, J. F., & Salas-Lopez, D. (2010). Developing a culturally competent health network: A planning framework and guide. *Journal of Healthcare Management*, *55*(3), 190–204.

Gill, A. C., Zhou, Y., Greely, J. T., Beasley, A. D., Purkiss, J., & Juneja, M. (2022). Longitudinal outcomes one year following implicit bias training in medical students. *Medical Teacher*, *44*(7), 744–751. doi:10.1080/0142159X.2021.2023120 PMID:35021935

Gofine, M., Mielenz, T. J., Vasan, S., & Lebwohl, B. (2018). Use of colorectal cancer screening among people with mobility disability. *Journal of Clinical Gastroenterology*, *52*(9), 789–795. doi:10.1097/MCG.0000000000000835 PMID:28723854

Gomez, L. E., & Bernet, P. (2019). Diversity improves performance and outcomes. *Journal of the National Medical Association*, *111*(4), 383–392. doi:10.1016/j.jnma.2019.01.006 PMID:30765101

Gonzaga, A. M., Marbin, J., & Terhune, K. (2022). Evidence-based inclusive graduate medical education recruitment strategies. *Journal of Graduate Medical Education*, *14*(1), 115–116. https://doi.org/10.4300/JGME-D-21-01134.1

Gonzaga, A., Appiah-Pippim, J., Onumah, C. M., & Yialamas, M. A. (2020). A framework for inclusive graduate medical education recruitment strategies: Meeting the ACGME standard for a diverse and inclusive workforce. *Academic Medicine*, *95*(5), 710–716. https://doi.org/10.1097/ACM.0000000000003073

Gonzalez, C. M., Lypson, M. L., & Sukhera, J. (2021). Twelve tips for teaching implicit bias recognition and management. *Medical Teacher*, *43*(12), 1368–1373. https://doi.org/10.1080/0142159X.2021.1879378

Gozu, A., Kern, D. E., & Wright, S. M. (2009). Similarities and differences between international medical graduates and U.S. medical graduates at six Maryland community-based internal medicine residency training programs. *Academic Medicine*, *84*(3), 385–390. doi:10.1097/ACM.0b013e318197321b PMID:19240453

Green, A. R., & Nze, C. (2017). Language-Based Inequity in Health Care: Who Is the "Poor Historian"? *AMA Journal of Ethics*, *19*(3), 263–271. doi:10.1001/journalofethics.2017.19.3.medu1-1703 PMID:28323607

Green, M. A., Evans, C. R., & Subramanian, S. V. (2017). Can intersectionality theory enrich population health research? *Social Science & Medicine*, *178*, 217–219. doi:10.1016/j.socscimed.2017.02.029 PMID:28238539

Greeson, J. K. P., Briggs, E. C., Kisiel, C. L., Layne, C. M., Ake, G. S., Ko, S. J., Gerrity, E. T., Steinberg, A. M., Howard, M. L., Pynoos, R. S., & Fairbank, J. A. (2011). Complex Trauma and Mental Health in Children and Adolescents Placed in Foster Care: Findings from the National Child Traumatic Stress Network. *Child Welfare*, *90*(6), 91–108. https://www.jstor.org/stable/48625371 PMID:22533044

Guiton, G., Chang, M. J., & Wilkerson, L. (2007). Student body diversity: Relationship to medical students' experiences and attitudes. *Academic Medicine*, *82*(Suppl), S85–S88. doi:10.1097/ACM.0b013e31813ffe1e

Gurchiek, K. (2019). *ERGs to effect change, spark innovation.* Society for Human Resource Management (SHRM). https://www.shrm.org/resourcesandtools/hr-topics/behavioral-competencies/global-and-cultural-effectiveness/pages/use-ergs-to-affect-change-spark-innovation.aspx

Hadinger, M. A. (2017). Underrepresented minorities in medical school admissions: A qualitative study. *Teaching and Learning in Medicine*, *29*(1), 31–41. https://doi.org/10.1080/10401334.2016.1220861

Hadziabdic, E., & Hjelm, K. (2014). Arabic-speaking migrants' experiences of the use of interpreters in healthcare: A qualitative explorative study. *International Journal for Equity in Health*, *13*(1), 49. doi:10.1186/1475-9276-13-49 PMID:24934755

Haghnegahdar, M., Sharma, P., Hubbard, K. P., & White, W. A. (2021). The Influence of Religious Belief on Burnout in Medical Students. *Missouri Medicine*, *118*(1), 63–67. PMID:33551488

Haley, C. M., & Brown, B. P. (2022). Implementation of diversity, equity, and inclusion dialogue for second-year dental students. *Journal of Dental Education*, *86*(5), 599–604. https://doi.org/10.1002/jdd.12862

Handy, J., & Davy, D. (2007). Gendered ageism: Older women's experiences of employment agency practices. *Asia Pacific Journal of Human Resources*, *45*(1), 85–99. doi:10.1177/1038411107073606

Hankivsky, O. (2022). *Intersectionality 101.* Institute for Intersectionality Research and Policy. https://resources.equityinitiative.org/handle/ei/433

Haque, O. S., Stein, M. A., & Marvit, A. (2021). Physician, Heal Thy Double Stigma: Doctors with Mental Illness and Structural Barriers to Disclosure. *The New England Journal of Medicine*, *384*(10), 888–891. doi:10.1056/NEJMp2031013 PMID:33705616

Harrison, T. (2021). Florence Nightingale's legacy on the role of men in community nursing. *British Journal of Community Nursing*, *26*(6), 302–306. doi:10.12968/bjcn.2021.26.6.302 PMID:34105367

Havranek, E. P., Mujahid, M. S., Barr, D. A., Blair, I. V., Cohen, M. S., Cruz-Flores, S., Davey-Smith, G., Dennison-Himmelfarb, C. R., Lauer, M. S., Lockwood, D. W., Rosal, M., & Yancy, C. W. (2015). Social Determinants of Risk and Outcomes for Cardiovascular Disease: A Scientific Statement From the American Heart Association. *Circulation*, *132*(9), 873–898. https://doi.org/10.1161/CIR.0000000000000228

Healthy People 2020 Overview of Health Disparities. Healthy People 2020 Final Review. (n.d.). doi:10.15620/cdc:111173

Herd, P., Mills, M. C., & Dowd, J. B. (2021). Reconstructing Sociogenomics Research: Dismantling Biological Race and Genetic Essentialism Narratives. *Journal of Health and Social Behavior*, *62*(3), 419–435. https://doi.org/10.1177/00221465211018682

Herrera, H., Alsaif, M., Khan, G., Barnes, N., & Rutter, P. (2019). Provision of Bilingual Dispensing Labels to Non-Native English Speakers: An Exploratory Study. *Pharmacy (Basel, Switzerland)*, *7*(1), 32. doi:10.3390/pharmacy7010032 PMID:30934609

HHS. (2021). Access and Functional Needs Toolkit: Integrating a Community Partner Network to Inform Risk Communication Strategies. U.S. Department of Health and Human Services (HHS), CDC.

Hollmann, P. (2021). Charting our first steps: An update on the AGS initiative to address the intersection of structural racism and ageism. *Geriatric Nursing (New York, N.Y.)*, *42*(4), 961–962. doi:10.1016/j.gerinurse.2021.06.025 PMID:34229872

Hommes, B., Borash, A. I., Hartwig, K., & DeGracia, D. (2018). American Sign Language Interpreters Perceptions of Barriers to Healthcare Communication in Deaf and Hard of Hearing Patients. *Journal of Community Health*, *43*(5), 956–961. doi:10.100710900-018-0511-3 PMID:29696596

Houkes, I., Winants, Y., Twellaar, M., & Verdonk, P. (2011). Development of burnout over time and the causal order of the three dimensions of burnout among male and female GPs. A three-wave panel study. *BMC Public Health*, *11*(1), 1–13. doi:10.1186/1471-2458-11-240 PMID:21501467

Hsieh, E. (2008). "I am not a robot!" Interpreters' views of their roles in health care settings. *Qualitative Health Research*, *18*(10), 1367–1383. doi:10.1177/1049732308323840 PMID:18832768

Hsieh, E. (2015). Not just "getting by": Factors influencing providers' choice of interpreters. *Journal of General Internal Medicine*, *30*(1), 75–82. doi:10.100711606-014-3066-8 PMID:25338731

Hsueh, L., Hirsh, A. T., Maupomé, G., & Stewart, J. C. (2021). Patient-Provider Language Concordance and Health Outcomes: A Systematic Review, Evidence Map, and Research Agenda. *Medical Care Research and Review: MCRR*, *78*(1), 3–23. doi:10.1177/1077558719860708 PMID:31291823

Huang, J., & Liu, R. (2020). Xenophobia in America in the age of coronavirus and beyond. *Journal of Vascular and Interventional Radiology*, *31*(7), 1187–1188. https://doi.org/10.1016/j.jvir.2020.04.020

Humans-are-999-genetically-identical. (n.d.). https://www.pbs.org/video/humans-are-999-genetically-identical-1lggn4/

Hung, R. (2007). Student perspectives on diversity and the cultural climate at a US medical school. *Academic Medicine*, *82*(2), 184–192.

Hunter, K., & Thompson, B. (2019). A Scoping review of Social Determinants of Health Curricula in Post-Graduate Medical Education. *Canadian Medical Education Journal*, *10*(3), e61–e71. doi:10.36834/cmej.61709 PMID:31388378

Hussain, S. (2020, February 3). Fear of coronavirus fuels racist sentiment targeting Asians. *Los Angeles Times*. https://www.latimes.com/california/story/2020-02-03/fear-panic-around-the-coronavirus-fuels-racist-sentiment

Hu, Y. Y., Ellis, R. J., Hewitt, D. B., Yang, A. D., Cheung, E. O., Moskowitz, J. T., Potts, J. R. III, Buyske, J., Hoyt, D. B., Nasca, T. J., & Bilimoria, K. Y. (2019). Discrimination, Abuse, Harassment, and Burnout in Surgical Residency Training. *The New England Journal of Medicine*, *381*(18), 1741–1752. doi:10.1056/NEJMsa1903759 PMID:31657887

Iezzoni, L. I. (2022). Cancer detection, diagnosis, and treatment for adults with disabilities. *The Lancet. Oncology*, *23*(4), e164–e173. doi:10.1016/S1470-2045(22)00018-3 PMID:35358465

Iezzoni, L. I., & Agaronnik, N. D. (2020). Healthcare disparities for individuals with disability: informing the practice. In *Disability as Diversity* (pp. 15–31). Springer. doi:10.1007/978-3-030-46187-4_2

Iezzoni, L. I., Kurtz, S. G., & Rao, S. R. (2015). Trends in mammography over time for women with and without chronic disability. *Journal of Women's Health*, *24*(7), 593–601. doi:10.1089/jwh.2014.5181 PMID:26083235

Iezzoni, L. I., Kurtz, S. G., & Rao, S. R. (2016). Trends in pap testing over time for women with and without chronic disability. *American Journal of Preventive Medicine*, *50*(2), 210–219. doi:10.1016/j.amepre.2015.06.031 PMID:26372417

Iezzoni, L. I., Ngo, L. H., Li, D., Roetzheim, R. G., Drews, R. E., & McCarthy, E. P. (2008). Treatment disparities for disabled medicare beneficiaries with stage I non-small cell lung cancer. *Archives of Physical Medicine and Rehabilitation*, *89*(4), 595–601. doi:10.1016/j.apmr.2007.09.042 PMID:18373987

Iezzoni, L. I., Rao, S. R., Ressalam, J., Bolcic-Jankovic, D., Agaronnik, N. D., Donelan, K., Lagu, T., & Campbell, E. G. (2021). Physicians' Perceptions Of People With Disability And Their Health Care: Study reports the results of a survey of physicians' perceptions of people with disability. *Health Affairs*, *40*(2), 297–306. doi:10.1377/hlthaff.2020.01452 PMID:33523739

Iezzoni, L. I., Rao, S. R., Ressalam, J., Bolcic-Jankovic, D., Agaronnik, N. D., Lagu, T., Pendo, E., & Campbell, E. G. (2022). US Physicians' Knowledge About The Americans With Disabilities Act And Accommodation Of Patients With Disability: Study examines what physicians know about the Americans With Disabilities Act and what is done to accommodate patients with a disability. *Health Affairs*, *41*(1), 96–104. doi:10.1377/hlthaff.2021.01136 PMID:34982624

Iezzoni, L. I., Rao, S. R., Ressalam, J., Bolcic-Jankovic, D., & Campbell, E. G. (2022). Incidence of accommodations for patients with significant vision limitations in physicians' offices in the US. *JAMA Ophthalmology*, *140*(1), 79–84. doi:10.1001/jamaophthalmol.2021.5072 PMID:34854912

Inoue, A. B. (2020). Teaching Antiracist Writing. *Journal of College Reading and Learning*, *50*(1), 1–23. doi:10.1080/10790195.2020.1787079

Institute of Medicine (US) Committee on Institutional and Policy-Level Strategies for Increasing the Diversity of the U.S. Healthcare Workforce. (2004). *In the Nation's Compelling Interest: Ensuring Diversity in the Health-Care Workforce.* National Academies Press (US). Available at https://www.ncbi.nlm.nih.gov/books/NBK216009/

Institute of Medicine. (2001). *Crossing the quality chasm: A new health care system for the 21st century*. National Academy Press.

Iversen, T. J., Larsen, L., & Solem, P. E. (2009). A conceptual analysis of Ageism. *Nordic Psychology*, *61*(3), 3, 4–22. doi:10.1027/1901-2276.61.3.4

Jacobs, E. A., Sadowski, L. S., & Rathouz, P. J. (2007). The impact of an enhanced interpreter service intervention on hospital costs and patient satisfaction. *Journal of General Internal Medicine*, *22*(S2, Suppl 2), 306–311. doi:10.100711606-007-0357-3 PMID:17957416

Jarus, T., Bezati, R., Trivett, S., Lee, M., Bulk, L. Y., Battalova, A., Mayer, Y., Murphy, S., Gerber, P., & Drynan, D. (2020). Professionalism and disabled clinicians: The client's perspective. *Disability & Society*, *35*(7), 1085–1102. doi:10.1080/09687599.2019.1669436

Jeung, R., & Nham, K. (2020). *Incidents of coronavirus-related discrimination*. A3PCON. https://www.asianpacificpolicyandplanningcouncil.org/wp-content/uploads/STOP_AAPI_HATE_MONTHLY_REPORT_4_23_20.pdf

Jilani, M. H., Javed, Z., Yahya, T., Valero-Elizondo, J., Khan, S. U., Kash, B., Blankstein, R., Virani, S. S., Blaha, M. J., Dubey, P., Hyder, A. A., Vahidy, F. S., Cainzos-Achirica, M., & Nasir, K. (2021). Social Determinants of Health and Cardiovascular Disease: Current State and Future Directions Towards Healthcare Equity. *Current Atherosclerosis Reports*, *23*(9), 55. https://doi.org/10.1007/s11883-021-00949-w

Johnson, C. (2022, February). *Physician Cultural Responsibility* [Unpublished Doctoral Study Manuscript]. Antioch University, Seattle, WA, United States.

Johnson, A., & Sandford, J. (2005). Written and verbal information versus verbal information only for patients being discharged from acute hospital settings to home: Systematic review. *Health Education Research, 20*(4), 423–429. doi:10.1093/her/cyg141 PMID:15572437

Johnson, J. L., Bottorff, J. L., Browne, A. J., Grewal, S., Hilton, B. A., & Clarke, H. (2004). Othering and being othered in the context of health care services. *Health Communication, 16*(2), 255–271. doi:10.1207/S15327027HC1602_7 PMID:15090288

Joint Commission. (2014). International Accreditation Standards for Hospitals. *Joint Commission.*

Jones, C. P. (2001). Invited commentary: "race," racism, and the practice of epidemiology. *American Journal of Epidemiology, 154*(4), 299–304. https://doi.org/10.1093/aje/154.4.299

Joseph, C., Garruba, M., & Melder, A. (2018). Patient satisfaction of telephone or video interpreter services compared with in-person services: A systematic review. *Australian Health Review, 42*(2), 168–177. doi:10.1071/AH16195 PMID:30021688

Juckett, G., & Unger, K. (2014). Appropriate use of medical interpreters. *American Family Physician, 90*(7), 476–480. PMID:25369625

Juster, F., & Edwards, K. (2001). A rotation in chronic-care pediatrics with a focus on children and their families in the community. *Academic Medicine, 76*(5), 568. doi:10.1097/00001888-200105000-00118 PMID:11346625

Kahsay, W. G., Negarandeh, R., Dehghan Nayeri, N., & Hasanpour, M. (2020). Sexual harassment against female nurses: A systematic review. *BMC Nursing, 19*(1), 58. doi:10.118612912-020-00450-w PMID:32612455

Kale, E., & Syed, H. R. (2010). Language barriers and the use of interpreters in the public health services. A questionnaire-based survey. *Patient Education and Counseling, 81*(2), 187–191. doi:10.1016/j.pec.2010.05.002 PMID:20542656

Kane, R. L., & Kane, R. A. (2005). Ageism in Healthcare and Long-Term Care. *Generations: Journal of the American Society on Aging, 29*(3), 49–54. https://www.jstor.org/stable/26555410

Karash, S., Solone, M., Chavez, J., & Shanafelt, T. (2019). Physician Work-Life Integration: Challenges and Strategies for Improvement. *Clinical Obstetrics and Gynecology, 62*(3), 455–465. doi:10.1097/GRF.0000000000000442 PMID:30950862

Karliner, L. S., Jacobs, E. A., Chen, A. H., & Mutha, S. (2007). Do professional interpreters improve clinical care for patients with limited English proficiency? A systematic review of the literature. *Health Services Research, 42*(2), 727–754. doi:10.1111/j.1475-6773.2006.00629.x PMID:17362215

Karliner, L. S., Pérez-Stable, E. J., & Gregorich, S. E. (2017). Convenient Access to Professional Interpreters in the Hospital Decreases Readmission Rates and Estimated Hospital Expenditures for Patients With Limited English Proficiency. *Medical Care, 55*(3), 199–206. doi:10.1097/MLR.0000000000000643 PMID:27579909

Kassam, R., Vaillancourt, L. R., & Collins, J. B. (2004). Pictographic instructions for medications: Do different cultures interpret them accurately? *International Journal of Pharmacy Practice, 12*(4), 199–209. doi:10.1211/0022357044698

Kawai, Y. (2005). Stereotyping Asian Americans: The Dialectic of the Model Minority and the Yellow Peril. *The Howard Journal of Communications, 16*(2), 109–130. https://doi.org/10.1080/10646170590948974

Kennedy, B. R., Mathis, C. C., & Woods, A. K. (2007). African Americans and their distrust of the health care system: Healthcare for diverse populations. *Journal of Cultural Diversity, 14*(2), 56–60. PMID:19175244

Kinayama, S., Karasawa, M., Curhan, K. B., Ryff, C. D., & Markus, H. R. (2010). Independence and interdependence predict health and wellbeing: Divergent patterns in the United States and Japan. *Frontiers in Psychology, 1*(163), 1–10. doi:10.3389/fpsyg.2010.00163 PMID:21833228

Knaak, S., Mantler, E., & Szeto, A. (2017). Mental illness-related stigma in healthcare: Barriers to access and care and evidence-based solutions. *Healthcare Management Forum / Canadian College of Health Service Executives = Forum Gestion Des Soins de Sante / College Canadien Des Directeurs de Services de Sante, 30*(2), 111–116.

Koff, M. D., & McGowan, J. J. (1999). MedSpanish: a language tool for the emergency department. In *Proceedings of the AMIA Symposium* (p. 565). American Medical Informatics Association.

Komaromy, M. (1996). The role of Black and Hispanic physicians in providing health care for underserved populations. *The New England Journal of Medicine*, *334*(2), 1305–1310.

Krahn, G. L., Walker, D. K., & Correa-De-Araujo, R. (2015, April). Persons with disabilities as an unrecognized health disparity population. *American Journal of Public Health*, *105*(S2, Suppl 2), S198–S206. doi:10.2105/AJPH.2014.302182 PMID:25689212

Kripalani, S., Robertson, R., Love-Ghaffari, M. H., Henderson, L. E., Praska, J., Strawder, A., Katz, M. G., & Jacobson, T. A. (2007). Development of an illustrated medication schedule as a low-literacy patient education tool. *Patient Education and Counseling*, *66*(3), 368–377. doi:10.1016/j.pec.2007.01.020 PMID:17344015

Kydd, A., & Fleming, A. (2015). Ageism and age discrimination in health care: Fact or fiction? A narrative review of the literature. *Maturitas*, *81*(4), 432–438. doi:10.1016/j.maturitas.2015.05.002 PMID:26044073

Lachance, C., & Wright, M. D. (2019). *Avoidance of physical restraint use among hospitalized older adults: a review of clinical effectiveness and guidelines*. CADTH.

Landrum, T. J., Tankersley, M., & Kauffman, J. M. (2003). What Is Special About Special Education for Students with Emotional or Behavioral Disorders? *The Journal of Special Education*, *37*(3), 148–156. doi:10.1177/00224669030370030401

Langness, S., Rajapuram, N., Marshall, M., Rahman, A. S., & Sammann, A. (2022). Risk factors associated with student distress in medical school: Associations with faculty support and availability of wellbeing resources. *Public Library of Science ONE*, *17*(4), e0265869. doi:10.1371/journal.pone.0265869 PMID:35395007

Lapinski, J., & Sexton, P. (2014). Still in the closet: The invisible minority in medical education. *BMC Medical Education*, *14*(1), 171. Advance online publication. doi:10.1186/1472-6920-14-171 PMID:25128252

LeBlanc, B. (2017). *Gender Performativity in Nursing: Men, Power, and the Construction of the Ideal Nurse* [Unpublished doctoral dissertation]. University of Ottawa, Ontario, Canada.

LEP.gov. (2020). *Source and Methodology*. Limited English Proficiency gov. https://www.lep.gov/source-and-methodology

Lett, E., Asabor, E., Beltrán, S., Cannon, A. M., & Arah, O. A. (2022). Conceptualizing, Contextualizing, and Operationalizing Race in Quantitative Health Sciences Research. *Annals of Family Medicine*, *20*(2), 157–163. https://doi.org/10.1370/afm.2792

Levy, A., & Perry, A. (2011). Outcomes in adolescents and adults with autism: A review of the literature. *Research in Autism Spectrum Disorders*, *5*(4), 1271–1282. doi:10.1016/j.rasd.2011.01.023

Levy, B. R. (2001). Eradication of ageism requires addressing the enemy within. *The Gerontologist*, *41*(5), 578–580. doi:10.1093/geront/41.5.578 PMID:11574700

Liaison Committee on Medical Education. (2022). *Functions and structure of a medical school*. https://lcme.org/publications/

Lie, D. (2006). Interpreter cases for cultural competency instruction. *MedEdPORTAL: the Journal of Teaching and Learning Resources*, *2*, 205. doi:10.15766/mep_2374-8265.205

Limbert, W., & Williams, W. R. (2014). Classism. In T. Teo (Ed.), *Encyclopedia of Critical Psychology*. Springer. doi:10.1007/978-1-4614-5583-7_43

Link, B. G., Struening, E. L., Rahav, M., Phelan, J. C., & Nuttbrock, L. (1997). On stigma and its consequences: Evidence from a longitudinal study of men with dual diagnoses of mental illness and substance abuse. *Journal of Health and Social Behavior*, *38*(2), 177–190. doi:10.2307/2955424 PMID:9212538

Locatis, C., Williamson, D., Gould-Kabler, C., Zone-Smith, L., Detzler, I., Roberson, J., & Ackerman, M. (2010). Comparing in-person, video, and telephonic medical interpretation. *Journal of General Internal Medicine*, *25*(4), 345–350. doi:10.100711606-009-1236-x PMID:20107916

Lott, B. (2012). The Social Psychology of Class and Classism. *The American Psychologist*, *67*(8), 650–658. doi:10.1037/a0029369 PMID:23163450

Magence, A., Gross, J., Wilson, J., Juster, F., Edwards, K., & Petersen, K. (2021). *Year one: Reflections on implementation of a disabilities curriculum for medical students*. AMA Research Challenge.

Magnan, S. (2017). *Social Determinants of Health 101 for Health Care: Five Plus Five. In NAM Perspectives*. National Academy of Medicine. doi:10.31478/201710c

Mahoney, S. (2022). *Caring for adults with intellectual and developmental disabilities*. AAMC. https://www.aamc.org/news-insights/caring-adults-intellectual-and-developmental-disabilities

Makadon, H. J. (2006). Improving health care for the lesbian and gay communities. *The New England Journal of Medicine*, *354*(9), 895–897. https://doi.org/10.1056/NEJMp058259

Malat, J. (2001). Social distance and patients' rating of healthcare providers. *Journal of Health and Social Behavior*, *42*(4), 360–372.

Malik, A., Qureshi, H., Abdul-Razakq, H., Yaqoob, Z., Zahra Javaid, F., Esmail, F., ... Latif, A. (2019). 'I decided not to go into surgery due to dress code': A cross-sectional study within the UK investigating experiences of female Muslim medical health professionals on bare below the elbows (BBE) policy and wearing headscarves (hijabs) in theatre. *BMJ Open*, *9*(3), e019954. Advance online publication. doi:10.1136/bmjopen-2017-019954 PMID:30898792

Malinen, S., & Johnston, L. (2013). Workplace ageism: Discovering hidden bias. *Experimental Aging Research*, *39*(4), 445–465. doi:10.1080/0361073X.2013.808111 PMID:23875840

Manderino, M. A., & Berkey, N. (1997). Verbal abuse of staff nurses by physicians. *Journal of Professional Nursing*, *13*(1), 48–55.

Margolius, S. W., Papp, K. K., Altose, M. D., & Wilson-Delfosse, A. L. (2020). Students perceive skills learned in pre-clerkship PBL valuable in core clinical rotations. *Medical Teacher*, *42*(8), 902–908. https://doi.org/10.1080/0142159X.2020.1762031

Marku, C. (2019). *The Art Of Setting Smart Goals Set Winning Goals and Live a Life of Abundance, Success and Achievement*. Amazon Digital Services LLC.

Marques, V. C., & Berry, G. R. (2021). Enhancing work-life balance using a resilience framework. *Business and Society Review*, *126*(3), 263–281. doi:10.1111/basr.12237

Marvaldi, M., Mallet, J., Dubertret, C., Moro, M. R., & Guessoum, S. B. (2021). Anxiety, depression, trauma-related, and sleep disorders among healthcare workers during the COVID-19 pandemic: A systematic review and meta-analysis. *Neuroscience and Biobehavioral Reviews*, *126*, 252–264. doi:10.1016/j.neubiorev.2021.03.024 PMID:33774085

Maslach, C., Jackson, S. E., & Leiter, M. P. (1997). *Maslach burnout inventory*. Scarecrow Education.

Maslach, C., Jackson, S. E., & Leiter, M. P. (2017). *Maslach Burnout Inventory Manual* (4th ed.). Mind Garden, Inc.

Masters, C., Robinson, D., Faulkner, S., Patterson, E., McIlraith, T., & Ansari, A. (2019). Addressing Biases in Patient Care with The 5Rs of Cultural Humility, a Clinician Coaching Tool. *Journal of General Internal Medicine*, *34*(4), 627–630. doi:10.100711606-018-4814-y PMID:30623383

Mata, D. A., Ramos, M. A., Bansal, N., Khan, R., Guille, C., Di Angelantonio, E., & Sen, S. (2015). Prevalence of Depression and Depressive Symptoms Among Resident Physicians: A Systematic Review and Meta-analysis. *Journal of the American Medical Association*, *314*(22), 2373–2383. doi:10.1001/jama.2015.15845 PMID:26647259

McChesney, K. Y. (2015). *Teaching Diversity: The Science You Need to Know to Explain Why Race Is Not Biological.* doi:10.1177/2158244015611712

McClintock, A. H., Fainstad, T. L., & Jauregui, J. (2021). Creating Psychological Safety in the Learning Environment: Straightforward Answers to a Longstanding Challenge. *Academic Medicine*, *96*(11S), S208–S209. https://doi.org/10.1097/ACM.0000000000004319

McDermott, R. C. (2018). *Rates of Depression and Anxiety in Physical Therapy and Occupational Therapy Students: A Cross-Profession Comparison study*. Educatationa; Leadership Conference. Jacksonville, Florida. https://aptaeducation.org/abstract-archive/view.cfm?id=2996450

McKinley, S. K., Wang, L. J., Gartland, R. M., Westfal, M. L., Costantino, C. L., Schwartz, D., Merrill, A. L., Petrusa, E., Lillemoe, K., & Phitayakorn, R. (2019). "Yes, I'm the Doctor": One Department's Approach to Assessing and Addressing Gender-Based Discrimination in the Modern Medical Training Era. *Academic Medicine*, *94*(11), 1691–1698. doi:10.1097/ACM.0000000000002845 PMID:31274522

McOwen, K. S., Whelan, A. J., & Farmakidis, A. L. (2020). Medical Education in the United States and Canada, 2020. *Academic Medicine* , *95*(9S), S2–S4. doi:10.1097/ACM.0000000000003497

Meeks, L. (2019). *The disabilities we don't see*. AAMC. https://www.aamc.org/news-insights/disabilities-we-dont-see

Meeks, L. M., Case, B., Herzer, K., Plegue, M., & Swenor, B. K. (2019). Change in prevalence of disabilities and accommodation practices among US medical schools, 2016 vs 2019. *Journal of the American Medical Association*, *322*(20), 2022–2024. doi:10.1001/jama.2019.15372 PMID:31769816

Meeks, L. M., Case, B., Plegue, M., Moreland, C. J., Jain, S., & Taylor, N. (2020). National prevalence of disability and clinical accommodations in medical education. *Journal of Medical Education and Curricular Development*, *7*, 2382120520965249. doi:10.1177/2382120520965249 PMID:33178890

Meeks, L. M., Herzer, K., & Jain, N. R. (2018). Removing barriers and facilitating access: Increasing the number of physicians with disabilities. *Academic Medicine*, *93*(4), 540–543. doi:10.1097/ACM.0000000000002112 PMID:30248081

Meeks, L. M., & Jain, N. (2018). *Accessibility, inclusion, and action in medical education: lived experiences of learners and physicians with disabilities*. Association of American Medical Colleges.

Meeks, L. M., Stergiopoulos, E., & Petersen, K. H. (2022). Institutional accountability for students with disabilities: A call for liaison committee on medical education action. *Academic Medicine*, *97*(3), 341–345. doi:10.1097/ACM.0000000000004471 PMID:34670236

Mellner, C., Aronsson, G., & Kecklund, G. (2014). Boundary Management Preferences, Boundary Control, and Work-Life Balance among Full-Time Employed Professionals in Knowledge-Intensive, Flexible Work. *Nordic Journal of Working Life Studies*, *4*(4), 7. doi:10.19154/njwls.v4i4.4705

Miller, A. N., Todd, A., Toledo, R., & Duvuuri, V. N. S. (2022). The Relationship of Ethnic, Racial, and Cultural Concordance to Physician–Patient Communication: A Mixed-Methods Systematic Review Protocol. *Health Communication*, 1–7. doi:10.1080/10410236.2022.2070449 PMID:35502565

Mills, J., Wand, T., & Fraser, J. A. (2018). Exploring the meaning and practice of self-care among palliative care nurses and doctors: A qualitative study. *BMC Palliative Care*, *17*(1), 63. doi:10.118612904-018-0318-0 PMID:29669559

Minichiello, V., Browne, J., & Kendig, H. (2000). Perceptions and consequences of ageism: Views of older people. *Ageing and Society*, *20*(3), 253–278. doi:10.1017/S0144686X99007710

Minkler, M., Fuller-Thomson, E., & Guralnik, J. M. (2006). Gradient of disability across the socioeconomic spectrum in the United States. *The New England Journal of Medicine*, *355*(7), 695–703. doi:10.1056/NEJMsa044316 PMID:16914705

Missouridou, E. (2017). Secondary Posttraumatic Stress and Nurses' Emotional Responses to Patient's Trauma. *Journal of Trauma Nursing*, *24*(2), 110–115. doi:10.1097/JTN.0000000000000274 PMID:28272184

Mitchell, D. L., Bennett, M. J., & Manfrin-Ledet, L. (2006). Spiritual development of nursing students: Developing competence to provide spiritual care to patients at the end of life. *The Journal of Nursing Education*, *45*, 365–370.

Molina, M. F., Landry, A. I., Chary, A. N., & Burnett-Bowie, S. M. (2020). Addressing the Elephant in the Room: Microaggressions in Medicine. *Annals of Emergency Medicine*, *76*(4), 387–391. doi:10.1016/j.annemergmed.2020.04.009 PMID:32456801

Morgantini, L. A., Naha, U., Wang, H., Francavilla, S., Acar, Ö., Flores, J. M., Crivellaro, S., Moreira, D., Abern, M., Eklund, M., Vigneswaran, H. T., & Weine, S. M. (2020). Factors contributing to healthcare professional burnout during the COVID-19 pandemic: A rapid turnaround global survey. *PLoS One*, *15*(9), e0238217. doi:10.1371/journal.pone.0238217 PMID:32881887

Moy, E., & Bartman, B. (1995). Physician race and care of minority and medically indigent patients. *Journal of the American Medical Association*, *273*(19), 1515–1520.

Murphy, C. (2021). *Equity vs. Equality: Here's the difference*. Health. Retrieved from https://www.health.com/mind-body/health-diversity-inclusion/equity-vs-equality

Murthy, V. H. (2022). Confronting Health Worker Burnout and Well-Being. *The New England Journal of Medicine*, *387*(7), 577–579. doi:10.1056/NEJMp2207252 PMID:35830683

Myers, K. A., Lindburg, J. J., & Nied, D. M. (2014). Allies for Inclusion: Disability and Equity in Higher Education: ASHE Volume 39, Number 5. John Wiley & Sons.

Nadal, K. L. K. R., Sissoko, G., Floyd, N., & Hines, D. (2021). The legacies of systemic and internalized oppression: Experiences of microaggressions, imposter phenomenon, and stereotype threat on historically marginalized groups. *New Ideas in Psychology, 63*.

Nadal, K. L., Wong, Y., Griffin, K. E., Davidoff, K., & Sriken, J. (2014). The adverse impact of racial microaggressions on college students' self-esteem. *Journal of College Student Development*, *55*(5), 461–474.

Nadal, K. L., Wong, Y., Griffin, K. E., Davidoff, K., & Sriken, J. (2014). The Adverse Impact of Racial Microaggressions on College Students' Self-Esteem. *Journal of College Student Development*, *55*(5), 461–474. doi:10.1353/csd.2014.0051

Nama, N., MacPherson, P., Sampson, M., & McMillan, H. J. (2017). Medical students' perception of lesbian, gay, bisexual, and transgender (LGBT) discrimination in their learning environment and their self-reported comfort level for caring for LGBT patients: A survey study. *Medical Education Online*, *22*(1), 1368850. doi:10.1080/10872981.2017.1368850 PMID:28853327

Nash, P., Taylor, T., & Levy, B. (2020). The Intersectionality of Ageism. *Innovation in Aging*, *4*(Suppl 1), 846–847. doi:10.1093/geroni/igaa057.3105

National Healthcare Quality and Disparities Report. (2022). Agency for Healthcare Research and Quality. AHRQ Pub. No. 22(23)-0030.

National Institute on Minority Health and Health Disparities. (n.d.). https://www.nimhd.nih.gov/about/overview/research-framework/nimhd-framework.html

National Institutes of Health. (2007). *Cultural Awareness Glossary of Key Terms*. https://www.niehs.nih.gov/news/events/pastmtg/hazmat/assets/2007/wtp_2007ntec_wruc_latino_tips_glossary_508.pdf

National Institutes of Health. (November 15, 2018). *Surgeon Chris McCulloh Stands Up to Disability*. National Institute of General Medical Sciences. https://biobeat.nigms.nih.gov/2018/11/surgeon-chris-mcculloh-stands-up-to-disability/

Nazar, M., Kendall, K., Day, L., & Nazar, H. (2015). Decolonising medical curricula through diversity education: Lessons from students. *Medical Teacher*, *37*(4), 385–393. doi:10.3109/0142159X.2014.947938 PMID:25156358

NCP Clinical Practice Guidelines for Quality Palliative Care. (2009). National Consensus Project. Available at: http://ww.nationalconsensusproject.org/guideline.pdf

Nedrow, A., Steckler, N. A., Hardman, J. (2012). Physician Resilience and Burnout: Can you make the switch. *Family Practice Management,* 25-30.

Neuhausen, K., Davis, A. C., Needleman, J., Brook, R. H., Zingmond, D., & Roby, D. H. (2014). Disproportionate-share hospital payment reductions may threaten the financial stability of safety-net hospitals. *Health Affairs (Project Hope)*, *33*(6), 988–996. doi:10.1377/hlthaff.2013.1222 PMID:24889948

New York Medical College. (June 30, 2022). *Expanded Disabilities Curriculum at New York Medical College Receives Enthusiastic Student Response*. New York Medical College. https://www.nymc.edu/news-and-events/news-archives/expanded-disabilities-curriculum-at-new-york-medical-college-receives-enthusiastic-student-response.php

Newman, C., Ng, C., Pacque-Margolis, S., & Frymus, D. (2016). Integration of gender-transformative interventions into health professional education reform for the 21st century: Implications of an expert review. *Human Resources for Health*, *14*(1), 14. doi:10.118612960-016-0109-8 PMID:27067144

Ngo-Metzger, Q., Sorkin, D. H., Phillips, R. S., Greenfield, S., Massagli, M. P., Clarridge, B., & Kaplan, S. H. (2007). Providing high-quality care for limited English proficient patients: The importance of language concordance and interpreter use. *Journal of General Internal Medicine*, *22*(S2, Suppl 2), 324–330. doi:10.100711606-007-0340-z PMID:17957419

Nimmon, L., & Stenfors-Hayes, T. (2016). The "Handling" of power in the physician-patient encounter: Perceptions from experienced physicians. *BMC Medical Education*, *16*(1), 114. doi:10.118612909-016-0634-0 PMID:27091146

Niu, N. N., Syed, Z. A., Krupat, E., Crutcher, B. N., Pelletier, S. R., & Shields, H. M. (2012). The impact of cross-cultural interactions on medical students' preparedness to care for diverse patients. *Academic Medicine*, *87*(11), 1530–1534.

Nondiscrimination in Health Programs and Activities, 42 CFR Parts 438, 440, and 460; 45 CFR Parts 80, 84, 86, 91, 92, 147, 155, and 156 (2022)

North, M. S., & Fiske, S. T. (2012). An inconvenienced youth? Ageism and its potential intergenerational roots. *Psychological Bulletin*, *138*(5), 982–997. doi:10.1037/a0027843 PMID:22448913

Notzer, N., Zisenwine, D., Oz, L., & Rak, Y. (2006, July). Overcoming the Tension between Scientific and Religious Views in Teaching Anatomical Dissection: The Israeli Experience. *Clinical Anatomy (New York, N.Y.), 19*(5), 442–447. doi:10.1002/ca.20312 PMID:16683239

Nouri, Z., Dill, M. J., Conrad, S. S., Moreland, C. J., & Meeks, L. M. (2021). Estimated Prevalence of US Physicians With Disabilities. *JAMA Network Open, 4*(3), e211254–e211254. doi:10.1001/jamanetworkopen.2021.1254 PMID:33710286

O'Keefe, V. M., Wingate, L. R., Cole, A. B., Hollingsworth, D. W., & Tucker, R. P. (2015). Seemingly Harmless Racial Communications Are Not So Harmless: Racial Microaggressions Lead to Suicidal Ideation by Way of Depression Symptoms. *Suicide & Life-Threatening Behavior, 45*(5), 567–576. https://doi.org/10.1111/sltb.12150

Office of the Surgeon General. (2005). *The Surgeon General's Call to Action to Improve the Health and Wellness of Persons with Disabilities*. U.S. Department of Health and Human Services, Office of the Surgeon General.

Okoro, C. A., Hollis, N. D., Cyrus, A. C., & Griffin-Blake, S. (2018). Prevalence of disabilities and health care access by disability status and type among adults—United States, 2016. *Morbidity and Mortality Weekly Report, 67*(32), 882–887. doi:10.15585/mmwr.mm6732a3 PMID:30114005

Oluo, I. (2019). So you want to talk about race. Academic Press.

Ortiz Reyes, M., & Sepúlveda Arroyo, L. (2020). The impact of recent demographic changes and migration patterns on education in Puerto Rico. In M. Slowey, H. Schuetze, & T. Zubrzycki (Eds.), *Inequality, Innovation and Reform in Higher Education* (pp. 59–69). Springer Nature Switzerland AG.

Pajarillo, E. J., & Korn, K. H. (2021). Equitable academic preparation: A structured onboarding program for incoming graduate nursing students. *Journal of Nursing Education and Practice, 11*(7), 1. Advance online publication. doi:10.5430/jnep.v11n7p1

Palmore, E. B. (1990). Ageism: Negative and positive. *Springer Publishing Company*. https://www.scirp.org/(S(oyulxb452alnt1aej1nfow45))/reference/ReferencesPapers.aspx?ReferenceID=1987593

Palmore, E. B., Branch, L., & Harris, D. K. (Eds.). (2005). *Encyclopedia of ageism*. Haworth Pastoral Press. doi:10.4324/9781315043975

Papantoniou, P. (2021). Are male nurses sexually harassed? A cross-sectional study in the Greek Health System. *BMC Nursing, 20*(1), 137. doi:10.118612912-021-00656-6 PMID:34372829

Paradies, Y., Ben, J., Denson, N., Elias, A., Priest, N., Pieterse, A., Gupta, A., Kelaher, M., & Gee, G. (2015). Racism as a Determinant of Health: A Systematic Review and Meta-Analysis. *PLoS One, 10*(9), e0138511. https://doi.org/10.1371/journal.pone.0138511

Parkhurst, D. C., Kayingo, G., & Fleming, S. (2017). Redesigning Physician Assistant Education to Promote Cognitive Diversity, Inclusion, and Health Care Equity. *The Journal of Physician Assistant Education: the Official Journal of the Physician Assistant Education Association, 28*(Suppl 1), S38–S42. https://doi.org/10.1097/JPA.0000000000000128

Pascoe, E. A., & Smart Richman, L. (2009). Perceived discrimination and health: A meta-analytic review. *Psychological Bulletin, 135*(4), 531–554. doi:10.1037/a0016059 PMID:19586161

Patel, E., Baxter, K. B., & Silverman, N. (2015). Leadership Practices for Interfaith Excellence in Higher Education. *Liberal Education, 101*, 48–53.

Patel, M., Swift, S., & Digesu, A. (2021). Mental health among clinicians: What do we know and what can we do? *International Urogynecology Journal and Pelvic Floor Dysfunction, 32*(5), 1055–1059. doi:10.100700192-021-04805-y PMID:33938962

Paul, D. P. III, & Skiba, M. (2016). Concierge Medicine: A Viable Business Model for (Some) Physicians of the Future? *The Health Care Manager*, *35*(1), 3–8. doi:10.1097/HCM.0000000000000088 PMID:27892907

Pelton, L. H. (2015). The continuing role of material factors in child maltreatment and placement. *Child Abuse & Neglect*, *41*, 30–39. doi:10.1016/j.chiabu.2014.08.001 PMID:25169149

Perdue, C. W., & Gurtman, M. B. (1990). Evidence for the automaticity of ageism. *Journal of Experimental Social Psychology*, *26*(3), 199–216. doi:10.1016/0022-1031(90)90035-K

Perron, R. (2018). *The Value of Experience: AARP Multicultural Work and Jobs Study.* AARP Research. https://www.aarp.org/research/topics/economics/info-2018/multicultural-work-jobs.html

Phelan, S. M., Burke, S. E., Hardeman, R. R., White, R. O., Przedworski, J., Dovidio, J. F., Perry, S. P., Plankey, M. A., Cunningham, B., Finstad, D. W., Yeazel, M., & van Ryn, M. (2017). Medical School Factors Associated with Changes in Implicit and Explicit Bias Against Gay and Lesbian People among 3492 Graduating Medical Students. *Journal of General Internal Medicine*, *32*(11), 1193–1201. doi:10.100711606-017-4127-6 PMID:28766125

Pierce, C. (1974). *Psychiatric problems of the black minority. Vol. American Handbook of Psychiatry*. Basic Books.

Pitre, C., Ladd, L., & Welch, J. (2017). Negotiating Work-Life Integration. *MedEdPORTAL: the Journal of Teaching and Learning Resources*, *5*(13), 10623. doi:10.15766/mep_2374-8265.10623 PMID:30800824

Poorsattar, S. P., Blake, C. M., & Manuel, S. P. (2021). Addressing Microaggressions In Academic Medicine. *Academic Medicine*, *96*(6), 927–927. doi:10.1097/ACM.0000000000004029 PMID:33656013

Porter, J. L., Townley, T., Huggett, K., & Warrier, R. (2008). An acculturization curriculum: Orienting international medical graduates to an internal medicine residency program. *Teaching and Learning in Medicine*, *20*(1), 37–43. doi:10.1080/10401330701542644 PMID:18444184

Posner, P., Ali, M., & Douglas, S. (2019). Religion and Spirituality Among Medical Students. In D. Zappetti & J. Avery (Eds.), *Medical Student Well-Being*. Springer. doi:10.1007/978-3-030-16558-1_6

Powell, P. S., Pazol, K., Wiggins, L. D., Daniels, J. L., Dichter, G. S., Bradley, C. B., Pretzel, R., Kloetzer, J., McKenzie, C., Scott, A., Robinson, B., Sims, A. S., Kasten, E. P., Fallin, M. D., Levy, S. E., Dietz, P. M., & Cogswell, M. E. (2021). Health Status and Health Care Use Among Adolescents Identified With and Without Autism in Early Childhood—Four US Sites, 2018–2020. *Morbidity and Mortality Weekly Report*, *70*(17), 605–611. doi:10.15585/mmwr.mm7017a1 PMID:33914722

Pratt-Chapman, M. L. (2020). Implementation of sexual and gender minority health curricula in health care professional schools: A qualitative study. *BMC Medical Education*, *20*(1), 138. https://doi.org/10.1186/s12909-020-02045-0

Prazeres, F., & Passos, L. (2021). Age discrimination at work against health-related professionals in Portugal. *Work (Reading, Mass.)*, *70*(3), 929–935. doi:10.3233/WOR-213612 PMID:34744039

Prejudice. (2022). In T. Grant (Ed.), *The Britannica Dictionary*. Retrieved from https://www.britannica.com/dictionary/prejudice

Puchalski, C., & Larson, D. (1998). Developing curricula in spirituality and medicine. *Academic Medicine*, *73*(9), 970–974. doi:10.1097/00001888-199809000-00015 PMID:9759099

Puzzanchera, C., Taylor, M., Kang, W., & Smith, J. (2022). *Disproportionality Rates for Children of Color in Foster Care Dashboard.* National Council of Juvenile and Family Court Judges. http://ncjj.org/AFCARS/Disproportionality_Dashboard.aspx

Rabie, T., Rossouw, L., & Machobane, B. F. (2020). Exploring occupational gender-role stereotypes of male nurses: A South African study. *International Journal of Nursing Practice, 12890.* Advance online publication. doi:10.1111/ijn.12890 PMID:32964584

Racism. (2022). In T. Grant (Ed.), *The Britannica Dictionary.* Retrieved from https://www.britannica.com/dictionary/racism

Rao, T. S., & Indla, V. (2010). Work, family or personal life: Why not all three? *Indian Journal of Psychiatry, 52*(4), 295–297. doi:10.4103/0019-5545.74301 PMID:21267360

Reith, T. P. (2018). Burnout in United States Healthcare Professionals: A Narrative Review. *Cureus, 10*(12), e3681. doi:10.7759/cureus.3681 PMID:30761233

Religious Advisors. (2022). Retrieved from Swarthmore: https://www.swarthmore.edu/interfaith-center/religious-advisors

Religious Landscape Study . (2022). Retrieved from Pew Research Center: https://www.pewresearch.org/religion/religious-landscape-study/educational-distribution/

Rhodes, M., & Moty, K. (2020). What is social essentialism and how does it develop? *Advances in Child Development and Behavior, 59,* 1–30. https://doi.org/10.1016/bs.acdb.2020.05.001

Ripp, J. A., Privitera, M. R., West, C. P., Leiter, R., Logio, L., Shapiro, J., & Bazari, H. (2017). Well-being in graduate medical education: A call for action. *Academic Medicine, 92*(7), 914–917. doi:10.1097/ACM.0000000000001735 PMID:28471780

Robards, F., Kang, M., Usherwood, T., & Sanci, L. (2018). How Marginalized Young People Access, Engage With, and Navigate Health-Care Systems in the Digital Age: Systematic Review. *The Journal of adolescent health: official publication of the Society for Adolescent Medicine, 62*(4), 365–381. doi:10.1016/j.jadohealth.2017.10.018

Robinson, D. (2022). Neurodiversity in medical education: How can we improve postgraduate learning for neurodiverse doctors? *Medical Teacher, 44*(5), 564–566. doi:10.1080/0142159X.2022.2039383 PMID:35236237

Rodriguez, J. E., Campbell, K. M., & Pololi, L. H. (2015). Addressing disparities in academic medicine: What of the minority tax? *BMC Medical Education, 15*(1), 6. doi:10.118612909-015-0290-9 PMID:25638211

Romanski, P. A., Bartz, D., Pelletier, A., & Johnson, N. R. (2020). The "invisible student": Neglect as a form of medical student mistreatment, a call to action. *Journal of Surgical Education, 77*(6), 1327–1330. doi:10.1016/j.jsurg.2020.05.013 PMID:32507361

Rose, D. (2000). Universal design for learning. *Journal of Special Education Technology, 15*(3), 45–49. doi:10.1177/016264340001500307

Rose, L., Aouad, M., Graham, L., Schoemaker, L., & Wagner, T. (2021). Association of Expanded Health Care Networks With Utilization Among Veterans Affairs Enrollees. *JAMA Network Open, 4*(10), e2131141. doi:10.1001/jamanetworkopen.2021.31141 PMID:34698845

Rössler, W. (2012). Stress, burnout, and job dissatisfaction in mental health workers. *European Archives of Psychiatry and Clinical Neuroscience, 262*(2), 65–69. doi:10.100700406-012-0353-4 PMID:22926058

Rostad, W. L., Ports, K. A., Tang, S., & Kelvins, J. (2020). Reducing the Number of Children Entering Foster Care: Effects of State Earned Income Tax Credits. *Child Maltreatment, 25*(4), 393–397. doi:10.1177/1077559519900922 PMID:31973550

Rotenstein, L. S., Ramos, M. A., Torre, M., Segal, J. B., Peluso, M. J., Guille, C., Sen, S., & Mata, D. A. (2016). Prevalence of Depression, Depressive Symptoms, and Suicidal Ideation Among Medical Students: A Systematic Review and Meta-Analysis. *Journal of the American Medical Association, 316*(21), 2214–2236. doi:10.1001/jama.2016.17324 PMID:27923088

Rotenstein, L. S., Torre, M., Ramos, M. A., Rosales, R. C., Guille, C., Sen, S., & Mata, D. A. (2018). Prevalence of burnout among physicians: A systematic review. *Journal of the American Medical Association, 320*(11), 1131–1150. doi:10.1001/jama.2018.12777 PMID:30326495

Rowe, D., Ng, Y. C., O'Keefe, L., & Crawford, D. (2017). Providers' Attitudes and Knowledge of Lesbian, Gay, Bisexual, and Transgender Health. *Federal Practitioner: For the Health Care Professionals of the VA, DoD, and PHS, 34*(11), 28–34. PMID:30766240

RTOERO. (2022). *Nuances of Ageism.* RTOERO. https://rtoero.ca/wp-content/uploads/2022/01/Nuances-of-ageism-whitepaper-RTOERO-2021.pdf

Rust, G., Nembhard, W. N., Nichols, M., Omole, F., Minor, P., Barosso, G., & Mayberry, R. (2004). Racial and ethnic disparities in the provision of epidural analgesia to Georgia Medicaid beneficiaries during labor and delivery. *American Journal of Obstetrics and Gynecology, 191*(2), 456–462. https://doi.org/10.1016/j.ajog.2004.03.005

Ruzycki, S. M., Daodu, O., Hernandez, S., & Lithgow, K. C. (2022). The contribution of undergraduate medical education dresscodes to systemic discrimination: A critical policy analysis. *Medical Education, 56*(9), 949–957. doi:10.1111/medu.14854 PMID:35688162

Ryus, C. R., Samuels, E. A., Wong, A. H., Hill, K. A., Huot, S., & Boatright, D. (2022). Burnout and Perception of Medical School Learning Environments Among Gay, Lesbian, and Bisexual Medical Students. *JAMA Network Open, 5*(4), E229596. doi:10.1001/jamanetworkopen.2022.9596 PMID:35486396

Sabin, J. A. (2022). Tackling Implicit Bias in Health Care. *The New England Journal of Medicine, 387*(2), 105–107. https://doi.org/10.1056/NEJMp2201180

Sagalowsky, S. T., Woodward, H., Evins, J., & Kessler, D. O. (2021). Responding to Microaggressions: Further Frameworks From Simulation Debriefing. *Annals of Emergency Medicine, 77*(3), 381–382. doi:10.1016/j.annemergmed.2020.10.006 PMID:33618815

Saha, S., Guiton, G., Wimmers, P. F., & Wilkerson, L. (2008). Student body racial and ethnic composition and diversity-related outcomes in US medical schools. *Journal of the American Medical Association, 300*(10), 1135–1145. https://doi.org/10.1001/jama.300.10.1135

Sakamoto, A., Takei, I., & Woo, H. (2012). The Myth of the Model Minority Myth. *Sociological Spectrum, 32*(4), 309–321. https://doi.org/10.1080/02732173.2012.664042

Saluja, B., & Bryant, Z. (2021). How Implicit Bias Contributes to Racial Disparities in Maternal Morbidity and Mortality in the United States. *Journal of Women's Health, 30*(2), 270–273. doi:10.1089/jwh.2020.8874

Samuels, E. A., Boatright, D. H., Wong, A. H., Cramer, L. D., Desai, M. M., Solotke, M. T., Latimore, D., & Gross, C. P. (2021). Association Between Sexual Orientation, Mistreatment, and Burnout Among US Medical Students. *JAMA Network Open, 4*(2), e2036136. doi:10.1001/jamanetworkopen.2020.36136 PMID:33528552

Samulowitz, A., Gremyr, I., Eriksson, E., & Hensing, G. (2018). "Brave Men" and "Emotional Women": A theory-guided literature review on gender bias in health care and gendered norms towards patients with chronic pain. *Pain Research & Management, 2018*, 1–14. doi:10.1155/2018/6358624 PMID:29682130

Sanchez, N. F., Rabatin, J., Sanchez, J. P., Hubbard, S., & Kalet, A. (2006). Medical students' ability to care for lesbian, gay, bisexual, and transgendered patients. *Family Medicine*, *38*(1), 21–27.

Sandra, F. (2016) *Intersectional discrimination in EU gender equality and non-discrimination law*. European Commission. https://data.europa.eu/doi/10.2838/241520

Saravia, N. G., & Miranda, J. F. (2004). Plumbing the brain drain. *Bulletin of the World Health Organization*, *82*(8), 608–615.

Sarcahmi, R., Rajael, S., & Aalaei, S. (2020). Evaluation of the relationship between religious beliefs and academic achievements of dental students. *Journal of Education and Health Promotion*, *9*(305), 305. Advance online publication. doi:10.4103/jehp.jehp_576_19 PMID:33426109

Sarmiento, C., Miller, S. R., Chang, E., Zazove, P., & Kumagai, A. K. (2016). From impairment to empowerment: A longitudinal medical school curriculum on disabilities. *Academic Medicine*, *91*(7), 954–957. doi:10.1097/ACM.0000000000000935 PMID:26422593

Say, L., Chou, D., Gemmill, A., Tunçalp, Ö., Moller, A. B., Daniels, J., Gülmezoglu, A. M., Temmerman, M., & Alkema, L. (2014). Global causes of maternal death: A WHO systematic analysis. *The Lancet. Global Health*, *2*(6), e323–e333. doi:10.1016/S2214-109X(14)70227-X PMID:25103301

Scambler, G. (2019). Sociology, Social Class, Health Inequalities, and the Avoidance of "Classism". *Front Sociol.*, *4*, 56. doi:10.3389/fsoc.2019.00056 PMID:33869379

Schenker, Y., Pérez-Stable, E. J., Nickleach, D., & Karliner, L. S. (2011). Patterns of interpreter use for hospitalized patients with limited English proficiency. *Journal of General Internal Medicine*, *26*(7), 712–717. doi:10.100711606-010-1619-z PMID:21336672

Schenker, Y., Wang, F., Selig, S. J., Ng, R., & Fernandez, A. (2007). The impact of language barriers on documentation of informed consent at a hospital with on-site interpreter services. *Journal of General Internal Medicine*, *22*(S2, Suppl 2), 294–299. doi:10.100711606-007-0359-1 PMID:17957414

Schneiderman, J. U., Smith, C., & Palinkas, L. A. (2012). The caregiver as gatekeeper for accessing health care for children in foster care: A qualitative study of kinship and unrelated caregivers. *Children and Youth Services Review*, *34*(10), 2123–2130. doi:10.1016/j.childyouth.2012.07.009 PMID:23139436

Schulz, R., & Sherwood, P. R. (2009). Physical and Mental Health Effects of Family Caregiving. *The American Journal of Nursing*, *108*(9), 23–27. doi:10.1097/01.NAJ.0000336406.45248.4c PMID:18797217

Schwartz, S. B., Smith, S. G., & Johnson, K. R. (2020). ADEA Faculty Diversity Toolkit: A Comprehensive Approach to Improving Diversity and Inclusion in Dental Education. *Journal of Dental Education*, *84*(3), 279–282. https://doi.org/10.1002/jdd.12143

Schwartz, S. P., Adair, K. C., Bae, J., Rehder, K. J., Shanafelt, T. D., Profit, J., & Sexton, J. B. (2019). Work-life balance behaviours cluster in work settings and relate to burnout and safety culture: A cross-sectional survey analysis. *BMJ Quality & Safety*, *8*(2), 142–150. doi:10.1136/bmjqs-2018-007933 PMID:30309912

Serna, D. C. (2019). Lifestyle Medicine in a Concierge Practice: My Journey. *American Journal of Lifestyle Medicine*, *13*(4), 367–370. doi:10.1177/1559827618821865 PMID:31285719

Sexton, J. B., Schwartz, S. P., Chadwick, W. A., Rehder, K. J., Bae, J., Bokovoy, J., Doram, K., Sotile, W., Adair, K. C., & Profit, J. (2017). The associations between work-life balance behaviors, teamwork climate and safety climate: Cross-sectional survey introducing the work-life climate scale, psychometric properties, benchmarking data and future directions. *BMJ Quality & Safety*, *26*(8), 632–640. doi:10.1136/bmjqs-2016-006032 PMID:28008006

Shain, M. (2009). Psychological safety at work: Emergence of a corporate and social agenda in Canada. *International Journal of Mental Health Promotion*, *11*(3), 42–48. doi:10.1080/14623730.2009.9721791

Shanafelt, T. D., Balch, C. M., Dyrbye, L., Bechamps, G., Russell, T., Satele, D., Rummans, T., Swartz, K., Novotny, P. J., Sloan, J., & Oreskovich, M. R. (2011). Special report: Suicidal ideation among American surgeons. *Archives of Surgery (Chicago, Ill.)*, *146*(1), 54–62. doi:10.1001/archsurg.2010.292 PMID:21242446

Shanafelt, T. D., Boone, S., Tan, L., Dyrbye, L. N., Sotile, W., Satele, D., West, C. P., Sloan, J., & Oreskovich, M. R. (2012). Burnout and Satisfaction with Work-Life Balance Among US Physicians Relative to the General US Population. *Archives of Internal Medicine*, *172*(18), 1377–1385. doi:10.1001/archinternmed.2012.3199 PMID:22911330

Shanafelt, T. D., Dyrbye, L. N., Sinsky, C., Trockel, M., Makowski, M. S., Tutty, M., Wang, H., Carlasare, L. E., & West, C. P. (2022). Imposter Phenomenon in US Physicians Relative to the US Working Population. *Mayo Clinic Proceedings*, *97*(11), 1981–1993. doi:10.1016/j.mayocp.2022.06.021 PMID:36116974

Shanafelt, T. D., West, C. P., Sinsky, C., Trockel, M., Tutty, M., Satele, D. V., Carlasare, L. E., & Dyrbye, L. N. (2019). Changes in Burnout and Satisfaction with Work-Life Integration in Physicians and the General US Working Population Between 2011 and 2017. *Mayo Clinic Proceedings*, *94*(9), 1681–1694. doi:10.1016/j.mayocp.2018.10.023 PMID:30803733

Shang, Z., Kim, J. Y., & Cheng, S. O. (2021). Discrimination experienced by Asian Canadian and Asian American health care workers during the COVID-19 pandemic: A qualitative study. *CMAJ Open*, *9*(4). https://doi.org/10.9778/cmajo.20210090

Shapiro, J. (2008). Walking a mile in their patients' shoes: Empathy and othering in medical students' education. *Philosophy, Ethics, and Humanities in Medicine; PEHM*, *3*(1), 1–11. doi:10.1186/1747-5341-3-10 PMID:18336719

Shea, G., & Solomon, C. A. (2020). *Leading successful change, revised and updated edition: 8 keys to making change work*. Wharton School Press.

Shen, M. J., Peterson, E. B., Costas-Muñiz, R., Hernandez, M. H., Jewell, S. T., Matsoukas, K., & Bylund, C. L. (2018). The Effects of Race and Racial Concordance on Patient-Physician Communication: A Systematic Review of the Literature. *Journal of Racial and Ethnic Health Disparities*, *5*(1), 117–140. https://doi.org/10.1007/s40615-017-0350-4

Sherman, D. (2004). Nurses' stress & burnout: How to care for yourself when caring for patients and their families experiencing life-threatening illness. *The American Journal of Nursing*, *104*(5), 52. doi:10.1097/00000446-200405000-00020 PMID:15166716

Shillcutt, S. (2022). *Brave Boundaries: Strategies to Say No, Stand Strong, and Take Control of your time: The Key to Living Empowered*. Health Communications Inc.

Shrider, E. A., Kollar, M., Chen, F., & Semega, J. (2021). *Income and poverty in the United States: 2020*. U.S. Census Bureau. https://www.census.gov/library/publications/2021/demo/p60-273.html

Silva, A., Adelman, R. D., Singh, V., Gupta, R., Moxley, J., Sobota, R. M., Tsai, S., Abel, B. T., & Reid, M. C. (2022). Healthcare Provider Perspectives Regarding Use of Medical Interpreters During End-of-Life Conversations With Limited English Proficient Patients. *The American Journal of Hospice & Palliative Care*, *39*(2), 220–227. doi:10.1177/10499091211015916 PMID:34000817

Simons, A. M., Koster, A., Groffen, D. A., & Bosma, H. (2017). Perceived classism and its relation with socioeconomic status, health, health behaviours and perceived inferiority: The Dutch Longitudinal Internet Studies for the Social Sciences (LISS) panel. *International Journal of Public Health*, *62*(4), 433–440. doi:10.100700038-016-0880-2 PMID:27572684

SinghR.VolnerK.MarloweD. (2022). *Provider Burnout.* https://www.ncbi.nlm.nih.gov/books/NBK538330/

Sivashanker, K., Couillard, C., Goldsmith, J., Walker, N., & Eappen, S. (2020). Addressing the caste system in U.S. healthcare in the era of COVID-19. *International Journal for Equity in Health*, *19*(1), 184. doi:10.118612939-020-01298-x PMID:33076929

Slaughter-Acey, J. C., Sealy-Jefferson, S., Helmkamp, L., Caldwell, C. H., Osypuk, T. L., Platt, R. W., Straughen, J. K., Dailey-Okezie, R. K., Abeysekara, P., & Misra, D. P. (2016). Racism in the form of micro aggressions and the risk of preterm birth among black women. *Annals of Epidemiology*, *26*(1), 7–13.e1. https://doi.org/10.1016/j.annepidem.2015.10.005

Smedley, B. D., Stith Butler, A., & Bristow, L. R. (Eds.). (2004). In the nation's compelling interest: Ensuring diversity in the health-care workforce. National Academies Press (US).

Smedley, B. D., Stith, A. Y., & Nelson, A. R. (2003) Institute of Medicine (US) Committee on Understanding and Eliminating Racial and Ethnic Disparities in Health Care. In *Unequal Treatment: Confronting Racial and Ethnic Disparities in Health Care.* National Academies Press (US). https://www.ncbi.nlm.nih.gov/books/NBK220364/

Smeijers, A. S., Ens-Dokkum, M. H., van den Bogaerde, B., & Oudesluys-Murphy, A. M. (2011). Clinical practice: The approach to the deaf or hard-of-hearing paediatric patient. *European Journal of Pediatrics*, *170*(11), 1359–1363. doi:10.100700431-011-1530-6 PMID:21766166

Smith, D. L. (2009). Disparities in patient-physician communication for persons with a disability from the 2006 Medical Expenditure Panel Survey (MEPS). *Disability and Health Journal*, *2*(4), 206–215. doi:10.1016/j.dhjo.2009.06.002 PMID:21122761

Snyder, C. R., Wang, P. Z., & Truitt, A. R. (2018). Multiracial Patient Experiences With Racial Microaggressions in Health Care Settings. *Journal of Patient-Centered Research and Reviews*, *5*(3), 229–238. doi:10.17294/2330-0698.1626 PMID:31414007

Social-determinants-of-health-101-for-health-care-five-plus-five. (n.d.). https://nam.edu/social-determinants-of-health-101-for-health-care-five-plus-five/

Sonneville, K. R., & Lipson, S. K. (2018). Disparities in eating disorder diagnosis and treatment according to weight status, race/ethnicity, socioeconomic background, and sex among college students. *International Journal of Eating Disorders*, *51*(6), 518–526. https://doi.org/10.1002/eat.22846

Sotto-Santiado, A., Poll-Hunter, N., Trice, T., Buenconsejo-Lum, L., Golden, S., Howell, J., Jacobs, N., Lee, W., Mason, H., Ogunyemi, D., Crespon, W., & Lamba, S. (2022, January). A Framework for Developing Antiracist Medical Educators and Prationer-Scholars. *Academic Medicine*, *97*(1), 41–47. Advance online publication. doi:10.1097/ACM.0000000000004385

Sotto-Santiago, S., Mac, J., Duncan, F., & Smith, J. (2020). "I Didn't Know What to Say": Responding to Racism, Discrimination, and Microaggressions With the OWTFD Approach. *MedEdPORTAL: the Journal of Teaching and Learning Resources*, *16*, 10971. doi:10.15766/mep_2374-8265.10971 PMID:32754635

Souza, T. J. (2018). *Responding to Microaggressions in the Classroom: Taking Action.* Magna Publication. https://www.facultyfocus.com/articles/effective-classroom-management/responding-to-microaggressions-in-the-classroom/

Souza, T. J. (2016). *Managing Hot Moments in the Classroom: Concrete Strategies for Cooling Down Tension. Faculty Focus Special Report: Diversity and Inclusion in the College Classroom.* Magna Publication.

Spector, N. D., Asante, P. A., Marcelin, J. R., Poorman, J. A., Larson, A. R., Salles, A., Oxentenko, A. S., & Silver, J. K. (2019). Women in pediatrics: Progress, barriers, and opportunities for equity, diversity, and inclusion. *Pediatrics, 144*(5), e20192149. doi:10.1542/peds.2019-2149 PMID:31548337

Spector, P. E., Zhou, Z. E., & Che, X. X. (2014). Nurse exposure to physical and nonphysical violence, bullying, and sexual harassment: A quantitative review. *International Journal of Nursing Studies, 51*(1), 72–84. doi:10.1016/j.ijnurstu.2013.01.010 PMID:23433725

Spiritual Life Advisors. (2022). Retrieved from NYU: https://www.nyu.edu/students/communities-and-groups/student-diversity/spiritual-life/religious-and-spiritual-life-on-campus/chaplains-circle.html

Spoorthy, M. S., Pratapa, S. K., & Mahant, S. (2020). Mental health problems faced by healthcare workers due to the COVID-19 pandemic–A Review. *Asian Journal of Psychiatry, 51*, 102119. https://doi.org/10.1016/j.ajp.2020.102119

Staff and Advisors. (2022). Retrieved from DePauw University: https://www.depauw.edu/campus-life/spiritual-life/center/staff-and-advisors/

Stanley, D., Beament, T., Falconer, D., Haigh, M., Saunders, R., Stanley, K., Wall, P., & Nielson, S. (2016). The male of the species: A profile of men in nursing. *Journal of Advanced Nursing, 72*(5), 1155–1168. doi:10.1111/jan.12905 PMID:26799533

Stewart, M. A. (1995). Effective physician-patient communication and health outcomes: A review. *CMAJ. Canadian Medical Association Journal, 152*(9), 1423. PMID:7728691

Streed, C. G. J., Lunn, M. R., Siegel, J., & Obedin-Maliver, J. (2021). Meeting the Patient Care, Education, and Research Missions: Academic Medical Centers Must Comprehensively Address Sexual and Gender Minority Health. *Academic Medicine, 96*(6), 822–827. https://doi.org/10.1097/ACM.0000000000003703

Stypinska, J., & Turek, K. (2017). Hard and soft age discrimination: The dual nature of workplace discrimination. *European Journal of Ageing, 14*(1), 49–61. doi:10.100710433-016-0407-y PMID:28804394

Sue, D. W. (2010). *Microaggressions in everyday life: race, gender, and sexual orientation.* John Wiley & Sons Inc. https://www.wiley.com/en-us/Microaggressions+in+Everyday+Life%3A+Race%2C+Gender%2C+and+Sexual+Orientation-p-9780470491409

Sue, D. W., Alsaidi, S., Awad, M. N., Glaeser, E., Calle, C. Z., & Mendez, N. (2019). Disarming racial microaggressions: Microintervention strategies for targets, White allies, and bystanders. *The American Psychologist, 74*(1), 128–142. doi:10.1037/amp0000296 PMID:30652905

Sue, D. W., Capodilupo, C. M., Torino, G. C., Bucceri, J. M., Holder, A. M., Nadal, K. L., & Esquilin, M. (2007). Racial microaggressions in everyday life: Implications for clinical practice. *The American Psychologist, 62*(4), 271–286. https://doi.org/10.1037/0003-066X.62.4.271

Suen, L. W., Makam, A. N., Snyder, H. R., Repplinger, D., Kushel, M. B., Martin, M., & Nguyen, O. K. (2022). National Prevalence of Alcohol and Other Substance Use Disorders Among Emergency Department Visits and Hospitalizations: NHAMCS 2014-2018. *Journal of General Internal Medicine, 37*(10), 2420–2428. doi:10.100711606-021-07069-w PMID:34518978

Sullivan, W. F., Diepstra, H., Heng, J., Ally, S., Bradley, E., Casson, I., Hennen, B., Kelly, M., Korossy, M., McNeil, K., Abells, D., Amaria, K., Boyd, K., Gemmill, M., Grier, E., Kennie-Kaulbach, N., Ketchell, M., Ladouceur, J., Lepp, A., Lunsky, Y., McMillan, S., Niel, U., Sacks, S., Shea, S., Stringer, K., Sue, K., & Witherbee, S. (2018). Primary care of adults with intellectual and developmental disabilities. *2018 Canadian consensus guidelines, 64*(4), 254-279.

Swartz, M. S. (2006). "Conscience clauses" or "unconscionable clauses": Personal beliefs versus professional responsibilities. *Yale Journal of Health Policy, Law, and Ethics*, *6*(2), 269–350. PMID:17133969

Symons, A. B., McGuigan, D., & Akl, E. A. (2009). A curriculum to teach medical students to care for people with disabilities: Development and initial implementation. *BMC Medical Education*, *9*(1), 1–7. doi:10.1186/1472-6920-9-1 PMID:20042110

Tang, S. Y., Browne, A. J., Mussell, B., Smye, V. L., & Rodney, P. (2015). 'Underclassism' and access to healthcare in urban centres. *Sociology of Health & Illness*, *37*(5), 698–714. doi:10.1111/1467-9566.12236 PMID:25720520

Tarn, D. M., & … . (2005). Trust in one's physician: The role of ethnic match, autonomy, acculturation, and religiosity among Japanese and Japanese Americans. *Annals of Family Medicine*, *3*(4), 339–347.

Ten ways to support learners with dyslexia . (n.d.). Cambridge English. Retrieved September 30, 2022, from https://www.cambridgeenglish.org/blog/ten-ways-to-support-learners-with-dyslexia/

Tervalon, M., & Murray-Garcia, J. (1998). Cultural Humility Versus Cultural Compentence: A critical distinction in defining physician training outcomes in multicultural education. *Journal of Health Care for the Poor and Underserved*, *9*(2), 117–125. doi:10.1353/hpu.2010.0233 PMID:10073197

The Informed Patient. (n.d.). *A podcast connecting you with health, science and medicine*. https://www.upstate.edu/informed/2022/051322-caruso-brown-podcast.php

The Joint Commission. PC.02.02.13. 3.7.0.0 ed. (2011). Available at: https://www.jointcommission.org/assets/1/6/LTC_Core_PC.pdf

The UDL guidelines . (2022, September 2). UDL. Retrieved September 30, 2022, from https://udlguidelines.cast.org/

The United States Department of Justice . (2022). Retrieved from Types of educational opportunities discrimination: https://www.justice.gov/crt/types-educational-opportunities-discrimination

Thomas, C. M., Bertram, E., & Johnson, D. (2009). The SBAR communication technique: Teaching nursing students professional communication skills. *Nurse Educator*, *34*(4), 176–180. doi:10.1097/NNE.0b013e3181aaba54 PMID:19574858

Thornicroft, G., Rose, D., & Kassam, A. (2007). Discrimination in health care against people with mental illness. *International Review of Psychiatry (Abingdon, England)*, *19*(2), 113–122. doi:10.1080/09540260701278937 PMID:17464789

Ting, X., Yong, B., Yin, L., & Mi, T. (2016). Patient perception and the barriers to practicing patient-centered communication: A survey and in-depth interview of Chinese patients and physicians. *Patient Education and Counseling*, *99*(3), 364–369. doi:10.1016/j.pec.2015.07.019 PMID:26776708

Tips from students . (n.d.). Yale Dyslexia. Retrieved September 30, 2022, from https://dyslexia.yale.edu/resources/dyslexic-kids-adults/tips-from-students/

Tonkin, E. (2017). *The Importance of Medical Interpreters*. The American Journal of Psychiatry Online Resident's Journal., doi:10.1176/appi.ajp-rj.2017.120806

Torres, M. B., Salles, A., & Cochran, A. (2019). Recognizing and Reacting to Microaggressions in Medicine and Surgery. *JAMA Surgery*, *154*(9), 868–872. https://doi.org/10.1001/jamasurg.2019.1648

Tran, A. (2020, May 22). Hero and villain: An Asian American doctor's perspective on being viewed as the solution and the problem. *The Hill*. https://thehill.com/changing-america/opinion/499156-hero-and-villain-an-asian-american-doctors-perspective-on-being

Tsai, J. (2022). How Should Educators and Publishers Eliminate Racial Essentialism? *AMA Journal of Ethics*, *24*(3), E201–E211. https://doi.org/10.1001/amajethics.2022.201

Tsai, J. W., & Muindi, F. (2016). Towards sustaining a culture of mental health and wellness for trainees in the biosciences. *Nature Biotechnology*, *34*(3), 353–355. doi:10.1038/nbt.3490 PMID:26963557

Tung, Y.-J., Lo, K. K. H., Ho, R. C. M., & Tam, W. S. W. (2018). Prevalence of depression among nursing students: A systematic review and meta-analysis. *Nurse Education Today*, *63*, 119–129. doi:10.1016/j.nedt.2018.01.009 PMID:29432998

U.S Centers for Medicare & Medicaid Services. (2016) *Medicare.gov: the official U.S. government site for Medicare*. Medicare. http://medicare.gov

U.S. Census Bureau. (2020). Selected Social Characteristics in the United States [Retrieved from]. *Matrix (Stuttgart, Germany)*, DP02.

U.S. Department of Health and Human Services. (in press). *Disparities: Healthy People 2030*. U.S. Department of Health and Human Services, Office of Disease Prevention and Health Promotion.

U.S. Department of Labor. (2022) Age *Discrimination*. USDL. https://www.dol.gov/general/topic/discrimination/agedisc#:~:text=The%20Age%20Discrimination%20in%20Employment,conditions%20or%20privileges%20of%20employment

U.S. Equal Employment Opportunity Commission. (2022) *Age Discrimination | U.S. Equal Employment Opportunity Commission*. EEOC. https://www.eeoc.gov/age-discrimination#:~:text=Age%20discrimination%20involves%20treating%20an,are%20age%2040%20or%20older

UN Women. (2015). *Beijing Declaration and Platform for Action*. United Nations Entity for Gender Equality and the Empowerment of Women (UN Women). https://www.unwomen.org/en/digital-library/publications/2015/01/beijing-declaration

United States Census Bureau. (2022). *CS 5-Year Estimates Public Use Microdata Sample*. USCB. https://data.census.gov/mdat/#/search?ds=ACSPUMS5Y2018&cv=ENG%282,3,4%29&wt=PWGTP

United States Department of Justice. (2022). *Justice Department and HHS Issue Guidance on Nondiscrimination in Telehealth the Week of the 32nd Anniversay of the Americans with Disabilities Act*. USDJ. https://www.justice.gov/opa/pr/justice-department-and-hhs-issue-guidance-nondiscrimination-telehealth-week-32nd-anniversary

United States Holocaust Memorial Museum. (2020). *Documenting Numbers Of Victims Of The Holocaust And Nazi Persecution*. https://encyclopedia.ushmm.org/content/en/article/documenting-numbers-of-victims-of-the-holocaust-and-nazi-persecution

US Census Bureau. (2020). *2020 Census*. https://www.census.gov/programs-surveys/decennial-census/decade/2020/2020-census-main.html

USDA mapping food deserts in the US. (n.d.). https://www.ers.usda.gov/amber-waves/2011/december/data-feature-mapping-food-deserts-in-the-us/accessed

USDHHS. (2012). *Healthy People 2010 Final Review*. U.S. Department of Health and Human Services, National Center for Heatlh Statistics.

USDJ. (2022). *2020 FBI Hate Crimes Statistics*. The United States Department of Justice. https://www.justice.gov/crs/highlights/2020-hate-crimes-statistics

USFG. (2001) Guidance to Federal Financial Assistance Recipients Regarding Title VI Prohibition Against National Origin Discrimination Affecting Limited English Proficient Persons. 67 FR 4968

van Ryn, M., Hardeman, R., Phelan, S. M., Burgess, D. J., Dovidio, J. F., Herrin, J., Burke, S. E., Nelson, D. B., Perry, S., Yeazel, M., & Przedworski, J. M. (2015). Medical School Experiences Associated with Change in Implicit Racial Bias Among 3547 Students: A Medical Student CHANGES Study Report. *Journal of General Internal Medicine*, *30*(12), 1748–1756. https://doi.org/10.1007/s11606-015-3447-7

Van Wicklin, S. A. (2020). Ageism in Nursing. *Plastic surgical nursing: official journal of the American Society of Plastic and Reconstructive Surgical Nurses*, *40*(1), 20–24. doi:10.1097/PSN.0000000000000290

Vanderwoerd, J. R. (2016). The promise and perils of anti-oppressive practice for Christians in social work education. *Social Work & Christianity*, *43*(2), 153–188.

Velázquez-Estrada, A. (2016). *Perfil del migrante 2014*. Instituto de Estadísticas de Puerto Rico. https://estadisticas.pr/files/Publicaciones/Perfil_del_Migrante_2014_0.pdf

Villarroel, M. A., & Terlizzi, E. P. (2020). Symptoms of Depression Among Adults: United States, 2019. *NCHS Data Brief*, *379*, 1–8. PMID:33054920

Villegas, S., Rosenthal, J. A., O'Brien, K., & Pecora, P. (2011). Health outcomes for adults in family foster care as children: An analysis by ethnicity. *Children and Youth Services Review*, *33*(1), 110–117. doi:10.1016/j.childyouth.2010.08.020

Vogan, C. L., McKimm, J., Da Silva, A. L., & Grant, A. (2014). Twelve tips for providing effective student support in undergraduate medical education. *Medical Teacher*, *36*(6), 480–485. https://doi.org/10.3109/0142159X.2014.907488

Vyas, D. A., Eisenstein, L. G., & Jones, D. S. (2020). Hidden in Plain Sight - Reconsidering the Use of Race Correction in Clinical Algorithms. *The New England Journal of Medicine*, *383*(9), 874–882. https://doi.org/10.1056/NEJMms2004740

Walker, A. (2020, May 3). News outlets contribute to anti-Asian racism with careless stock photos on coronavirus coverage. *Media Matters for America*. https://www.mediamatters.org/coronavirus-covid-19/news-outlets-contribute-anti-asian-racism-careless-stock-photos-coronavirus

Wan, W. (2021). *Burned out by the pandemic, 3 in 10 health-care workers consider leaving the profession*. https://www.washingtonpost.com/health/2021/04/22/health-workers-covid-quit/

Warner, N. S., Njathi-Ori, C. W., & O'Brien, E. K. (2020). The GRIT (Gather, Restate, Inquire, Talk It Out) Framework for Addressing Microaggressions. *JAMA Surgery*, *155*(2), 178–179. doi:10.1001/jamasurg.2019.4427 PMID:31774484

Wasserman, M., Renfrew, M. R., Green, A. R., Lopez, L., Tan-McGrory, A., Brach, C., & Betancourt, J. R. (2014). Identifying and preventing medical errors in patients with limited English proficiency: Key findings and tools for the field. *Journal for Healthcare Quality*, *36*(3), 5–16. doi:10.1111/jhq.12065 PMID:24629098

Watt, K., Abbott, P., & Reath, J. (2016). Developing cultural competence in general practitioners: An integrative review of the literature. *BMC Family Practice*, *17*(1), 158. doi:10.118612875-016-0560-6 PMID:27846805

West, C. P., Dyrbye, L. N., Erwin, P. J., & Shanafelt, T. D. (2016). Interventions to prevent and reduce physician burnout: A systematic review and meta-analysis. *Lancet*, *388*(10057), 2272–2281. doi:10.1016/S0140-6736(16)31279-X PMID:27692469

West, C. P., Dyrbye, L. N., & Shanafelt, T. D. (2018). Physician burnout: Contributors, consequences and solutions. *Journal of Internal Medicine*, *283*(6), 516–529. doi:10.1111/joim.12752 PMID:29505159

West, C. P., Dyrbye, L. N., Sinsky, C., Trockel, M., Tutty, M., Nedelec, L., Carlasare, L. E., & Shanafelt, T. D. (2020). Resilience and Burnout Among Physicians and the General US Working Population. *JAMA Network Open, 3*(7), e209385. doi:10.1001/jamanetworkopen.2020.9385 PMID:32614425

West, C. P., Shanafelt, T. D., & Kolars, J. C. (2011). Quality of life, burnout, educational debt, and medical knowledge among internal medicine residents. *Journal of the American Medical Association, 306*(9), 952–960. doi:10.1001/jama.2011.1247 PMID:21900135

White, P. H., Cooley, W. C., Boudreau, A. D. A., Cyr, M., Davis, B. E., Dreyfus, D. E., Forlenza, E., Friedland, A., Greenlee, C., Mann, M., McManus, M., Meleis, A. I., & Pickler, L.Transitions Clinical Report Authoring Group. (2018). Supporting the Health Care Transition From Adolescence to Adulthood in the Medical Home. *Pediatrics, 142*(5), e20182587. doi:10.1542/peds.2018-2587 PMID:30348754

Whitgob, E. E., Blankenburg, R. L., & Bogetz, A. L. (2016). The Discriminatory Patient and Family: Strategies to Address Discrimination Towards Trainees. *Academic medicine: journal of the Association of American Medical Colleges, 91*(11). 10.1097/ACM.0000000000001357

Whitla, D. K., Orfield, G., Silen, W., Teperow, C., Howard, C., & Reede, J. (2003). Educational benefits of diversity in medical school: A survey of students. *Academic Medicine, 78*(5), 460–466. https://doi.org/10.1097/00001888-200305000-00007

WHO. (n.d.). *Mental disorders*. WHO. https://www.who.int/news-room/fact-sheets/detail/mental-disorders

Wilkerson, I. (2020). *Caste: The Origins of Our Discontents*. Random House.

Wilkin, T. (2015). Clinical Practice. Primary Care for Men Who Have Sex with Men. *The New England Journal of Medicine, 373*(9), 854–862. https://doi.org/10.1056/NEJMcp1401303

Williams, D. A., Berger, J. B., & McClendon, S. A. (2005). Toward a model of inclusive excellence and change in post-secondary institutions. Washington, DC: Association of American Colleges and Universities.

Williams, D. R., Lawrence, J. A., & Davis, B. A. (2019). Racism and Health: Evidence and Needed Research. *Annual Review of Public Health, 40*, 105–125. https://doi.org/10.1146/annurev-publhealth-040218-043750

Williams, E. S., Rathert, C., & Buttigieg, S. C. (2019). The Personal and Professional Consequences of Physician Burnout: A Systematic Review of the Literature. *Medical Care Research and Review: MCRR, 77*(5), 371–386. doi:10.1177/1077558719856787 PMID:31216940

Wilson, E., Chen, A. H., Grumbach, K., Wang, F., & Fernandez, A. (2005). Effects of limited English proficiency and physician language on health care comprehension. *Journal of General Internal Medicine, 20*(9), 800–806. doi:10.1111/j.1525-1497.2005.0174.x PMID:16117746

Winkelmann, A., & Güldner, F. H. (2004). Cadavers as teachers: The dissecting room experience in Thailand. *BMJ (Clinical Research Ed.), 329*(7480), 1455–1457. doi:10.1136/bmj.329.7480.1455 PMID:15604182

Wociechowski, M. (2015). *Male Nurses Confronting Stereotypes and Discrimination: Part 1, The Issues*. https://minoritynurse.com/male-nurses-confronting-stereotypes-and-discrimination-part-1-the-issues/

World Health Organization. (November 24, 2021). *Disability and health*. WHO. https://www.who.int/news-room/fact-sheets/detail/disability-and-health

Wright, D. (2000). Educational support for nursing and midwifery students with dyslexia. *Nursing Standard, 14*(41), 35.

Wright, A. A., & Katz, I. T. (2018). Beyond Burnout— Redesigning Care to Restore Meaning and Sanity for Physicians. *The New England Journal of Medicine*, *378*(4), 309–311. doi:10.1056/NEJMp1716845 PMID:29365301

Xu, H., Stjernswärd, S., & Glasdam, S. (2021). Psychosocial experiences of frontline nurses working in hospital-based settings during the COVID-19 pandemic: A qualitative systematic review. *Int J Nurs Stud Adv*, *3*, 100037. doi:10.1016/j.ijnsa.2021.100037 PMID:34308373

Yang, L. H., Wong, L. Y., Grivel, M. M., & Hasin, D. S. (2017). Stigma and substance use disorders: An international phenomenon. *Current Opinion in Psychiatry*, *30*(5), 378–388. doi:10.1097/YCO.0000000000000351 PMID:28700360

Yousuf, Y., & Yu, J. C. (2021). Improving Representation of Skin of Color in a Medical School Preclerkship Dermatology Curriculum. *Medical Science Educator*, *32*(1), 27–30. https://doi.org/10.1007/s40670-021-01473-x

Yudell, M., Roberts, D., DeSalle, R., & Tishkoff, S. (2016). Science and Society. Taking race out of human genetics. *Science*, *351*(6273), 564–565. https://doi.org/10.1126/science.aac4951

Zeng-Treitler, Q., Kim, H., Rosemblat, G., & Keselman, A. (2010). Can multilingual machine translation help make medical record content more comprehensible to patients? *Studies in Health Technology and Informatics*, *160*(Pt 1), 73–77. PMID:20841653

About the Contributors

Chasity Beth O'Malley has more than 20 years of experience as an educator in higher education. She has worked closely with student populations of varying ages, genders, abilities, races, and, ethnicities. She is currently working in the Boonshoft School of Medicine at Wright State University in Dayton, Ohio, as an Associate Professor in Medical Education. While relatively new to the field of Diversity, Equity, and Inclusion, she has been successful in obtaining extramural funding to facilitate curricular changes related to DEI topics and in reporting on the findings and successes of DEI focused curricular interventions for the past several years.

Arkene Levy is a Jamaican Native who moved to South Florida in 2015. She currently serves as an Associate Professor of Pharmacology and Director of Diversity Equity and Inclusion for the Dr Kiran C Patel College of Allopathic Medicine at Nova Southeastern University in sunny Florida. In her role as DEI Director, Arkene has mentored students in research related to health disparities, race equity and lesbian, gay, bisexual, transgender, questioning, queer, intersex (LGBTQI+) cultural competency. She has presented and published her DEI work at the regional and national level including the International Association of Medical Sciences Educators (IAMSE) and Association of American Medical Colleges (AAMC) National conferences. Arkene is currently a member of the AAMC Group on Diversity and Southern Group on Educational Affairs, as well as IAMSE. She is a founding member of the DEI working group for the Florida Council of Deans and also serves as Co-Co-Chair of the South Florida Community Coalition which focuses on opioid and substance use prevention education for at-risk youth. Dr Levy is currently PI and Co-PI for several DEI-related grants including a Florida Blue foundation grant for opioid abuse prevention awareness and IAMSE curricular innovation grants focused on LGBTQ Proficiency and mitigating imposter phenomenon in diverse medical student populations.

Amanda Chase is an Associate Professor of Medical Education with Nova Southeastern University Dr. Kiran C. Patel College of Allopathic Medicine where she contributes to global course design and case writing for an integrated, case-based learning curriculum. She earned her Ph.D. in Cellular and Molecular Medicine at Johns Hopkins University School of Medicine and completed postdoctoral research on viral immunology at the Centers for Disease Control and Prevention. Dr. Chase has ten years of experience as a medical educator and has collaborated with teams of educators to build innovative curriculum and assessment models for two new medical schools. Currently, she serves as the Cardiovascular, Pulmonary, and Renal Course Co-Director and Interprofessional Collaboration Thread Director. Her educational research focuses on enhancing strategic learning through the integration and assessment of communication skills, with a particular focus on role play. Dr. Chase is actively involved in educator mentoring and committee tasks through the International Association of Medical Science Educators.

Samiksha Prasad is the Assistant Professor in Medical Education at the Dr. Kiran C. Patel College of Allopathic Medicine, Nova Southeastern University. She has been using multiple learning modalities within integrated, preclinical medical education curricula. Dr. Prasad serves as the Director of curriculum thread and course blocks. Dr. Prasad is highly engaged in student mentoring. She serves as a medical student advisor and mentors students for research. She has actively conducted funded research on several diversity-centered topics and published in peer-reviewed journals. She has also been involved in community engagements that focus on encouraging health and sciences. Dr. Prasad has been on the editorial board for peer-reviewed journals and grant decision committees. Dr. Prasad earned her Bachelor's in Technology degree in Biotechnology (Genetic Engineering) from Sam Higginbottom Institute of Agriculture Technology and Sciences, India. She obtained her Ph.D. degree in the Department of Microbiology and Cell Science at the University of Florida, USA. She continued on at the University of Florida to complete Post-Doctoral research on Parasitic Proteomics and Immunology, where her research was focused on host-pathogen interactions. During this time, she also taught undergraduate, graduate, and medical science courses at multiple institutions including the University of Florida, Santa Fe College, and Polk State College in Florida, USA.

* * *

Omair Abbasi is Assistant Professor, Florida Atlantic University Charles E. Schmidt College of Medicine and Assistant Professor, University of Miami Miller School of Medicine.

Andreia Alexander received her MD/PhD from the Indiana University School of Medicine in 2014. She then went on to complete her residency in Emergency Medicine at Rutgers New Jersey Medical School. She is currently an Assistant Professor of Emergency Medicine, Assistant Program Director for the Emergency Medicine Residency, and Co-Director of the Health Equity Pathway at Indiana University. She works clinically with Indiana University Health. Her clinical interests include resident education, improving Emergency Department care for sexual and reproductive health (SRH) issues, and raising awareness of systemic racism and implicit biases in ED clinical practice. Her research focuses on decreasing SRH inequities and the implementation of diversity, equity, and inclusion interventions in graduate medical education.

Thura Al-Khayat, MD, joined Dr. Kiran C. Patel College of Allopathic Medicine in August 2021 as an Assistant Professor at the Department of Medical Education. At NSU MD, she co-directs the Practice of Medicine (POM) course1&2 for the M1class. She also conducts OBGYN didactic sessions for the M3 class and serves as an advisor for a group of M3-M4 students, in addition to other duties. Prior to this current position, Dr. Al-Khayat served as an Assistant Professor of OBGYN and Medical Skills at California Northstate University, College of Medicine (CNSUCOM). At CNSUCOM she primarily served as a Course Director for both the M1 and M2 Medical Skills courses. She also co-directed the Reproductive Medicine course for the M2 class, in addition to serving as the College of Medicine Interprofessional Education (IPE) representative, and co-chair of the IPE committee at CNSUCOM. Overseas, Dr. Al-Khayat practiced as an OBGYN Specialist for almost a decade after completing her OBGYN residency in 2004. Dr. Al-Khayat has special interest in Healthcare Simulations and IPE. In affiliation with the Health Sciences Simulation Center at Broward College, she developed workshops in

Healthcare Simulations for NSU MD faculty as part of faculty development. She participated in several scholarly activities including curriculum development, IPE, and OBGYN.

Delores Amorelli, EdD, is an Assistant Professor in the Department of Clinical Science and the Director of Faculty Educator Development at the Kaiser Permanent Bernard J. Tyson School of Medicine (KPSOM), where she oversees the school's program to support faculty in their continual professional growth as educators, including efforts to advance skills in teaching, assessment, curriculum development, leadership, and mentoring, and helps to foster vibrant communities of practice among didactic and clinical faculty. She has 15 years of experience in higher education as an administrator and a faculty member. Prior to her role at KPSOM, Dr. Amorelli worked at Columbia University, where she helped launch new academic programs and new courses from vision to implementation and developed a faculty development program centered on inclusive teaching and equitable assessment. Her research interests include the professional identity formation of educators, using quality improvement frameworks to enhance curriculum design, and evaluating faculty connection and sense of belonging at higher education institutions.

Melissa Armas is an Assistant Professor of Medical Education and has experience teaching undergraduate, graduate, and medical students. She has taught in the pre-clerkship and clerkship curriculum in topics related to basic sciences, public health, and ethics using multiple learning modalities. Dr. Armas serves as a medical student advisor, and she is involved in research that includes diversity centered topics such as health disparities and health equity in the foster care community. Her research interests include areas such as ethics, health disparities, and social determinants of health. Dr. Armas earned her Bachelor of Science degree in Biology and her Master of Public Health degree from the University of South Florida, USA. She obtained her Ph.D. degree in Medical Sciences with a concentration in Molecular Cell Biology from the University of Florida, USA. Her research focused on Colorectal cancer and the role of Long-Patch Base Excision Repair.

Christina Brown-Wujick is an alumna of the University of South Florida where she received her M.A. degree in Sociology, M.Ed. in College Student Affairs, and Ph.D. in Curriculum & Instruction with an emphasis in higher education administration. She is currently employed as an Assistant Professor at the Dr. Kiran C. Patel College of Osteopathic Medicine (KPCOM) where she serves as the Director of its Graduate Certificate in Health Professions Preparation (post-bac) program, works as a Medical Education faculty advisor for the Doctor of Osteopathic Medicine program, and leads other KPCOM initiatives on the Tampa Bay campus for Undergraduate, Graduate, Technology and Community Education.

Kate Carnevale received her PhD in Biochemistry from the Florida State University in Tallahassee, FL in 2018. She is currently serving as an Assistant Professor of Medical Education at the Kiran C. Patel College of Allopathic Medicine at Nova Southeastern University in Fort Lauderdale, FL, where she has directed the Brain, Body and Behavior second year medical student systems block course for the last three years, as well as participated in active learning modalities such as team and problem based learning for first and second year students. Her training is in biochemistry, cell biology, and the biological applications of nanomaterials. Since joining NSU, she has expanded her research interests into public health and medical education, specifically health equity and student success. She currently has funded projects in stem cell engineering with peptide coated nanoparticles and foster care health advocacy. Dr.

Carnevale takes joy in training students in research as well as teaching biochemistry to professional students in medical, dental, optometry and biomedical science programs, as well as undergraduate nutrition students at NSU.

Monica Chavan, MA, is a fourth-year medical student at Case Western Reserve University whose academic interests include bioethics, curriculum development, and promoting diversity, equity, and inclusion at all levels of medical education. She intends to pursue residency training in interventional and diagnostic radiology.

Colleen Croniger is a faculty member in the department of Nutrition at Case Western Reserve University. She is the Assistant Dean of Basic Science Education for CWRU School of Medicine. Dr. Croniger has been actively involved in curriculum development for over 20 years. She co-leads Block 3 (nutrition, biochemistry, and gastroenterology) for the first-year medical students at CWRU. In addition, she teaches undergraduates and graduate student metabolism. Dr. Croniger has received several awards for teaching, The John S Diekhoff Award and The Kaiser-Permanente Award for Excellence in Teaching. Dr. Croniger has participated in the Harvard Macy Institute Program for Educators in Health Professions and just completed the AMA Health System Science Fellowship. Dr. Croniger continues to work on curriculum development with CWRU faculty to enhance the current curriculum.

Gabriella Dauer, born and raised in Miami Beach, Florida, is a board certified Pediatrician and board eligible Pediatric Hospitalist. She attended medical school at the University of Miami Miller school of Medicine and completed her Pediatric Residency at the Children's Hospital at Montefiore of Albert Einstein in New York City. She continued her passion for academic medicine as a Pediatric Hospitalist with Boston Children's Health Physicians at Maria Fareri Children's Hospital where she served as the Assistant Program Director for the Pediatric Residency Program and Director of Resident Education for Hospital Medicine, furthering program curricula and resident wellness while caring for her inpatient teams. Dr. Dauer also dedicated her time to teaching medical students as Assistant Professor of Pediatrics at New York Medical College where she was inducted into Alpha Omega Alpha for her medical education efforts. Training and working in urban quaternary care hospitals in Miami and the Bronx has furthered her passion of caring and advocating for underserved and underrepresented children and families. Dr. Dauer is also interested in complex child pathophysiology and care, clinical reasoning education, physician wellbeing and resiliency training, and hospital quality metrics and throughput.

William Dawson, originally from Rochester, New York, graduated from Brown University with a Computer Science and Economics degree and from Duke University School of Medicine with a Master of Biomedical Science degree. At Nova Southeastern University's Kiran C. Patel College of Allopathic Medicine, he is pursuing his interest in behavioral and substance use addiction.

Britney Farmer is the Chief of the Child and Family Behavioral Health Services (CAFBHS) at Martin Army Community Hospital. Stationed at Fort Benning in Columbus, Georgia, this clinic serves spouses and children of active-duty services members and military retirees. Dr. Farmer graduated medical school from The Ohio State University in 2014. She completed her residency training for general psychiatry and a child/adolescent psychiatry fellowship at Tripler Army Medical Center in Honolulu,

Hawaii in 2019. Currently, Dr. Farmer is an Assistant Professor in the department of Psychiatry at the Uniformed Services University of Health Sciences. Her special interests, within her pediatric population, include learning disabilities, developmental delays and the intersection of behavioral health and school systems. She has proudly served in the United States Army for the last eight years and is looking forward to her next grand adventure.

Eric Gertner, M.D., M.P.H., F.A.C.P., is a general internist and an Associate Medical Director for Population Health and Patient-Centered Medical Homes with Lehigh Valley Physicians Group in Allentown, Pennsylvania. He received his undergraduate degree from Princeton University, and his Doctor of Medicine from UMDNJ – Robert Wood Johnson Medical School (Rutgers). He completed his residency in internal medicine at the Medical College of Pennsylvania, and a Master's Degree in Public Health at the Drexel School of Public Health. He was inducted as a Fellow of the American College of Physicians in 2002. He was appointed as Clinical Professor in the Department of Internal Medicine at the University of South Florida, Morsani College of Medicine in 2014. Dr. Gertner has been actively involved in cultural competency, health equity and diversity for many years. He served as Chair of the Council on Patient Advocacy and the Workgroup on Cultural Competency and Medical Diversity for the Pennsylvania Medical Society from 2006-2012. At Lehigh Valley Health Network, Dr. Gertner co-chaired the Cultural Awareness Leadership Council, overseeing the development and implementation of a strategic plan for cultural awareness, including education around cultural competence, disparity reduction, and recruitment and retention of a diverse workforce. He was a member of the Lehigh Valley Board of Health. A native of Lakewood NJ, Dr. Gertner has published research in reducing disparities in health care and promoting quality medical care for everyone.

Daniel P. Griffin is the Assistant Dean of Pre-Clerkship Curriculum and an Associate Professor of Medical Education at Nova Southeastern University Dr. Kiran C. Patel College of Allopathic Medicine (NSU MD). He has extensive experience in active learning such as problem-based learning (PBL), case-based learning (CBL), and team-based learning (TBL). He has been fortunate to have had opportunities to take educational programs at two new medical schools to full implementation. As he develops curricula and programs, he strives to stay at the forefront of advances in medical education and administration, and to develop and disseminate best practices. He has a history of and is actively involved in promoting diversity, equity, and inclusion in medical school training and processes; and executing projects designed to innovate curriculum delivery methods.

Margaret Hadinger serves as the Director of Academic and Student Affairs at OnlineMedEd. She previously served as Designated Institutional Official and Director of Medical Education at Lehigh Valley Health Network in Allentown, PA, and as Affiliate Assistant Professor at the University of South Florida Morsani College of Medicine.

Cory Horowitz achieved his Bachelor's degree in Psychology from Cornell University in 2014. Following this he worked with Teach For America as a high school science teacher for two years. He then went on to achieve his medical doctorate from the University of Oklahoma School of Community Medicine in 2020. He is now completing his psychiatry residency at the Memorial Healthcare System.

Christen D. Johnson, MD, MPH, FAAFP, is a champion for health equity and Board Certified Family Physician practicing Family Medicine at a Federally qualified health center in Columbus, Ohio. She attended Wright State University where she acquired a B.A. in Biological Sciences, followed by her M.D. and MPH from Wright State University Boonshoft School of Medicine, and completed residency in the Urban Track at The Ohio State University Family Medicine Residency Program in Columbus, Ohio. Dr. Johnson is currently pursuing a Doctorate of Education in Antiracist and Multicultural Education and serves as the Faculty Lead for Cultural Competency and Race in Medicine Curriculum at Wright State University Boonshoft school of Medicine. She lives the phrase "To whom much is given, much is required" through her career in leadership and dedication to serving the most vulnerable communities. Her research interests include health disparities, medical education, and antiracist medicine and have facilitated numerous local, regional, and national research presentations, and publications in peer-reviewed journals, textbooks, and grants. Dr. Johnson has also been honored with multiple opportunities including serving as the 2016-2017 National President of the Student National Medical Association, a 2021 American Academy of Family Physicians Health Equity Fellow, as well as several scholarships and awards including the National Health Service Corps Scholarship, the 2017 NBC Black 28 under 28, and the 2020 National Minority Quality Forum 40 Under 40 Leaders in Health.

Heejung Kim, originally from New York, graduated from Wellesley College with a Bachelor of Arts in Neuroscience. She has mostly become involved in the field of Geriatric Psychiatry with a specific focus on Tech and Aging, most notably contributing to a chapter in the American Psychiatric Publishing Comprehensive textbook of Geriatric Psychiatry. During medical school, she has continued her interests in behavioral health with a focus on substance abuse and dementia research. Her invited conferences include the American Association of Geriatric Psychiatry, Harvard Psychiatry Research Day as well as American Association for Geriatric Psychiatry.

Kevin Kuang, originally from Chelmsford, Massachusetts, graduated from Boston University with a Bachelor of Arts (with Honors) in Biology, Cum Laude. He is currently a medical student at Nova Southeastern University Dr. Kiran C. Patel College of Allopathic Medicine. Throughout his time, he has worked in several biomedical fields including gene therapy, muscular dystrophy, and melanoma. Some of his invited conferences include the Society of Investigative Dermatology 2020, Academy for Professionalism in Health Care 2022, and US-Korea Conference 2022. In medical school, he is president of several clubs, and was elected as a first year mentor.

Jason Lambrese is a child and adolescent psychiatrist, an Assistant Professor of Medicine and Assistant Dean for Student Affairs, Case Western Reserve University School of Medicine. He directs the Behavioral Sciences course at the Cleveland Clinic Lerner College of Medicine and is a faculty mentor for the CaseMed Pride student group. He is the faculty lead on the LGBTQ+ curricular integration action group.

Nicole Lawson is the inaugural Faculty Director of Inclusive Curriculum Assistant Professor in the Health Systems Science department, and Lead of Equity, Inclusion, and Diversity curricular content at the Kaiser Permanente School of Medicine. This role builds on her expertise in curriculum development and instructional design as well as cultural anthropology, focusing on curricular EID to guide the development of the school's inclusive curriculum strategy and resources. This work includes supporting faculty in session design, creating faculty development programming on EID, and building evaluation and development tools to support EID integration. Prior to joining the School of Medicine, Dr. Lawson worked in instructional design Loyola Marymount University School of Education. She earned a Bachelor's of Arts degree in Anthropology from Yale University, and an MA and PhD from UCLA in cultural anthropology. Her scholarship continues to explore cultural and epistemological diversity in environmental STEM education, with a focus on place-based learning.

Jed Mangal is a board certified internist and psychiatrist. He has a research and clinical interest in psychosomatic medicine. He is passionate about health professions education and improving interprofessional teams.

Yael Mauer, MD, MPH, completed her medical degree from Rutgers University, her Internal Medicine residency training at MetroHealtth Medical Center / Case Western Reserve University, and her Master of Public Health at the Medical College of Wisconsin. She is currently a Staff Physician at the Cleveland Clinic Foundation, an Assistant Professor of Medicine at the Cleveland Clinic Lerner College of Medicine, and Core Faculty at the Cleveland Clinic Internal Medicine Residency Program.

Jocelyn Mitchell-Williams, M.D., Ph.D., is the Associate Dean for Medical Education and an Associate Professor of Obstetrics and Gynecology at Cooper Medical School of Rowan University (CMSRU) in Camden, New Jersey. Dr. Mitchell-Williams earned her Bachelor of Science degree in Electrical Engineering and her Doctor of Philosophy degree in Biomedical Engineering from Rutgers University – College of Engineering. She spent two years working in neuroscience bench research before returning to the classroom to earn her medical degree at Rutgers University - Robert Wood Johnson Medical School. She went on to complete her residency in the field of Obstetrics and Gynecology at Cooper University Health Care based in Camden, New Jersey, where she has been on staff for the past 25 years. Dr. Mitchell-Williams is also a Fellow for the American College of Obstetrics and Gynecology and a 2020 graduate of the Hedwig van Ameringen Executive Leadership in Academic Medicine (ELAM) Program of Drexel University. Dr. Mitchell-Williams joined Rowan University in 2010 as part of the founding leadership for the medical school (CMSRU). In the Camden community, she continues to serve not only as a practicing obstetrician/gynecologist, but also a community volunteer, educator, and advocate for vulnerable populations. She serves on the board for several non-profit organizations, including the Camden Coalition for Healthcare Providers and Volunteers of America, Delaware Valley. She has a special interest in addressing bias, racism, and health disparities, especially regarding their impact on persons of color, LGBTQ+ communities, and other underserved populations. In her current administrative position, Dr. Mitchell-Williams oversees the medical education program at CMSRU, including curricular development, simulation center activities, library services, and student/faculty assessment. Prior to this role, she served for 11 years as the Associate Dean for Diversity and Community Affairs at CMSRU, where she led efforts to improve the health outreach for disadvantaged communities, including the creation of a pipeline to medical professions, diversity and anti-racism training, and community service programs. She has received foundation, state, and federal grants to support her diversity and community education programs. She helped lead CMSRU to national recognition as the recipient of the Association of American Medical College's (AAMC) Spencer Foreman Award for community engagement. She has delivered numerous talks on implicit bias in medicine, micro-aggressions in medical education, and cultural competency. She has received several awards for her commitment to service, including the Crystal Award from the National Association for the Advancement of Colored People (NAACP) for her influence and professionalism with youth in the community.

Maria Claudia Moncaliano is a fourth-year medical student at Case Western Reserve University. She completed her undergraduate studies at Johns Hopkins University in Molecular and Cellular Biology. During medical school, Ms. Moncaliano has engaged in community service, advocacy, and education about the social determinants of health and Diversity, Equity, and Inclusion in healthcare. She is passionate about medical education and providing high quality and culturally sensitive care to underserved patient populations.

Joseph Napolitano is the Vice President for Network Operations and Nursing Liaison Services for Lehigh Valley Health Network. He is responsible for the overall recruitment and retention of nurses across a 13 hospital, horizontally and vertically integrated, health care network with 20,000+ team members. Dr. Napolitano also serves as adjunct faculty at Cedar Crest College and DeSales University schools of nursing. He is the former chair of the Pennsylvania State Board of Nursing and served in senior roles on the boards of The Wellness Community – Greater Lehigh Valley and The Hillside School. Napolitano is the current Chair of the Pennsylvania Action Coalition and an affiliate scholar for Virginia Commonwealth University's Langston's Center for Innovation in Quality and Safety. Napolitano previously held leadership roles at The Dorothy Rider Pool Health Care Trust, The Hospital of the University of Pennsylvania, and Memorial Sloan-Kettering Cancer Center. Dr. Napolitano holds a BA from Skidmore College, an MPH from Yale University, a BSN and MSN from the University of Pennsylvania and a PhD from New York University.

Nicole Novotny received her MD from the University of Mississippi Medical Center in 2018. She then went on to complete her residency in Emergency Medicine as well as her fellowship in Medical Simulation at Indiana University. She currently practices Emergency Medicine in New Orleans, Louisiana at Ochsner Medical Center where she serves as the Director for Emergency Medicine Simulation and core faculty for the Emergency Medicine Residency Program. Her research interests include incorporating diversity, equity and inclusion in simulation.

Amie Ogunsakin is a clinical endocrinologist at the University of Iowa Hospitals and Clinics. Her interests focus on healthcare disparities in diabetes, obesity and transgender care.

María de los A. Ortiz Reyes has over 25 years of experience in the higher education area in Puerto Rico, Latin America, USA, Europe and Asia. A tenured faculty and researcher in the Educational Leadership Program at University of Puerto Rico, Rio Piedras Campus, is also Consultant in Accreditation, Evaluation/assessment and accountability and internationalization. Author and experienced speaker at local and international scenarios, entrepreneur, and laureate poet. Have been Visiting Professor at the National Autonomous University in Honduras, the University of New Delhi in India and University of Bahrain in Middle East. Member of the Board of Directors of Carlos Albizu University and The Teachers Hospital (Hospital del Maestro de P.R.).

Kristina H. Petersen is an Associate Professor of Biochemistry & Molecular Biology Department and the Assistant Dean of Academic Support Programs at New York Medical College. Since arriving at NYMC in 2014, she received three Student Senate Awards for enhancement of student life, six mentoring/teaching awards, and was inducted into the Alpha Omega Alpha Honor Medical Society. In 2021 and 2022, the NYMC AOA Chapter nominated her for the Robert J. Glaser Distinguished Teaching Award. Dr. Petersen leads a team that focuses on all aspects of academic support, including supporting students who receive accommodations. Her research focuses on efficacy of programs and teaching interventions in supporting medical student success. Kristina is a co-author on several articles and chapters on disability inclusion. She has served on the Board of the Coalition for Disabilities in Health Sciences Education since 2019; she is currently the President through 2024.

Vijay Rajput grew up in Mumbai, India, and received his medical school training in India before moving to the United States. He practiced academic hospital medicine in Camden New Jersey for 22 years. He has authored or co-authored more than 110 papers, abstracts, and book chapters. He has presented more than two hundred seminars, workshops, and grand rounds at regional, national, and international conferences. Dr. Rajput serves on editorial boards and reviewers on several journals. Dr. Rajput has received several grants from HRSA and Arnold P. Gold Foundation in the last 15 years. He was supported for Literature and medicine, ethics OSCEs, and Hidden curriculum in medical education. Over the last 25 years, Dr. Rajput has received more than fifteen "Excellence in Teaching" awards from students, residents, and national organizations like ACGME, ACP, and SHM. He was awarded the ACGME Parker J. Palmer "Courage to Teach Award"— the most prestigious teaching award in 2011. He was inducted into the UMDNJ's Master Educator Guild in 2005. Dr. Rajput enjoyed teaching at the bedside with patients and learners engaged in patient-centered discussion. His primary areas of interest are bedside teaching, professionalism, ethics, and humanism in medicine as well as, student well-being, mentoring, and curriculum development.

Kathleen Robinson is an Endocrinology Associate at the University of Iowa. She completed her MD/PhD at the University of Wisconsin in 2016, and her Internal Medicine residency and Endocrinology Fellowship at the University of Iowa in 2019 and 2022 respectively. Her doctoral work examined the history of the "Fat Acceptance Movement" and how the medicalization of high body weight presents both opportunities and challenges for those labeled as having obesity. Currently, she works with an interdisciplinary team to develop methods to measure and reduce weight stigma in health care.

Judith Sabino serves as the chief diversity equity and inclusion liaison at Lehigh Valley Health Network in Allentown, PA.

Taru Saigal is Clinical Assistant Professor Director, Language Concordant Care Member, Diversity Committee, Department of Internal Medicine, The Ohio State University.

Amal Shibli-Rahhal is a professor of Internal Medicine/Endocrinology at the University of Iowa Carver College of Medicine where she also serves as Associate Dean for Student Affairs and Curriculum. Her interests include diversity, equity and inclusion in medical education.

Sherrica Taylor obtained her bachelor's degree from the University of South Florida, M.S. in Higher Education-College Administration and Leadership from Kaplan University and her PhD in Education with a focus on Leadership in Higher Education from Northcentral University. She currently serves as the Vice Chair/Assistant Professor of Medical Education at Nova Southeastern University's Kiran C. Patel College of Osteopathic Medicine. She also serves on various committees and councils focused on diversity, equity, inclusion and belonging including the AACOM's Council on Diversity and Equity and Nova Southeastern' s Belonging, Equity, Diversity and Inclusion Council.

Amy Wilson-Delfosse, PhD, is Professor of Pharmacology and Associate Dean for Curriculum at Case Western Reserve University School of Medicine. She also serves as the Senior Director of the Aquifer Sciences Initiative at Aquifer. Dr. Wilson-Delfosse received her Bachelor's degree in Chemistry from The College of Wooster, her Ph.D. in Pharmacology from Vanderbilt University and completed a postdoctoral fellowship at the Weis Center for Research at the Geisinger Clinic in Danville, Pennsylvania. Her basic science research interests have been focused in the area of Ras-related GTPase biology and Parkinson's Disease. Her work in this area has been funded by the NIH, the National Parkinson's Foundation, and the Michael J. Fox Foundation. In 2004, Dr. Wilson-Delfosse combined her basic science research career with medical education administrative leadership and has gradually transitioned her research interests exclusively into the area of medical education. She has published in multiple areas of education and has a particular interest in developing strategies to promote integration of basic science with clinical medicine. Dr. Wilson-Delfosse was president of the International Association of Medical Science Educators from 2011-2015 and was recognized by the Association of American Medical Colleges for her accomplishments in medical education with the prestigious Alpha Omega Alpha Robert J. Glaser Distinguished Teacher Award in 2012.

Algevis Wrench was born and raised in Venezuela and moved to Florida in 2000. She currently serves as an Assistant Professor of Medical Education and Microbiology for the Dr. Kiran C. Patel College of Allopathic Medicine at Nova Southeastern University. During this time, Dr. Wrench has been highly engaged in student mentoring and bringing awareness to diversity, equity, and inclusion topics. She serves as co-advisor for the Latino Medical Student Association (LMSA) chapter. Dr. Wrench is currently PI for several curricular innovation grants including an International Association of Medical Sciences Educators (IAMSE) grant focused on the development of an imposter phenomenon mitigation toolkit for medical students in diverse populations.

Monica Yepes-Rios is Assistant Dean, Diversity, Equity and Inclusion and Associate Professor, Case Western Reserve University School of Medicine / Cleveland Clinic Lerner College of Medicine. She is an Internal Medicine Physician at the Cleveland Clinic, Ohio City Hispanic Clinic, and the West Region Medical Director for Community Health Strategies. Dr. Yepes-Rios has over 25 years of experience in medical education and internal medicine clinical practice with a special interest in education to promote thriving and equitable learning environments and the care of underserved communities. She completed her Internal Medicine Residency at The George Washington University Medical Center, and is a Robert Wood Johnson Clinical Scholar, Yale University. She earned her bachelor's degree from Duke University and medical degree from the George Washington University School of Medicine.

Index

N

O

P

Q

R

S

T

U

V

W

Recommended Reference Books

IGI Global's reference books are available in three unique pricing formats:
Print Only, E-Book Only, or Print + E-Book.

Shipping fees may apply.

www.igi-global.com

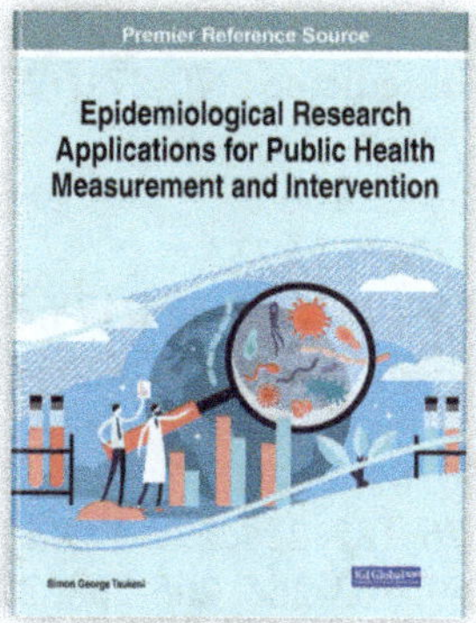

ISBN: 9781799844143
EISBN: 9781799844150
© 2021; 214 pp.
List Price: US$ **295**

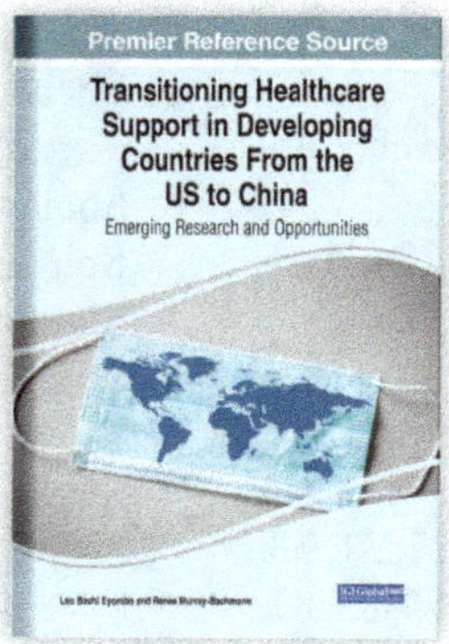

ISBN: 9781799844501
EISBN: 9781799844518
© 2021; 135 pp.
List Price: US$ **245**

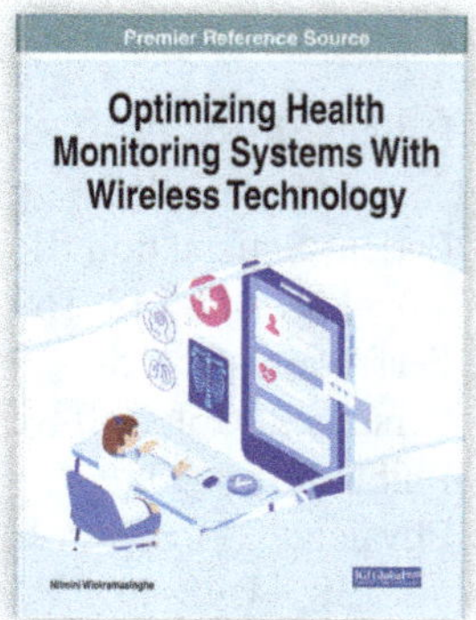

ISBN: 9781522560678
EISBN: 9781522560685
© 2021; 338 pp.
List Price: US$ **265**

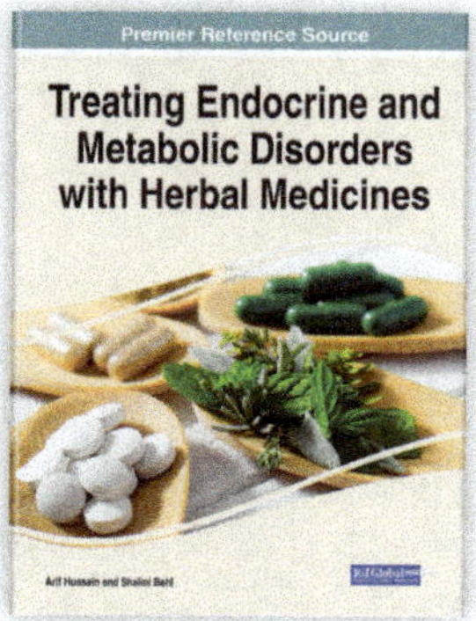

ISBN: 9781799848080
EISBN: 9781799848097
© 2021; 489 pp.
List Price: US$ **295**

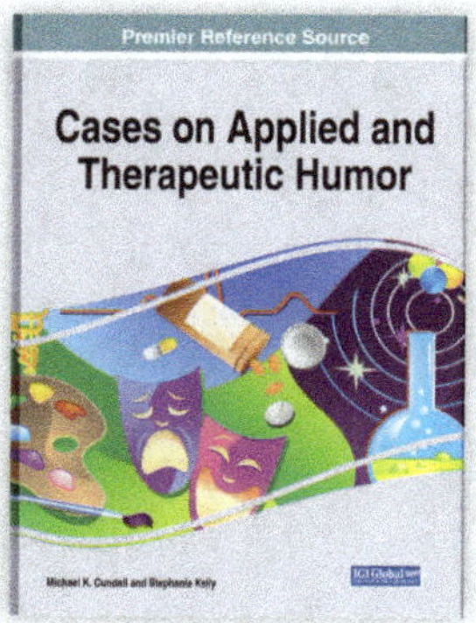

ISBN: 9781799845287
EISBN: 9781799845294
© 2021; 267 pp.
List Price: US$ **255**

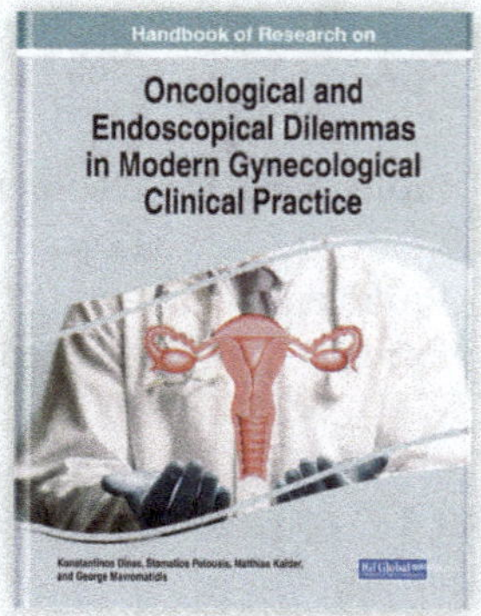

ISBN: 9781799842132
EISBN: 9781799842149
© 2021; 460 pp.
List Price: US$ **385**

Do you want to stay current on the latest research trends, product announcements, news, and special offers?
Join IGI Global's mailing list to receive customized recommendations, exclusive discounts, and more.
Sign up at: **www.igi-global.com/newsletters.**

Publisher of Timely, Peer-Reviewed Inclusive Research Since 1988

IGI Global
PUBLISHER of TIMELY KNOWLEDGE

www.igi-global.com Sign up at www.igi-global.com/newsletters facebook.com/igiglobal twitter.com/igiglobal linkedin.com/igiglobal

www.ingramcontent.com/pod-product-compliance
Lightning Source LLC
LaVergne TN
LVHW080535300926
849162LV00007B/1610